Prostate Cancer

Editor

CHRISTOPHER J. SWEENEY

HEMATOLOGY/ONCOLOGY CLINICS OF NORTH AMERICA

www.hemonc.theclinics.com

Consulting Editors
GEORGE P. CANELLOS
H. FRANKLIN BUNN

December 2013 • Volume 27 • Number 6

ELSEVIER

1600 John F. Kennedy Boulevard • Suite 1800 • Philadelphia, Pennsylvania, 19103-2899

http://www.theclinics.com

HEMATOLOGY/ONCOLOGY CLINICS OF NORTH AMERICA Volume 27, Number 6
December 2013 ISSN 0889-8588, ISBN 13: 978-0-323-22722-3

Editor: Patrick Manley
Developmental Editor: Donald Mumford

Hematology/Oncology Clinics (ISSN 0889-8588) is published bimonthly by Elsevier Inc., 360 Park Avenue South, New York, NY 10010-1710. Months of issue are February, April, June, August, October, and December. Business and Editorial Offices: 1600 John F. Kennedy Blvd., Ste. 1800, Philadelphia, PA 19103–2899. Customer Service Office: 3251 Riverport Lane, Maryland Heights, MO 63043. Periodicals postage paid at New York, NY and at additional mailing offices. Subscription prices are $385.00 per year (domestic individuals), $633.00 per year (domestic institutions), $190.00 per year (domestic students/residents), $440.00 per year (Canadian individuals), $783.00 per year (Canadian institutions) $520.00 per year (international individuals), $783.00 per year (international institutions), and $255.00 per year (international and Canadian students/residents). International air speed delivery is included in all *Clinics* subscription prices. All prices are subject to change without notice. **POSTMASTER:** Send address changes to *Hematology/Oncology Clinics of North America*, Elsevier Health Sciences Division, Subscription Customer Service, 3251 Riverport Lane, Maryland Heights, MO 63043. Customer Service (orders, claims, online, change of address): Elsevier Health Sciences Division, Subscription Customer Service, 3251 Riverport Lane, Maryland Heights, MO 63043. Tel: 1-800-654-2452 (U.S. and Canada); 314-447-8871 (outside U.S. and Canada). Fax: 314-447-8029. E-mail: journalscustomerservice-usa@elsevier.com (for print support); journalsonlinesupport-usa@elsevier.com (for online support).

Reprints. For copies of 100 or more, of articles in this publication, please contact the Commercial Reprints Department, Elsevier Inc., 360 Park Avenue South, New York, New York 10010-1710; Tel.: 212-633-3874, Fax: 212-633-3820, E-mail: reprints@elsevier.com.

Hematology/Oncology Clinics of North America is covered in *MEDLINE/PubMed (Index Medicus), EMBASE/ Excerpta Medica, and BIOSIS.*

Printed and bound by CPI Group (UK) Ltd, Croydon, CR0 4YY

Transferred to digital print 2012

Contributors

CONSULTING EDITORS

GEORGE P. CANELLOS, MD
William Rosenberg Professor of Medicine, Department of Medical Oncology, Dana-Farber Cancer Institute, Boston, Massachusetts

H. FRANKLIN BUNN, MD
Professor of Medicine, Division of Hematology, Brigham and Women's Hospital, Harvard Medical School, Boston, Massachusetts

EDITOR

CHRISTOPHER J. SWEENEY, MBBS
Dana-Farber Cancer Institute, Associate Professor of Medicine, Harvard Medical School, Boston, Massachusetts

AUTHORS

NEERAJ AGARWAL, MD
Assistant Professor of Medicine, Co-Leader, Genitourinary Oncology Multidisciplinary Program, Huntsman Cancer Institute, University of Utah, Salt Lake City, Utah

EMMANUEL S. ANTONARAKIS, MD
Assistant Professor of Oncology, Prostate Cancer Research Program, Sidney Kimmel Comprehensive Cancer Center at Johns Hopkins, Baltimore, Maryland

TUDOR BORZA, MD
Urologic Surgical Resident, Division of Urology, Department of Surgery, Brigham and Women's Hospital, Boston, Massachusetts

MICHAEL A. CARDUCCI, MD
AEGON Professor in Prostate Cancer Research, Prostate Cancer Research Program, Sidney Kimmel Comprehensive Cancer Center at Johns Hopkins, Baltimore, Maryland

TONI K. CHOUEIRI, MD
Associate Professor of Medicine, Lank Center for Genitourinary Oncology, Department of Medical Oncology, Dana-Farber Cancer Institute, Brigham and Women's Hospital, Harvard Medical School, Boston, Massachusetts

JOHANN DE BONO, MBChB, FRCP, MSc, PhD, FMedSci
Professor, Prostate Cancer Targeted Therapy Group and Drug Development Unit, The Royal Marsden NHS Foundation Trust, The Institute of Cancer Research, Sutton, Surrey, United Kingdom

MARIO A. EISENBERGER, MD
R. Dale Hughes Professor of Oncology, Prostate Cancer Research Program, Sidney Kimmel Comprehensive Cancer Center at Johns Hopkins, Baltimore, Maryland

L. MICHAEL GLODÉ, MD
Professor of Medicine and Robert Rifkin Chair, Division of Medical Oncology, University of Colorado Anschutz Medical Campus, Aurora, Colorado

MASOOM A. HAIDER, MD
Professor, Department of Medical Imaging, Sunnybrook Health Sciences Centre, University of Toronto, Toronto, Ontario, Canada

MAHA HUSSAIN, MD, FACP
Cis Maisel Professor of Oncology, Professor of Medicine and Urology, Associate Director for Clinical Research, Co-Leader, Prostate Cancer Program, University of Michigan Comprehensive Cancer Center, University of Michigan, Ann Arbor, Michigan

JASON P. IZARD, MD, MPH
Department of Urology, University of Washington School of Medicine, Seattle, Washington

RICHARD KHOR, MBBS, FRANZCR
Division of Radiation Oncology and Cancer Imaging, Peter MacCallum Cancer Centre, Victoria, Australia

ADAM S. KIBEL, MD
Chief of Urologic Surgery, Division of Urology, Department of Surgery, Brigham and Women's Hospital, Boston, Massachusetts

RAMDEV KONIJETI, MD
Urologic Oncology Fellow, Division of Urology, Department of Surgery, Brigham and Women's Hospital, Boston, Massachusetts

ELAINE T. LAM, MD
Assistant Professor of Medicine, Division of Medical Oncology, University of Colorado Anschutz Medical Campus, Aurora, Colorado

DANIEL W. LIN, MD
Department of Urology, University of Washington School of Medicine; Division of Public Health Sciences, Fred Hutchinson Cancer Research Center, Seattle, Washington

DAVID LORENTE, MD
Doctor, Prostate Cancer Targeted Therapy Group, The Royal Marsden NHS Foundation Trust, The Institute of Cancer Research, Sutton, Surrey, United Kingdom

RANA R. MCKAY, MD
Clinical Oncology Fellow, Lank Center for Genitourinary Oncology, Department of Medical Oncology, Dana-Farber Cancer Institute, Brigham and Women's Hospital, Harvard Medical School, Boston, Massachusetts

AURELIUS OMLIN, MD
Doctor, Prostate Cancer Targeted Therapy Group, The Royal Marsden NHS Foundation Trust, The Institute of Cancer Research, Sutton, Surrey, United Kingdom

CHANNING J. PALLER, MD
Assistant Professor of Oncology, Prostate Cancer Research Program, Sidney Kimmel Comprehensive Cancer Center at Johns Hopkins, Baltimore, Maryland

CARMEL PEZARO, MBChB, FRACP, DMedSc
Doctor, Prostate Cancer Targeted Therapy Group, The Royal Marsden NHS Foundation Trust, The Institute of Cancer Research, Sutton, Surrey, United Kingdom

MARY-ELLEN TAPLIN, MD
Associate Professor of Medicine, Lank Center for Genitourinary Oncology, Department of Medical Oncology, Dana-Farber Cancer Institute, Brigham and Women's Hospital, Harvard Medical School, Boston, Massachusetts

SCOTT WILLIAMS, MD, FRANZCR
Division of Radiation Oncology and Cancer Imaging, Peter MacCallum Cancer Centre, Victoria, Australia

JONATHAN L. WRIGHT, MD, MS
Department of Urology, University of Washington School of Medicine; Division of Public Health Sciences, Fred Hutchinson Cancer Research Center, Seattle, Washington

KATHERINE ZUKOTYNSKI, MD
Assistant Professor, Department of Medical Imaging, Sunnybrook Health Sciences Centre, University of Toronto, Toronto, Ontario, Canada; Visiting Assistant Professor, Department of Radiology, Brigham and Women's Hospital, Harvard Medical School, Boston, Massachusetts

Contents

HEMATOLOGY/ONCOLOGY
CLINICS OF NORTH AMERICA

FORTHCOMING ISSUES

February 2014
Hodgkin's Lymphoma
Volker Diehl, MD and
Peter Borchmann, MD, *Editors*

April 2014
Sickle Cell Disease
Elliott Vichinsky, MD, *Editor*

June 2014
Iron Disorders
Matthew M. Heeney, MD and
Alan Cohen, MD, *Editors*

RECENT ISSUES

October 2013
Sarcoma
Andrew Wagner, MD, *Editor*

August 2013
Breast Cancer
Harold J. Burstein, MD, *Editor*

June 2013
Disorders of the Platelets
A. Koneti Rao, MD, *Editor*

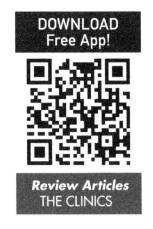

Preface

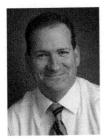

Christopher J. Sweeney, MBBS
Editor

In this edition of *Hematology/Oncology Clinics of North America*, a multidisciplinary team has compiled an issue that details the state of the art of prostate-cancer care. The edition spans the issues from PSA screening and management of early-stage cancer to castration-resistant disease. At each part of the disease spectrum, it has become abundantly clear that a multidisciplinary team is required to ensure the most appropriate treatment is administered to the right patient at the right time. The options range from surveillance for an older patient with low-grade, low-volume disease to multimodality therapy (eg, hormonal therapy and radiation for high-grade, high-volume disease) to palliative yet life-prolonging systemic therapies for patients who present with metastatic disease. This edition provides clinicians with the requisite knowledge about advances in our understanding of the role of surgery, radiation, imaging as well as systemic therapy for prostate cancer. This edition therefore provides information relevant to primary care physicians, urologists, radiation oncologists, medical oncologists, and radiologists.

The articles have been laid out to basically follow the different disease states a patient may face. Specifically, the first three articles detail management approaches (surveillance, surgery, radiation) for patients with clinically localized disease and emphasize the need to individualize recommendations to a given patient's unique situation (nature of their cancer and life expectancy). These articles are followed by discussions on strategies to augment localized therapies (ie, adjuvant therapies). The next article discusses the management of patients with biochemical recurrence after radiation or surgery and the subsequent article discusses data relevant to patients with radiographically evident metastatic disease that are about to commence androgen deprivation. The last stage of prostate cancer is castration-resistant disease and the role of new generation hormonal therapies, radiopharmaceuticals, immunotherapy, and chemotherapy, is discussed along with a review of novel agents in late stages of clinical development. In addition an article reviewing the important issue of bone health in prostate cancer discusses strategies for prevention of both treatment-induced bone loss and cancer-related skeletal morbidities. Finally, given the advances in strategies to image both localized and metastatic disease, an article is presented

Hematol Oncol Clin N Am 27 (2013) xi–xii
http://dx.doi.org/10.1016/j.hoc.2013.10.006
0889-8588/13/$ – see front matter © 2013 Elsevier Inc. All rights reserved.

hemonc.theclinics.com

that details the current and potential future use of imaging to guide treatment decisions.

In short, the theme running through each of these articles is that advances in technologies (surgery, radiation, imaging, understanding of biology and drug development) have improved our ability to deliver cancer care that minimizes morbidity and maximizes efficacy. However, a multidisciplinary team is required to achieve these goals and this edition gives each team member access to a comprehensive review of their colleagues' field. This edition therefore provides a "one-stop shop" and up-to-date reference to ensure each member of the multidisciplinary team is well informed and can provide their patients with the most appropriate and individualized treatment plans at all points along the disease spectrum.

Christopher J. Sweeney, MBBS
Dana-Farber Cancer Institute
Harvard Medical School
450 Brookline Avenue
D1230
Boston, MA 02215, USA

E-mail address:
christopher_sweeney@dfci.harvard.edu

Early Detection, PSA Screening, and Management of Overdiagnosis

Tudor Borza, MD, Ramdev Konijeti, MD, Adam S. Kibel, MD*

KEYWORDS

- Prostate cancer • PSA screening • Early detection • Overdiagnosis
- Active surveillance

KEY POINTS

- Prostate cancer diagnosis and treatment rates have increased significantly since the introduction of prostate-specific antigen (PSA) screening.
- Although it was initially thought that most prostate cancers would lead to death or significant morbidity, recent randomized trials have demonstrated that many patients with screening-detected prostate cancer will not die of their disease.
- Modifications to PSA screening, screening guideline statements, and novel screening markers have been developed to minimize the risk and morbidity associated with this overdiagnosis and overtreatment.
- Active surveillance protocols, in which patients with localized, low-risk prostate cancer are systematically monitored with the goal of deferring treatment until signs of disease progression arise, may also lead to lower treatment rates in men who are unlikely to benefit.

INTRODUCTION

Prostate cancer is the most commonly diagnosed cancer in men with an expected 238 600 new cases and 28 000 deaths in 2013 accounting for the second leading cause of cancer death in US men.[1] Over the past 20 years, a clinical focus has been on early detection using prostate-specific antigen (PSA) screening to find cancer before it becomes incurable. The result has been a dramatic increase in diagnosis accompanied by a decrease in mortality of almost 3.7% per year since 1994.[1] Recently, however, the utility of PSA screening has come into question because of an increase in diagnosis of cancers that are unlikely to cause significant harm to patients during their

Disclosures: Borza T and Konijeti R, no disclosures to report; Kibel AS, Sanofi-Aventis, Dendreon, Myriad.
Department of Surgery, Division of Urology, Brigham and Women's Hospital, 45 Francis Street, Boston, MA 02115, USA
* Corresponding author.
E-mail address: akibel@partners.org

Hematol Oncol Clin N Am 27 (2013) 1091–1110
http://dx.doi.org/10.1016/j.hoc.2013.08.002
0889-8588/13/$ – see front matter © 2013 Elsevier Inc. All rights reserved.

lifetime. Although controversy exists as to the effect of PSA screening on mortality, what is unquestioned is that a relatively large number of patients must be screened in order to prevent one cancer-related death.[2,3] As a result, efforts are focused on screening men most likely to benefit, development of new tests designed to aid in screening, and limiting treatment in men at low risk for dying of cancer. Herein, the authors review recent data on PSA screening, the rationale for new recommendations, novel screening tests, and the role of active surveillance in the management of this disease.

PSA SCREENING

PSA was introduced in the late 1980s as a screening tool for prostate cancer.[4] The initial recommendations were that all men older than 50 years undergo yearly screening with PSA and digital rectal examination (DRE), and screening should begin at 40 years of age for men at a higher risk. This screening paradigm led to a dramatic increase in the number of cases from about 100 per 100 000 US men in the pre-PSA era to approximately 160 per 100 000 US men subsequently.[1] In addition, a dramatic stage migration has been noted. Currently, 85% of prostate cancers diagnosed in the United States are clinically localized. Before PSA testing, as many as two-thirds of patients with apparently clinically localized disease were found to have pathologically advanced disease at the time of prostatectomy[5] and approximately one-third were found to have lymph node metastatic disease.[6] The number of patients presenting with locally advanced disease (stage T3 or T4) has decreased from 19.2% in the pre-PSA era to only 4.4% a decade later.[7] The rate of metastatic disease at presentation has also been greatly affected by PSA screening. Scosyrev and colleagues[8] performed an analysis of Surveillance Epidemiology and End Results (SEER) data and demonstrated a 3-fold decrease in the age-specific and race-specific observed annual incidence rates of metastatic prostate cancer at diagnosis in 2008 compared with the expected rates based on the incidence between 1983 and 1985.

Although initially it was thought that most of the tumors diagnosed by PSA screening had the potential to cause harm, there has been a realization over time that many of these tumors were similar to those detected in autopsy series and thought to be clinically insignificant. Incidental tumors were first appreciated in autopsy studies that demonstrated histologic evidence of prostate cancer in 1 in 3 men older than 50 years, with up to 80% of these tumors being clinically insignificant because of their limited size and grade.[9–12] These studies illustrated the high latent disease prevalence, thus, allowing for potential overdiagnosis by screening tests.

Selecting a threshold for normal PSA has also proven difficult because significant cancer has been shown to occur even with low PSA values. The Prostate Cancer Prevention Trial (PCPT) randomized men with PSA of less than 4 ng/mL to receiving finasteride or placebo to investigate whether finasteride prevented prostate cancer.[13] The study incorporated an end-of-study biopsy for all patients, including men on placebo, which allowed a more full understanding of prostate cancer risk in men with a normal PSA. Cancer was identified at the end-of-study biopsy in 15.2% of men with normal annual PSA and DRE over a 7-year interval. These tumors were not all clinically indolent because Gleason 7 or higher cancer was found in 2.3% of these patients. In men with a PSA between 2.1 and 4.0 ng/mL, 24.7% had prostate cancer and 5.2% had Gleason 7 or higher cancer. Even a PSA cutoff of 1.1 ng/mL would miss cancers because 25% of all cancers and 18% of Gleason 7 to 10 cancers were found in patients with PSA of less than this value.[14] It is clear from this data that there is no level of PSA that can be thought of as truly normal or abnormal.

Clinical trial data on the utility of PSA screening also have mixed results. Despite the decreases in prostate cancer mortality and rates of advanced disease at presentation[1,5–8] during the era of PSA screening and aggressive therapy, data emerged demonstrating that patients with localized prostate cancer at diagnosis had high non–prostate cancer–specific mortality if left untreated, raising the possibility that treatment in these patients would not have provided a benefit.[15] These seemingly contradictory findings highlighted the clear need for prospective, randomized controlled trials investigating the utility of PSA screening.

RANDOMIZED CONTROLLED TRIALS OF PSA SCREENING

Although the debate on PSA screening has continued for a decade or more, the recent publication of randomized trials has brought this discussion into the public eye. The Prostate, Lung, Colorectal, and Ovarian (PLCO) Cancer Screening Trial enrolled 76 693 men between 55 and 74 years of age and randomized them to annual PSA screening for 6 years and DRE for 4 years or usual care as the control group.[3] The study demonstrated no significant difference in prostate cancer mortality between the intervention cohort (screened) and the control cohort (usual care) at the 13-year follow-up. There were 4250 cancers detected it the screening group compared with 3815 cancers in the control group, resulting in a relative increase of 12% (relative risk [RR] 1.12, 95% confidence interval [CI] 1.07–1.17). A total of 158 prostate cancer deaths occurred in the screened arm and 145 deaths in the control arm, corresponding to a statistically insignificant difference in cumulative prostate cancer mortality rates of 3.7 and 3.4 deaths per 10 000 person-years, respectively (RR 1.09, 95% CI 0.87–1.36). There were some flaws in the PLCO trial. There was significant screening before randomization, with 45% of the total control cohort having a PSA before enrollment. Contamination was also a significant problem, with 52% in the control group undergoing at least one PSA test during the study. In addition, 15% of men in the screening group did not undergo PSA testing during the trial. As a result, the study lost power. Lastly, the study was designed to test PSA screening in the community. PSA was obtained; the results were sent to the primary care physician; and recommendations were made. However, neither biopsy nor treatment was mandated. As a consequence, an elevated PSA did not uniformly lead to biopsy and the diagnosis of cancer did not lead to treatment, which further decreased the ability of the study to detect a difference.

The European Randomized Study of Screening for Prostate Cancer (ERSPC) was a larger study that randomized 182 160 men between 50 and 74 years of age to PSA screening every 4 years or a control group that did not undergo screening.[2] Importantly, an elevated PSA (defined as 3.0 ng/mL or more) uniformly led to biopsy and treatment was strongly encouraged. At a median 11-year follow-up, the incidence of prostate cancer in the screening group was 9.6% compared with 6.0% in the control group. There were 299 prostate cancer deaths in the screening group and 462 prostate cancer deaths in the control group, with death rates of 0.39 and 0.50 per 1000 person-years, respectively. This finding corresponded to an overall RR reduction of 21% in the screened group (RR 0.79, 95% CI 0.68–0.91) but an absolute difference in overall mortality of only 1.07 deaths per 1000 men randomized. When looking at prostate cancer deaths occurring in years 10 and 11 of the follow-up, an even more pronounced RR reduction of 38% was detected (RR 0.62, 95% CI 0.45–0.85). Although this study did demonstrate a clear advantage, it is important to point out that the number needed to screen was 1055 men to detect 37 cancers to prevent one prostate cancer death.

A third cohort reported was a subgroup of the ERSPC trial. It was reported separately because the trial predates the larger ERSPC trial and, as a result, was considered a separate study. This study randomized 19 904 men aged 50 to 64 years to PSA screening at 2-year intervals or no screening.[16] Although the study population was smaller, the follow-up was longer. At the 14-year follow-up, 1138 cancers were detected in the screening group and 718 in the control group, resulting in a cumulative incidence of 12.7% versus 8.2% (hazard ratio [HR] 1.64, 95% CI 1.50–1.80). There were 78 prostate cancer deaths in the screening group and 44 in the control group, for an absolute risk reduction of 0.4%. This finding corresponded to a 44% reduction in death rate (RR 0.56, 95% CI 0.39–0.82). In this trial, the number needed to be screened was much more reasonable; 293 men would need to be screened to diagnose 12 prostate cancers and to prevent one prostate death.

These trials demonstrate that PSA screening invariably leads to a higher rate of detection of prostate cancer with some of the trials demonstrating a reduction in prostate cancer mortality.

PSA SCREENING MODIFICATIONS TO IMPROVE DETECTION

PSA is a glycoprotein produced by the epithelial cells that line the acini and ducts of the prostate gland. Any disruption of the normal prostatic architecture allows greater amounts of PSA to enter the general circulation. Therefore, many prostatic diseases, including benign prostatic hyperplasia, prostatitis, urinary tract infection, and urinary retention, have been shown to persistently elevate the PSA and should be treated before screening.[4,17,18] In addition, DRE and ejaculation may also lead to small, transient increases in serum PSA that persist for approximately 2 days.[19,20] Lastly, major manipulations of the genitourinary tract, such as prostate biopsy, transurethral resection of the prostate, and cystoscopy, have been shown to cause more dramatic elevations of PSA in the range of 6 to 8 ng/mL and result in persistently elevated levels for up to 4 weeks.[18] For this reason, PSA testing should be postponed until an adequate time period has elapsed. Because of these confounders, it is not surprising that modifications are needed to improve its ability to detect cancer.

Because of the known shortcomings of PSA testing, efforts have been underway for the past decades to improve PSA-based screening. These efforts can be placed into 4 broad categories: (1) PSA refinements, (2) novel tests, (3) prediction tools, and (4) risk-based screening. All of these modifications have been shown to improve the detection of cancer; but, unfortunately, most of them have a limited ability to detect aggressive disease.

PSA REFINEMENTS
PSA Velocity

Because PSA increases more rapidly in the setting of prostate cancer, PSA velocity has been proposed as an adjunct to improve PSA performance. This method involves obtaining at least 3 serial readings over an 18-month period to calculate the rate of increase in PSA.[21] Carter and colleagues[22] were the first to demonstrate this relationship. They found that a PSA velocity greater than 0.75 ng/mL/y was associated with an increased risk of cancer diagnosis and had a specificity of 90% compared with 60% if a PSA cutoff of 4.0 ng/mL alone was used. PSA velocity has been investigated in multiple settings since.[23–25] The most pertinent to screening is a second article by Carter and colleagues,[25] which examined PSA levels and the rate of risk decades before diagnosis in the Baltimore Longitudinal Study. They found that a PSA velocity greater than 0.35 ng/mL/y tested 10 to

15 years before the diagnosis of prostate cancer was associated with significantly worse cancer-specific survival and a higher RR of prostate cancer death (RR 4.7, 95% CI 1.3–16.5, $P = .02$). Not all studies have demonstrated a benefit to the use of PSA velocity. Pinsky and colleagues[26] examined PSA velocity as a predictor of aggressive disease in the PLCO trial. They failed to find an association with an advanced pathologic stage and, therefore, concluded that PSA velocity added little to the accuracy of PSA alone. In the ERSPC trial, subgroup analysis demonstrated that PSA velocity was not a predictor of positive biopsy when adjusting for PSA.[27] Similarly in the PCPT,[28] the PSA velocity did not add clinically important information to PSA testing alone in men. However, this trial showed that for men with PSA less than 4.0 ng/mL and normal DRE, a PSA velocity of 0.35 ng/mL/y was a predictor of cancer but would lead to a higher number of unnecessary biopsies, with nearly 1 in 7 men being biopsied. It is important to note that, with the exception of the data from Carter and colleagues, all PSA values were obtained relatively close to the diagnosis of prostate cancer. Therefore, it is possible that PSA velocity decades before diagnosis may be of clinical utility; but short-term fluctuations do not provide additional information.

Free PSA

PSA circulates in the blood in 2 fractions. Complexed PSA is bound to other plasma proteins and free PSA circulates unbound. Because benign prostatic tissue produces more free PSA than prostate cancer in the serum, patients with prostate cancer will have lower free/total PSA ratios.[29] A large, multicenter prospective trial in men between 50 and 75 years of age with PSA levels of 4.0 to 10.0 ng/mL and normal DRE found that a free PSA of 25% or more reduced unnecessary biopsies by 20%.[30] If the free PSA cutoff was set to 10%, the biopsy detection rate increased to 56%, more than doubling the reported positive biopsy rate. On multivariate analysis, the percentage of free PSA was an independent predictor of prostate cancer (odds ratio [OR] 3.2, 95% CI 2.5–4.1, $P<.001$) and had a stronger association than age (OR 1.2, 95% CI 0.92–1.55) or total PSA level (OR 1.0, 95% CI 0.92–1.11). However, the investigators also reported an 8% chance of prostate cancer among men with free PSA greater than 25%. A meta-analysis of 41 studies found that in men with PSA between 4.0 and 10.0 ng/mL, free PSA was of clinical value at the extremes of its range (less than 7%–10% or greater than 20%–25%).[31] For free PSA less than 7% to 10%, sensitivity was approximately 40% and specificity ranged between 72% and 92%. If the threshold of 20% to 25% free PSA was used, sensitivity would be increased to 90% to 95%.

Complexed PSA

Complexed PSA has also been investigated as an adjunct to total PSA. Most trials have studied the performance of complexed PSA in men with intermediate PSA values (4.0–10.0 ng/mL). These studies have demonstrated an increase in specificity and, thus, a decrease in unnecessary biopsies.[32–34] Partin and colleagues[32] conducted a large, multi-institutional prospective trial and showed a complexed PSA specificity of 13.3% compared with only 8.6% for total PSA in men with total PSA between 4.0 and 10.0 ng/mL. This finding was less specific than the specificity of free PSA at 21.5%. When looking at patients with a total PSA between 2.0 and 6.0 ng/mL, complexed PSA was more specific than total or free PSA. However, the investigators concluded that complexed PSA offered little additional benefit to total PSA in the differentiation of benign and malignant disease.

PSA Density

Prostate cancer has been reported to produce up to 10 times more PSA per volume of tissue than benign conditions.[3,35] For this reason, PSA density has been proposed as a way to improve PSA performance. A prospective multicenter clinical trial of nearly 5000 men demonstrated that using the accepted PSA density cutoff of 0.15 ng/mL/cm³ had better specificity than PSA alone; however, this threshold missed 47% of the tumors detected by PSA alone in men with a PSA range of 4.0 to 10.0 ng/mL or abnormal DRE.[36]

All of the aforementioned modifications to PSA seem to be able to improve the sensitivity or specificity of the standard PSA test but depend highly on the cutoff values used and the subsets of the populations in which they were evaluated.

RISK-BASED SCREENING

Applying PSA screening to a higher-risk population is another way of improving the performance of PSA testing. African American ethnicity and a family history of prostate cancer have been shown to be significant risk factors for the development of prostate cancer.[37–41] Race-specific incidence of prostate cancer has been shown to be significantly higher for African Americans as compared with Caucasians.[38] African American men also have a younger age of diagnosis,[39] higher-grade disease,[42] and increased risk of death.[40] Family history is also a strong risk factor. Data from 2 meta analyses demonstrated a RR risk of prostate cancer of 2.0 to 3.5 for men with a family history of prostate cancer,[41,43] depending on the degree of relatedness and number of affected relatives. Brandt and colleagues[44] used the Swedish Family Cancer Database to estimate the age-specific risk of prostate cancer according to the number of affected relatives. The investigators reported that HRs of prostate cancer diagnosis increased with the number of affected relatives and decreased with increasing age, with the highest hazard ratios in men younger than 65 years with 3 affected brothers (HR approximately 23) and lowest ratio in men aged 65 to 74 years with an affected father (HR approximately 1.8). For this reason, men at an increased risk for disease, particularly aggressive disease, should be a focus for prostate cancer screening.

Another strategy is to obtain a PSA early in life and allow that to determine risk and, therefore, subsequent need for additional testing. Although not a randomized controlled trial, a recent case-control study evaluating a total of 21 277 Swedish men aged 27 to 52 years who provided blood samples at baseline and 4922 men invited to provide a second sample 6 years later revealed that the measurement of the PSA concentration in early midlife can identify a small group of men at an increased risk of prostate cancer metastasis several decades later.[45] At a median 27 years of follow-up, 44% of the deaths were noted to occur in men with PSA concentrations in the highest 10th percentile (PSA ≥ 1.6 ng/mL) at 45 to 49 years of age, with a similar proportion for 51 to 55 years of age. For patients with PSA less than the median (0.68 ng/mL for 45–49 years of age and 0.85 ng/mL for 51–55 years of age), the 15-year risk of metastatic disease was 0.09% at 45 to 49 years of age and 0.28% at 51 to 55 years of age. These results supported the use of only 3 lifetime PSA tests (mid to late 40s, early 50s, and 60 years of age) for at least of half of the men who are less than the medians.

PREDICTION TOOLS

Several multivariate prediction tools for assessing the individualized risk of prostate cancer have been developed.[42,46–49] These tools provide individualized, evidence-based information with the aim of decreasing overdiagnosis through decreasing the number of unnecessary biopsies. One of the most commonly used tools is the PCPT risk calculator (http://deb.uthscsa.edu/URORiskCalc/Pages/uroriskcalc.jsp).[42] It is based on serum PSA, family history, DRE, and prior biopsy data. The study reported an area under the curve (AUC) of 0.70 for the calculator compared with 0.68 for PSA alone. A postulated reason for the relatively small benefit of the calculator over PSA alone was the impact on the predictive value of PSA level on systematically biopsied patients as opposed to the use of a cutoff level. The PCPT risk calculator has been externally validated with accuracies between 0.57 and 0.74.[50,51] It has also been shown to underestimate the risk of high-grade disease.[52] The ERSPC risk calculator (www.prostatecancer-riskcalculator.com) is another commonly used assessment tool.[46] It comprises 6 steps based on 6 different logistic regression models and estimates the risk of positive biopsy according to serum PSA, prostate volume, DRE, outcome of transrectal ultrasound, and previous biopsy results. External validation studies demonstrated AUCs between 0.71 and 0.80.[53,54] Trottier and colleagues[55] compared the PCPT with the ERSPC risk calculators and demonstrated that the ERSPC calculator was superior with an AUC of 0.71 compared with 0.63 for the PCPT calculator and 0.55 for PSA alone.

NOVEL SCREENING TESTS

The controversy around PSA screening for prostate cancer has demonstrated the need for a more reliable prostate cancer screening marker. Many novel markers are currently under investigation, with prostate cancer antigen 3 (PCA3), Prostate Health Index, and TMPRSS2:ERG gene fusion among the most studied.

PCA3

The PCA3 gene was identified in 1999. PCA3 is a noncoding RNA whose expression is restricted to the prostate and noted to be highly overexpressed in prostate cancer tissue as compared with normal or hyperplastic prostate tissues.[56] PCA3 mRNA can be detected in first-catch urine samples following attentive DRE. PCA3 mRNA and PSA mRNA in these samples are quantified and the ratio of PCA3/PSA is reported. Deras and colleagues[57] demonstrated that an increasing PCA3 score correlated with an increased risk of positive biopsy and was independent of prostate volume, serum PSA, and number of prior biopsies. A logistic regression algorithm using PCA3, serum PSA, prostate volume, and DRE resulted in an increased AUC from 0.69 for PCA3 alone to 0.75 ($P = .0002$). Both of these were superior to serum PSA alone, which had an AUC of 0.58. Aubin and colleagues[58] investigated the performance of PCA3 in the Reduction by Dutasteride of Prostate Cancer Events (REDUCE) trial cohort. The REDUCE trial was a prostate cancer risk reduction study in men taking dutasteride.[59] The study enrolled men with an increased risk of prostate cancer (aged 50–75 years, serum PSA 2.5–10.0 ng/mL [defined as intermediate PSA], and negative biopsy at baseline). Men were randomized to daily dutasteride or placebo, and biopsies were performed at 2 and 4 years. PCA3 scores were measured before year 2 and year 4 biopsies from 1072 and 1140 subjects in the placebo arm of the trial, respectively. PCA3 was found to be predictive of the biopsy outcome in patients with a previously negative biopsy, whereas PSA and free PSA were not. A meta-analysis of the utility of the PCA3 score from 11 clinical trials in men with PSA between 2.5 and 10.0 ng/mL or negative prior biopsy reported a sensitivity of 53% to 84% and a specificity of 71% to 80% for the intermediate PSA group and a sensitivity of 47% to 58% and a specificity of 71% to 72%

for the negative biopsy group.[60] PCA3 performance was superior to both PSA and free PSA. Based on this data, PCA3 has been approved by the Food and Drug Administration (FDA) for screening in men with clinical suspicion of prostate cancer and a previously negative prostate biopsy. The PCA3 assay involves the collection of whole urine following aggressive DRE. Using PCA3 and PSA mRNA levels, a PCA3 score is generated using the following formula: (PCA3 mRNA)/(PSA mRNA) × 1000. Based on the aforementioned data, a PCA3 score greater than 35 is considered abnormal.

Prostate Health Index

The prostate health index (PHI) is a composite number using PSA, free PSA, and [-2] proPSA. The [-2]proPSA is a precursor to PSA[61] and has been noted to have a higher sensitivity and specificity for the detection of prostate cancer than PSA or free PSA alone.[62] A study of 892 men with no history of prostate cancer, normal DRE, and PSA between 2.0 and 10.0 ng/mL demonstrated that the PHI had a higher sensitivity and specificity than PSA or free PSA. An increasing PHI was associated with a 4.7-fold increased risk of prostate cancer and a 1.61-fold increased risk of Gleason score greater than or equal to 4 + 3 = 7 disease on biopsy.[63] The study concluded that the use of the PHI may be a useful screening tool and decrease unnecessary biopsies in men older than 50 years with normal DRE and intermediate PSA. The PHI has been FDA approved for this indication.

TMPRSS2:ERG Gene Fusion

The gene fusion of the TMPRSS2 prostate-specific gene to the ERG transcription factor on chromosome 21q forms an oncogenic rearrangement that has been identified in half of prostate cancers and more than 40% of lymph node metastases indicating that the TMPRSS2:ERG fusion is associated with clinical features for prostate cancer progression compared with tumors that lack the TMPRSS2:ERG rearrangement.[64,65] A urine assay similar to PCA3 was developed and evaluated in a multicenter trial of 1312 men with elevated PSA.[66] Urine TMPRSS2:ERG was associated with indicators of clinically significant cancer at biopsy and prostatectomy. Importantly, because upwards of 50% of tumors do not express a fusion, the absence of a fusion by assay does not mean that cancer is not present. As a result, the investigators have used an assay that also incorporates PCA3. Men in the highest and lowest of 3 TMPRSS2:ERG+PCA3 score groups had markedly different rates of cancer, clinically significant cancer by Epstein criteria, and high-grade cancer. The study concluded that the TMPRSS2:ERG+PCA3 score enhances the utility of serum PSA for predicting the presence of clinically significant cancer on biopsy.

CURRENT SCREENING GUIDELINES

Various national organizations have developed guidelines to aid clinicians in the diagnosis of prostate cancer, particularly with regard to screening and the use of PSA. These results are summarized in **Table 1**. Questions raised by the aforementioned large randomized trials have led to a national debate on the benefits of PSA screening and recommendations have been modified. Guideline panels develop analysis criteria a priori. The result is that similar data can be used to draw different conclusions and can lead to different recommendations.

In its 2012 updated statement, the US Preventative Services Task Force (USPSTF) recommended that PSA not be used to routinely screen men for prostate cancer, concluding that there is moderate certainty that the benefits of screening do not outweigh the harms.[67] This recommendation was based largely on data from the

Table 1
Prostate cancer screening guidelines from the American Cancer Society, National Comprehensive Cancer Network, and the American Urological Association

	Screening Modality	Age to Commence Screening	Age to Terminate Screening	Screening Frequency	Triggers for Biopsy
ACS	PSA ± DRE	50 y[a]	Life expectancy <10 y	Annually if PSA ≥2.5 ng/mL, every 2 y otherwise	PSA ≥4.0 ng/mL[b]
NCCN	PSA and DRE	40 y[c]	75 y or significant comorbidities	Annually after 50 y[d]	1. PSA >2.5 ng/mL or PSA velocity ≥0.35 ng/mL/y 2. PSA 4–10 ng/mL 3. PSA >10 ng/mL[e]
AUA	PSA and DRE	55 y[f]	70 y[g] or life expectancy <10–15 y	Every 2 y or more	PSA ≥4.0 ng/mL[h]

Abbreviations: ACS, American Cancer Society; AUA, American Urological Association; NCCN, National Comprehensive Cancer Network.
[a] For average-risk men. Screening should commence at 40 to 45 years of age in high-risk men (first-degree relatives with prostate cancer diagnosed before 65 years of age or black men).
[b] Individualized decision for biopsy in men with PSA between 2.5 and 4.0 ng/mL.
[c] Initial screening performed to guide frequency of subsequent screening regimen.
[d] Screening frequency for 40 to 50 years of age is based on risk factors.
[e] Biopsy should be considered for scenario 1. It should be done in scenario 2 OR free to total PSA should be checked. Biopsy should be performed for scenario 3.
[f] High-risk men aged 40 to 55 years may undergo screening on an individualized basis.
[g] Some men older than 70 years in excellent health may continue to benefit from screening.
[h] A higher biopsy threshold (eg, 10 ng/mL) should be used in men older than 70 years.

PLCO and ERSPC trials.[2,3] The USPSTF did, however, advise that men requesting screening should be supported in making an informed decision. In addition, the task force did not address the issue of screening in high-risk groups, such as men with a family history of prostate cancer or African Americans.

The American Cancer Society (ACS) recommends involving men in the decision process before initiating screening.[68] Men should have sufficient information regarding the risks and benefits of screening and treatment in order to make an informed, shared decision. For men that decide to be screened, testing with PSA with or without DRE should begin at 50 years of age for average-risk men. Screening should not be offered to men with a life expectancy of less than 10 years. Screening should continue annually in men with an initial PSA of 2.5 ng/mL or greater and every 2 years in men with a lower PSA. Patients at a high risk of developing prostate cancer (men with first-degree relatives with prostate cancer diagnosed before 65 years of age or black men) should have screening initiated at 40 to 45 years of age. The ACS also recommends that the biopsy threshold should remain at 4.0 ng/mL and an individualized decision should be made if PSA is between 2.5 and 4.0 ng/mL.

The American Urological Association (AUA) recommends against screening of men younger than 40 years because of low clinical prevalence and the fact that autopsy data show that most prostate cancers in this age group are low grade.[69] Routine screening in men aged 40 to 54 years is also not recommended. This guideline is based on the fact that the randomized controlled trials[2,3] did not include men younger than 55 years, the extremely low probability of dying from prostate cancer before

55 years of age, and the large number of patients needing to be screened to prevent one death. Furthermore, they argue that screening in this age group will result in longer lead times and expose patients to extended time at risk for harm from treatment. Men younger than 55 years at a higher-than-average risk should undergo screening on an individualized basis and only after an informed, shared decision is made. Shared decision making, including discussion of life expectancy, prostate cancer risk based on race and family history, and the degree to which screening will influence risk is recommended in men aged 55 to 69 years considering PSA screening and proceeding with testing based on the patients' values and preferences because this is the age group whereby screening seems to be of greatest benefit. In this age group, the benefit of preventing one prostate cancer death per 1000 people screened must be weighed against the harms of screening and treatment. In men who wish to proceed with screening, an interval of 2 years or more is recommended over annual screening. The increased screening period is an attempt to preserve the benefits of screening and reduce overdiagnosis and false positives. It is based on data from the randomized controlled trials showing that screening at 2- to 4-year intervals was not inferior to annual screening and that more than 95% of cancers detected at 4-year screening intervals had curable pathologic features.

The AUA recommends against routine PSA screening in men 70 years of age and older or those with a life expectancy of less than 10 to 15 years but recognizes that some men older than 70 years and in excellent health may benefit from screening. An informed shared decision to undergo screening may be made in these men. In this age group, there is no evidence for a benefit to screening or treatment of localized prostate cancer. Additionally, they recommend a higher biopsy threshold (eg, 10 ng/mL) based on evidence that this subgroup is most likely to benefit from treatment and discontinuation of screening in men with PSA less than 3 ng/mL because these men are unlikely to develop lethal cancer, in this age group.

The National Comprehensive Cancer Network (NCCN) recommends initial screening with PSA and DRE at 40 years of after performing an individualized risk assessment and a thorough risk/benefit discussion.[70] Men with risk factors (African American men, those with a family history, men with a PSA ≥1 ng/mL, and those taking 5-alpha reductase inhibitors) should be rescreened after 1 year. If the PSA is greater than 1 ng/mL, then annual PSA and DRE screening should be continued. If the PSA is 1 ng/mL or less, then additional screening should be deferred until 45 years of age. Men without risk factors should be rescreened at 45 years of age. If rescreened at 45 years of age, if the PSA is less than 1 ng/mL, then annual screening with PSA and DRE is recommended starting at 50 years of age. Patients with a PSA of 1 ng/mL or more at 45 years of age should continue annual screening with PSA and DRE. The recommendation of early PSA screening (<50 years of age) is based on evidence that PSA elevation of more than 1.0 ng/mL in this age group identifies men at a high risk of developing clinically significant prostate cancer over the subsequent 30 years[71] and allows for decreased screening in lower-risk men. A biopsy should be considered in men with a PSA greater than 2.5 ng/mL or with PSA velocity of 0.35 ng/mL/y or more at the time of initial screening. Men with a PSA level between 4 and 10 ng/mL should get a biopsy or free to total PSA with biopsy for low free to total PSA ratio. A biopsy should be performed if the PSA is more than 10 ng/mL on the initial screening. PSA velocity is recommended for use as an adjunct to PSA alone based on data from the Baltimore Longitudinal Study of Aging.[25] The NCCN recommends that screening in men older than 75 years or those with significant comorbidities should be considered on an individual basis because it has been shown that treatment of prostate cancer in this population is not likely to improve survival.[72,73]

Although serum PSA testing remains the most widely used screening test for prostate cancer, it seems that the test is plagued by many shortcomings. Most notably, the relatively low specificity at the generally accepted biopsy threshold of 4.0 ng/mL leads to many unnecessary biopsies and its inability to discriminate between aggressive and indolent cancers, which leads to the detection and treatment of many cancers that would have otherwise have remained clinically occult.

OVERDIAGNOSIS IN PROSTATE CANCER

Overdiagnosis is defined as the detection of cancer that would otherwise not become clinically overt over a patient's lifetime or not lead to cancer-related death. Overdiagnosis is of particular importance in prostate cancer because of the high incidence of the disease and its low mortality rate. Although this is relatively easy to define for a population of patients, it can be hard to define for the individual. The lifetime risk of being diagnosed with prostate cancer is 21% in the United States, whereas the risk of death is approximately 3%.[1] A contemporary autopsy study of 1056 individuals dying of other causes demonstrated evidence of prostate cancer in 44% to 77% of men aged 50 to 79 years, with the incidence increasing with age.[9] This study also demonstrated a prostate cancer incidence of 8% to 31% in men aged 20 to 39 years, demonstrating the early age of onset and the long latency period seen in prostate cancer. Additional autopsy studies have shown similar results.[10–12]

The question raised is if tumors detected in routine screening are similar to these autopsy studies. Draisma and colleagues[74] investigated the rates of overdiagnosis in a subset of the ERSPC study. Overdiagnosis was defined as diagnosis of cancers that would have otherwise not have been detected during a person's lifetime in the absence of screening based on natural history data in prostate cancer. Modeling analysis of the Rotterdam section of the ERSPC estimated a lead time of 12.3 years (range 11.6–14.1 years) and overdiagnosis of 27% (range 24%–37%) for a single screening test at 55 years of age. The degree of overdiagnosis was heavily influenced by age and increased to 56% (range 53%–61%) by 75 years of age. In the age group of 55 to 67 years, overdiagnosis was estimated at 48% (range 44%–55%); the lead time was 11.2 years (range 10.8–12.1 years) with every 4-year screening as performed in the ERSPC[2]; and there was a 50% (range 46%–57%) rate of overdiagnosis with annual screening as in the PLCO trial.[3] Etzioni and colleagues[75] performed a similar analysis using SEER registry data from 1988 to 1998. Overdiagnosis was defined in an identical fashion as the Draisma study.[74] By comparing their model-generated predicted incidence of prostate cancer with actual SEER registry rates, they demonstrated significant overdiagnosis with variation based on race. For men aged 60 to 84 years, overdiagnosis was approximated to occur in 28.8% of white men and 43.8% of black men screened with PSA and lead times were 5 to 7 years.

High rates of overdiagnosis in prostate cancer are of concern because patients choose to undergo treatment most of the time. Despite a decrease in risk category of disease at the time of diagnosis, approximately 90% of men still elect some type of intervention, including surgery, radiation therapy, or androgen deprivation.[76]

IMPACT OF OVERDIAGNOSIS

PSA screening and the diagnosis of prostate cancer have been shown to have a detrimental effect on mental health and lead to anxiety and depression.[77] Prostate cancer diagnosis has adverse physical effects, such as an increase in cardiovascular events (RR 1.3, 95% CI 1.3–1.3) and suicide rates (RR 2.6, 95% CI 2.1–3.0).[78]

Because an elevated PSA often leads to prostate biopsy, the morbidity of this procedure must also be considered. Commonly reported adverse events after prostate biopsy included pain, low-grade fever, hematuria, hematochezia, and hematospermia.[79] Significant hemorrhage or infection was thought to occur in 1% to 4% of patients following biopsy.[80–82] However, recent data suggests that hospital admission for serious infection may be increasing because of the emergence of fluoroquinolone-resistant and multidrug-resistant bacteria.[83–85] Sepsis leading to death is the most feared complication. Analysis of the ERSPC trial data demonstrated a 4.2% fever and hospital admission rate following prostate biopsy as compared with 0.8% in the control group; however, no deaths were reported.[86] A population-based study in Canada reported a mortality rate of 0.09% in the 30 days following prostate biopsy, but the causes of death could not be ascertained.[87] This study did report an increase in the 30-day hospitalization rate from 1.0% in 1996 to 4.1% in 2005.

Prostate cancer overdiagnosis seems to expose most patients to the risks of treatment; in the United States, overdiagnosis is closely associated with overtreatment. This point is demonstrated by aggressive treatment in 91% of men in the PLCO trial[3] and 92.5% in the Cancer of the Prostate Strategic Urologic Research Endeavor Trial.[88]

Treatment of patients with indolent disease[89] or significant comorbidities[90] is unlikely to yield a mortality benefit and can result in a significant decrease in quality of life. Sanda and colleagues[91] reported urinary, bowel, and sexual quality-of-life outcomes among men undergoing radical prostatectomy, external beam radiation, or brachytherapy for prostate cancer. Patient-reported outcomes were collected before and after therapy in 1201 men and 625 spouses. Patients reported a significant decrease in quality of life caused by persistent urinary, sexual, and bowel dysfunction. Patients in the brachytherapy group reported long-standing urinary irritation and bowel and sexual symptoms. Radical prostatectomy was associated with decreased sexual function, somewhat mitigated if nerve sparing was performed, and increased urinary incontinence but improved urinary irritation and obstructive symptoms. Bowel dysfunction, particularly rectal urgency, frequency, pain, fecal incontinence, and hematochezia, was seen in both the brachytherapy and external-beam-radiation groups. Adjuvant hormone therapy was found to exacerbate the adverse effects of radiation therapy and brachytherapy.

Although patients at risk for death from disease clearly benefit from treatment, these adverse affects illustrate the need of minimizing overdiagnosis and the resultant overtreatment of clinically insignificant disease.

WATCHFUL WAITING AND OBSERVATION

A critical issue surrounding screening is treatment. Although it is not the focus of this review, if no effective treatment exists or if treatment is not performed, then screening will have little to no benefit. Recent mortality data from 2 large randomized trials comparing watchful waiting, whereby men are advised to defer treatment until symptoms develop and commence androgen deprivation at that time, with radical prostatectomy in men with localized prostate cancer indicate that there is a subset of men who have a survival benefit from treatment.[73,89] Bill-Axelson and colleagues[73] randomized 695 men with localized prostate cancer to watchful waiting or radical prostatectomy. At a median 12.8 years of follow-up, there were 166 deaths out of 347 men in the radical-prostatectomy group and 201 deaths out of 348 men in the watchful-waiting group ($P = .007$). There were 55 cancer-specific deaths in the surgery group and 81 in the watchful-waiting group, accounting for a cumulative incidence of death from prostate cancer of 14.6% versus 20.7%, respectively, (95% CI

0.2–12.0) and an RR with surgery of 0.62 (95% CI 0.44–0.87, $P = .01$). The survival benefit was observed even among men with low-risk prostate cancer but not in men older than 65 years of age. The number needed to treat to avert one death was 15 for the overall cohort and 7 for men younger than 65 years. In a similar study, Wilt and colleagues[89] randomized 731 men with localized prostate cancer to radical prostatectomy or observation. During a median follow-up of 10 years, there were 171 deaths out of 364 men in the radical-prostatectomy group and 183 deaths out of 367 men in the observation group (HR 0.88, 95% CI 0.7–1.08, $P = .22$). There were 21 cancer-specific deaths in the surgery group and 31 in the observation group (HR 0.63, 95% CI 0.36–1.09, $P = .09$). Thus, this study did not demonstrate a significant benefit for the overall cohort. However, for men with a PSA greater than 10 ng/mL and for men with aggressive prostate cancer, surgery reduced prostate cancer mortality (5.6% vs 12.8%, $P = .02$, and 9.1% vs 17.5%, $P = .04$, respectively). The results of this subgroup analysis are similar to those reported in the Scandinavian study.[73] These results along with the 21% survival benefit reported in the ERSPC trial[2] indicate that there are a significant proportion of men in which screening may be beneficial.

The current dilemma lies in identifying men who will benefit from treatment, thus, separating overdiagnosis from overtreatment and minimizing the adverse effects for patients who do not stand to gain from aggressive intervention. This outcome may be achieved by improved selection of patients in whom treatment should be pursued based on a better understanding of the natural history of the disease and the risk factors associated with progression to clinically significant cancer or death. For this reason, active surveillance has largely supplanted watchful waiting.[92,93]

ACTIVE SURVEILLANCE

Clearly, if we could define with certainty men with cancer of no clinical impact, we would refrain from treating them. The problem is that men with low-risk disease, who are not treated, do have an appreciable risk of dying of prostate cancer.[15] As a result, the focus has shifted from expectant management to close follow-up and intervention if the cancer becomes more aggressive. Active surveillance is a strategy for the management of low-risk prostate cancer (low volume, Gleason score, and clinical stage) whereby men are carefully observed with serial PSA testing, repeat biopsies, and other tests intended to identify early disease progression and allow for deferment of treatment.[92–94] This strategy differs significantly from watchful waiting, which is generally used in older men with significant comorbidity. It relies on the presumption that lead time from diagnosis to clinical progression is usually long for low-risk disease and that treatment of cancer at the first signs of higher-risk disease will likely fall well within the window of opportunity for cure.

Several institutions have reported active surveillance protocols,[92–100] with a total of nearly 2900 men accrued in all series. Each cohort includes slightly different inclusion criteria reflecting variations of low-grade (Gleason score 3 + 3), low-volume disease (number or percentage of total cores and clinical stage) with low PSA (PSA<10 ng/mL). Some protocols include a higher PSA (up to 15 ng/mL) and small focus of Gleason 4, particularly in elderly patients. However, most studies would exclude these patients; studies examining intermediate-risk patients have found a higher progression rate.[101] Protocols differ by institution but generally include periodic PSA and DRE as well as periodic repeat prostate biopsy. There is also a lack of uniformity in the definition of progression to higher-risk disease. Common triggers for treatment include biochemical progression (PSA more than the predefined threshold for biopsy, high PSA velocity, or rapid PSA doubling time), increase in tumor volume (based on the number or percent of involved biopsy cores), increase in Gleason score (presence of Gleason pattern 4), and increased clinical stage (DRE or imaging). The median ages range from 62 to 70 years, and the median follow-up ranges from 2 to 7 years, with no cohort mature enough to draw definitive conclusions regarding mortality risks. In these series, 14% to 41% of men will progress from surveillance to active treatment. This proportion depends on how stringently patients are evaluated, the initial inclusion criteria, the specified indications for radical treatment, and patient and clinician preferences.

Most patients are reclassified as higher risk by upgrading at the time of repeat biopsy. It is thought that this is caused, in large part, by undersampling at the time of the initial biopsy.[93,99] For this reason, early confirmatory biopsy should be considered in cases when the initial biopsy was less than 12 cores or was of questionable quality. Overall, prostate cancer mortality is reported to be in the range of 0% to 1%, but the median follow-up is relatively short.[94] The Toronto group reported outcomes of 450 men at the longest median follow-up of 6.8 years.[98] The median age for this group was 70 years. The overall survival was 78.6%, and the 10-year prostate cancer actuarial survival was 97.2%. Thirty percent of patients were reclassified and treated radically. In this group, half of the patients had PSA failure, representing 15% of the overall cohort. Overall, the RR for non–prostate cancer death was 19 times higher than for prostate cancer mortality.

These findings demonstrate that active surveillance seems to be a valid treatment option for patients with low-risk prostate cancer and offers an opportunity to limit intervention to patients that will benefit most from radical treatment. More widespread adoption of active surveillance is likely to lead to a significant decrease in the rates of overtreatment. However, given the relatively short follow-up, these cohorts should be followed closely to determine if this management strategy remains effective over time. In addition, the average age in these cohorts is relatively old. Utilization of active surveillance in younger patients should be approached cautiously.

SUMMARY

PSA-based screening has led to a dramatic change in the diagnosis and management of prostate cancer. There is a shift away from mass screening toward a more focused approach in younger, healthier men. There should be a particular focus on men at risk of aggressive disease. In addition, because of the high overdiagnosis rates, treatment should be tailored to those at risk for dying of disease. In particular, patients with low-risk disease should be offered active surveillance.

REFERENCES

1. Siegel R, Naishadham D, Jemal A. Cancer statistics, 2013. CA Cancer J Clin 2013;63:11–30.
2. Schroder FH, Hugosson J, Roobol MJ, et al. Prostate cancer mortality at 11 years of follow-up. N Engl J Med 2012;366:981–90.
3. Andriole GL, Crawford D, Grubb RL 3rd, et al. Prostate cancer screening in the randomized prostate, lung, colorectal, and ovarian cancer screening trial: mortality results after 13 years of follow-up. J Natl Cancer Inst 2012;104:125–32.
4. Catalona WJ, Smith DS, Ratliff TL, et al. Measurement of prostate-specific antigen in serum as a screening test for prostate cancer. N Engl J Med 1991;324: 1156–61.
5. Thompson IM, Ernst JJ, Gangai MP, et al. Adenocarcinoma of the prostate: results of routine urological screening. J Urol 1984;132:690.

6. McLaughlin AP, Saltzstein SL, McCullough DL, et al. Prostatic carcinoma: incidence and location of unsuspected lymphatic metastases. J Urol 1976; 115:89.
7. Paquette EL, Sun L, Paquette LR, et al. Improved prostate cancer-specific survival and other disease parameters: impact of prostate-specific antigen testing. Urology 2002;60:756.
8. Scosyrev E, Wu G, Mohile S, et al. Prostate-specific antigen screening for prostate cancer and the risk of overt metastatic disease at presentation. Cancer 2012;118:5768–76.
9. Powell IJ, Bock CH, Ruterbusch JJ, et al. Evidence supports a faster growth rate and/or earlier transformation to clinically significant cancer in black than in white American men, and influences racial progression and mortality disparity. J Urol 2010;183:1792–7.
10. Yatani R, Chigusa I, Akazaki K, et al. Geographic pathology of latent prostatic carcinoma. Int J Cancer 1982;29:611–6.
11. Scardino PT, Weaver R, Hudson MA. Early detection of prostate cancer. Hum Pathol 1992;23:211–22.
12. Stamatiou K, Alevizos A, Agapitos E, et al. Incidence of impalpable carcinoma of the prostate and of non-malignant and precarcinomatous lesions in Greek male population: an autopsy study. Prostate 2006;66:1319–28.
13. Thompson IM, Pauler DK, Goodman PJ, et al. Prevalence of prostate cancer among men with a prostate-specific antigen level<or =4.0 ng per milliliter. N Engl J Med 2004;350:2239.
14. Thompson IM, Ankerst DP, Chi C, et al. Operating characteristics of prostate-specific antigen in men with an initial PSA level of 3.0 ng/mL or lower. JAMA 2005;294:66.
15. Albertsen PC, Hanley JA, Fine J. 20-year outcomes following conservative management of clinically localized prostate cancer. JAMA 2005;293:2095–101.
16. Hugossan J, Carlsson S, Aus G, et al. Mortality results from the Goteborg randomised population-based prostate-cancer screening trial. Lancet Oncol 2010; 11:725–32.
17. Nadler RB, Humphrey PA, Smith DS, et al. Effect of inflammation and benign prostatic hyperplasia on elevated serum prostate specific antigen levels. J Urol 1995;154:407.
18. Tchetgen MB, Oesterling JE. The effect of prostatitis, urinary retention, ejaculation, and ambulation on the serum prostate-specific antigen concentration. Urol Clin North Am 1997;24:283.
19. Chybowski FM, Bergstralh EJ, Oesterling JE. The effect of digital rectal examination on the serum prostate specific antigen concentration: results of a randomized study. J Urol 1992;148:83.
20. Herschman JD, Smith DS, Catalona WJ. Effect of ejaculation on serum total and free prostate-specific antigen concentrations. Urology 1997;50:239.
21. D'Amico AV, Chen MH, Roehl KA, et al. Preoperative PSA velocity and the risk of death from prostate cancer after radical prostatectomy. N Engl J Med 2004;351: 125.
22. Carter HB, Pearson JD, Metter J, et al. Longitudinal evaluation of prostate specific antigen levels in men with and without prostate disease. JAMA 1992;267: 2215.
23. Moul JW, Sun L, Hotaling JM, et al. Age adjusted prostate specific antigen and prostate specific antigen velocity cut points in prostate cancer screening. J Urol 2007;177:499.

24. Loeb S, Roehl KA, Yu X, et al. Use of prostate-specific antigen velocity to follow up patients with isolated high-grade prostatic intraepithelial neoplasia on prostate biopsy. Urology 2007;69:108.
25. Carter HB, Ferrucci L, Kettermann A, et al. Detection of life-threatening prostate cancer with prostate-specific antigen velocity during a window of curability. J Natl Cancer Inst 2006;98:1521.
26. Pinsky PF, Andriole G, Crawford ED, et al. Prostate-specific antigen velocity and prostate cancer Gleason grade and stage. Cancer 2007;109:1689.
27. Raaijmakers R, Wildhagen MF, Ito K, et al. Prostate-specific antigen change in the European Randomized Study of Screening for Prostate Cancer, section Rotterdam. Urology 2004;63:316.
28. Vickers AJ, Till C, Tangen CM, et al. An empirical evaluation of guidelines on prostate-specific antigen velocity in prostate cancer detection. J Natl Cancer Inst 2011;103:462.
29. Jung K, Meyer A, Lein M, et al. Ratio of free-to-total prostate specific antigen in serum cannot distinguish patients with prostate cancer from those with chronic inflammation of the prostate. J Urol 1998;159:1595.
30. Catalona WJ, Partin AW, Slawin KM, et al. Use of the percentage of free prostate specific antigen to enhance differentiation of prostate cancer from benign prostatic diseases. JAMA 1998;279:1542.
31. Lee R, Localio AR, Armstrong K, et al. A meta-analysis of the performance characteristics of the free prostate-specific antigen test. Urology 2006;67:762.
32. Partin AW, Brawer MK, Bartsch G, et al. Complexed prostate specific antigen improves specificity for prostate cancer detection: results of a prospective multicenter clinical trial. J Urol 2003;170:1787.
33. Horninger W, Cheli CD, Babaian RJ, et al. Complexed prostate-specific antigen for early detection of prostate cancer in men with serum prostate-specific antigen levels of 2 to 4 nanograms per milliliter. Urology 2002;60:31.
34. Djavan B, Remzi M, Zlotta AR, et al. Complexed prostate-specific antigen, complexed prostate-specific antigen density of total and transition zone, complexed/total prostate specific antigen ratio, free-to-total prostate-specific antigen ratio, density of total and transition zone prostate-specific antigen: results of the prospective multicenter European trial. Urology 2002;60:4.
35. Stamey TA, Kabalin JN, McNeal JE, et al. Prostate specific antigen in the diagnosis and treatment of adenocarcinoma of the prostate. II. Radical prostatectomy treated patients. J Urol 1989;141:1076.
36. Catalona WJ, Richie JP, deKernion JB, et al. Comparison of prostate specific antigen concentration versus prostate specific antigen density in the early detection of prostate cancer: receiver operating characteristic curves. J Urol 1994;152:2031.
37. Zhu X, Albertsen PC, Andriole GL, et al. Risk-based prostate cancer screening. Eur Urol 2011;61:652–61.
38. Bostwick DG, Burke HB, Djakiew D, et al. Human prostate cancer risk factors. Cancer 2004;101:2371–490.
39. Cotter MP, Gern RW, Ho GY, et al. Role of family history and ethnicity on the mode and age of prostate cancer presentation. Prostate 2002;50:216–21.
40. Hsieh K, Albertsen PC. Populations at high risk for prostate cancer. Urol Clin North Am 2003;30:669–76.
41. Bruner DW, Moore D, Parlanti A, et al. Relative risk of prostate cancer for men with affected relatives: systematic review and meta-analysis. Int J Cancer 2003;107:797–803.

42. Thompson IM, Ankerst DP, Chi C, et al. Assessing prostate cancer risk: results from the Prostate Cancer Prevention Trial. J Natl Cancer Inst 2006;98: 529–34.

43. Johns LE, Houlston RS. A systematic review and meta-analysis of familial prostate cancer risk. BJU Int 2003;91:789–94.

44. Brandt A, Bermejo JL, Sundquist J, et al. Age-specific risk of incident prostate cancer and risk of death from prostate cancer defined by the number of affected family members. Eur Urol 2010;58:275–80.

45. Vickers AJ, Ulmert D, Sjorberg DD, et al. Strategy of detection of prostate cancer based on relation between prostate specific antigen at age 40-55 and long term risk of metastasis: case-control study. BMJ 2013;346:f2023.

46. Kranse R, Roobol M, Schroder FH. A graphical device to represent the outcomes of a logistic regression analysis. Prostate 2008;68:1674–80.

47. Nam RK, Toi A, Klotz LH, et al. Assessing individual risk for prostate cancer. J Clin Oncol 2007;25:3582–8.

48. Kattan MW, Eastham JA, Wheeler TM, et al. Counseling men with prostate cancer: a nomogram for predicting the presence of small, moderately differentiated, confined tumors. J Urol 2003;170:1792–7.

49. Shariat SF, Kattan MW, Vickers AJ, et al. Critical review of prostate cancer predictive tools. Future Oncol 2009;5:1555–84.

50. Eyre SJ, Ankerst DP, Wei JT, et al. Validation in a multiple urology practice cohort of the Prostate Cancer Prevention Trial calculator for predicting prostate cancer detection. J Urol 2009;182:2653–8.

51. Nguyen CT, Yu C, Moussa A, et al. Performance of prostate cancer prevention trial risk calculator in a contemporary cohort screened for prostate cancer and diagnosed by extended prostate biopsy. J Urol 2010;183:529–33.

52. Ngo TC, Turnbull BB, Lavori PW, et al. The prostate cancer risk calculator from the Prostate Cancer Prevention Trial underestimates the risk of high grade cancer in contemporary referral patients. J Urol 2011;185:483–7.

53. Cavadas V, Osorio L, Sabell F, et al. Prostate Cancer Prevention Trial and European Randomized Study of Screening for Prostate Cancer risk calculators: a performance comparison in a contemporary screened cohort. Eur Urol 2010; 58:551–8.

54. Oliveira M, Marques V, Carvalho AP, et al. Head-to-head comparison of two online nomograms for prostate biopsy outcome prediction. BJU Int 2011;107: 1780–3.

55. Trottier G, Roobol MJ, Lawrentschuk N, et al. Comparison of risk calculators from the Prostate Cancer Prevention Trial and the European Randomized Study of Screening for Prostate Cancer in a contemporary Canadian cohort. BJU Int 2011;108:E237–44.

56. Hessels D, Schalken JA. The use of PCA3 in the diagnosis of prostate cancer. Nat Rev Urol 2009;6:255.

57. Deras IL, Aubin SM, Blase A, et al. PCA3: a molecular urine assay for predicting prostate biopsy outcome. J Urol 2008;179:1587–92.

58. Aubin SM, Reid J, Sarno MJ, et al. PCA3 molecular urine test for predicting repeat prostate biopsy outcome in populations at risk: validation in the placebo arm of the dutasteride REDUCE trial. J Urol 2010;184:1947–52.

59. Andriole GL, Bostwick DG, Brawley OW, et al. Effect of dutasteride on risk of prostate cancer. N Engl J Med 2010;362:1192.

60. Vlaeminck-Guillem V, Ruffion A, André J, et al. Urinary prostate cancer 3 test: toward the age of reason? Urology 2010;75:447–53.

61. Mikolajczyk SD, Grauer LS, Millar LS, et al. A precursor form of PSA (pPSA) is a component of the free PSA in prostate cancer serum. Urology 1997;50:710–4.

62. Skoll LJ, Wang Y, Feng Z, et al. [-2]proenzyme prostate specific antigen for prostate cancer detection: a national cancer institute early detection research network validation study. J Urol 2008;180:539–43.

63. Catalona WJ, Partin AW, Sanda MG, et al. A multicenter study of [-2]pro-prostate specific antigen combined with prostate specific antigen and free prostate specific antigen for prostate cancer detection in the 2.0 to 10.0 ng/ml prostate specific antigen range. J Urol 2011;185:1650–5.

64. Perner S, Demichelis F, Beroukhim R, et al. TMPRSS2:ERG fusion-associated deletions provide insight into the heterogeneity of prostate cancer. Cancer Res 2006;66:8337–41.

65. Mosquera JM, Mehra R, Regan MM, et al. Prevalence of TMPRSS2-ERG fusion prostate cancer among men undergoing prostate biopsy in the United States. Clin Cancer Res 2009;15:4706–11.

66. Tomlins SA, Aubin SM, Siddiqui J, et al. Urine TMPRSS2:ERG fusion transcript stratifies prostate cancer risk in men with elevated serum PSA. Sci Transl Med 2011;3:94ra72.

67. Moyer VA, US Preventative Services Task Force. Screening for prostate cancer: US Preventative Services Task Force recommendation statement. Ann Intern Med 2012;157:120–34.

68. Wolf AM, Wender RC, Etzioni RB, et al. American Cancer Society guideline for the early detection of prostate cancer: update 2010. CA Cancer J Clin 2010; 60:70.

69. Carter HB, Albertsen PC, Barry MJ, et al. Early detection of prostate cancer; AUA guideline. J Urol 2013;190:419–26.

70. NCCN guidelines version 1. 2011 Prostate cancer early detection. Available at: http://www.nccn.org/professionals/physician_gls/pdf/prostate_detection.pdf. Accessed December 12, 2012.

71. Lilja H, Cronin AM, Dahlin A, et al. Prediction of significant prostate cancer diagnosed 20-30 years later with a single measure of prostate-specific antigen at or before age 50. Cancer 2011;117:1210–9.

72. Crawford ED, Grubb R 3rd, Black A, et al. Comorbidity and mortality results from a randomized prostate cancer screening trial. J Clin Oncol 2011;29:355–61.

73. Bill-Axelson A, Holmberg L, Ruutu M, et al. Radical prostatectomy versus watchful waiting in early prostate cancer. N Engl J Med 2011;364:1708–17.

74. Draisma G, Boer R, Otto SJ, et al. Lead times and overdetection due to prostate-specific antigen screening: estimates from the European Randomized Study of Screening for Prostate Cancer. J Natl Cancer Inst 2003;95:868–78.

75. Etzioni R, Penson DF, Legler JM, et al. Overdiagnosis due to prostate-specific antigen screening: lessons from U.S. prostate cancer incidence trends. J Natl Cancer Inst 2002;94:981.

76. Cooperberg MR, Broering JM, Kantoff PW, et al. Contemporary trends in low risk prostate cancer: risk assessment and treatment. Sixth Cambridge Conference on Innovations and Challenges in Prostate Cancer. J Urol 2007;178:S14.

77. Klotz L. Active surveillance for prostate cancer: patient selection and management. Curr Oncol 2010;17:S11–7.

78. Fall K, Fang F, Mucci LA, et al. Immediate risk for cardiovascular events and suicide following a prostate cancer diagnosis: prospective cohort study. PLoS Med 2009;6:e1000197.

79. Rosario DJ, Lane JA, Metcalfe C, et al. Short term outcomes of prostate biopsy in men tested for cancer by prostate specific antigen: prospective evaluation within ProtecT study. BMJ 2012;344:d7894.
80. Rietbergen JB, Kruger AE, Kranse R, et al. Complications of transrectal ultrasound-guided systematic sextant biopsies of the prostate: evaluation of complication rates and risk factors within a population-based screening program. Urology 1997;49:875.
81. Lee-Elliott CE, Dundas D, Patel U. Randomized trial of lidocaine vs. lidocaine/bupivacaine periprostatic injection on longitudinal pain scores after prostate biopsy. J Urol 2004;171:247.
82. Ragavan N, Philip J, Balasubramanian SP, et al. A randomized, controlled trial comparing lidocaine periprostatic nerve block, diclofenac suppository and both for transrectal ultrasound guided biopsy of prostate. J Urol 2005; 174:510.
83. Minamida S, Satoh T, Tabata K, et al. Prevalence of fluoroquinolone-resistant Escherichia coli before and incidence of acute bacterial prostatitis after prostate biopsy. Urology 2011;78:1235.
84. Taylor AK, Zembower TR, Nadler RB, et al. Targeted antimicrobial prophylaxis using rectal swab cultures in men undergoing transrectal ultrasound guided prostate biopsy is associated with reduced incidence of postoperative infectious complications and cost of care. J Urol 2012;187:1275.
85. Lange D, Zappavigna C, Hamidizadeh R, et al. Bacterial sepsis after prostate biopsy–a new perspective. Urology 2009;74:1200.
86. Loeb S, van den Heuvel S, Zhu X, et al. Infectious complications and hospital admissions after prostate biopsy in a European randomized trial. Eur Urol 2012;61:1110–4.
87. Nam RK, Saskin R, Lee Y, et al. Increasing hospital admission rates for urological complications after transrectal ultrasound guided prostate biopsy. J Urol 2010;183:963.
88. Cooperberg MR, Broering JM, Carroll PR. Time trends and local variation in primary treatment of localized prostate cancer. J Clin Oncol 2010;28:1117–23.
89. Wilt TJ, Brawer MK, Jones KM, et al. Radical prostatectomy versus observation for localized prostate cancer. N Engl J Med 2012;367:203–13.
90. Albertsen PC, Moore DF, Shih W, et al. Impact of comorbidity on survival among men with localized prostate cancer. J Clin Oncol 2011;29:1335–41.
91. Sanda MG, Dunn RL, Michalski J, et al. Quality of life and satisfaction with outcome among prostate-cancer survivors. N Engl J Med 2008;358:1250–61.
92. Cooperberg MR, Carroll PR, Klotz L. Active surveillance for prostate cancer: progress and promise. J Clin Oncol 2011;29:3669–76.
93. Klotz L. Active surveillance for favorable-risk prostate cancer: background, patient selection, triggers for intervention, and outcomes. Curr Urol Rep 2012; 13:153–9.
94. Dall'Era MA, Albertsen PC, Bangma C, et al. Active surveillance for prostate cancer: a systematic review of the literature. Eur Urol 2012;62:976–83.
95. van As NJ, Norman AR, Thomas K, et al. Predicting the probability of deferred radical treatment for localised prostate cancer managed by active surveillance. Eur Urol 2008;54:1297–305.
96. Soloway MS, Soloway CT, Eldefrawy A, et al. Careful selection and close monitoring of low-risk prostate cancer patients on active surveillance minimizes the need for treatment. Eur Urol 2010;58:831–5.

97. Tosoian JJ, Trock BJ, Landis P, et al. Active surveillance program for prostate cancer: an update of the Johns Hopkins experience. J Clin Oncol 2011;29: 2185–90.

98. Klotz L, Zhang L, Lam A, et al. Clinical results of long-term follow-up of a large, active surveillance cohort with localized prostate cancer. J Clin Oncol 2010;28: 126–31.

99. Berglund RK, Masaterson TA, Vora KC, et al. Pathologic upgrading and up staging with immediate repeat biopsy in patients eligible for active surveillance. J Urol 2008;180:1964–7.

100. van den Bergh RC, Vasarainen H, van der Poel HG, et al. Short-term outcomes of the prospective multicentre 'Prostate Cancer Research International: Active Surveillance' study. BJU Int 2010;105:956–62.

101. Cooperberg MR, Cowan JE, Reese AC, et al. Outcomes of active surveillance for men with intermediate-risk prostate cancer. J Clin Oncol 2011;29(2):228–34.

Surgical Management of Prostate Cancer

Jonathan L. Wright, MD, MS[a,b], Jason P. Izard, MD, MPH[a],
Daniel W. Lin, MD[a,b],*

KEYWORDS

- Prostate cancer • Radical prostatectomy • Pelvic lymph node dissection
- Surgical margin • Neoadjuvant therapy • Cryotherapy
- High-intensity focused ultrasound • Nerve sparing

KEY POINTS

- An individual's health state, not absolute age, should be utilized when determining fitness for radical prostatectomy.
- When performing a pelvic lymph node dissection for prostate cancer, an extended lymph node dissection should be performed.
- Nerve sparing selection should not compromise the oncologic goal of complete excision of the tumor with negative surgical margins.
- Multimodal therapy is often required for men with high risk prostate cancer.

INTRODUCTION

Prostate cancer (PCa) is the most common cancer diagnosis in men, with 238,590 estimated cases diagnosed in 2013.[1] PCa incidence increases with age, with the highest rates seen in men aged 70 to 80 years. Despite the low PCa case-fatality rate, the established overdiagnosis attributed to prostate-specific antigen (PSA) screening,[2] and the fact that most men with PCa will die of other causes, the majority of men still opt for surgical management of newly diagnosed PCa.[3] This article addresses various surgical and ablative approaches to local control of the primary tumor. A structured debate of the relative efficacies of the various treatments is beyond the scope of this article. Rather, here the authors address surgical aspects germane to the management of men with low-risk and high-risk PCa; the role of lymph node dissection (LND), surgical margins, and neoadjuvant therapy in localized PCa; and the content of published literature on surgical ablative therapies for PCa.

[a] Department of Urology, University of Washington School of Medicine, 1959 Northeast Pacific, Seattle, WA 98195, USA; [b] Division of Public Health Sciences, Fred Hutchinson Cancer Research Center, 1100 Fairview Avenue North, Seattle, WA 98109, USA
* Corresponding author. Department of Urology, University of Washington, 1959 Northeast Pacific, Box 356510, Seattle, WA 98195.
E-mail address: dlin@uw.edu

Hematol Oncol Clin N Am 27 (2013) 1111–1135
http://dx.doi.org/10.1016/j.hoc.2013.08.010
0889-8588/13/$ – see front matter © 2013 Elsevier Inc. All rights reserved.

PATIENT SELECTION

Historically, men with a life expectancy of longer than 10 years and localized disease were considered eligible for radical prostatectomy (RP). However, many clinicians may not accurately predict life expectancy in men with localized PCa.[4,5] Consequently life-expectancy tables, which provide the median survival for a man at a given age, are often consulted. Because life tables do not take into consideration an individual's comorbidities, they may not accurately predict overall survival in men with different severities of comorbidity. For example, a 70-year-old man in the healthiest quartile has a life expectancy of more than 18 years, compared with an estimated life expectancy of less than 7 years for a 70-year-old in the lowest quartile health state (**Fig. 1**).[6]

Nomograms incorporating comorbidities to predict life expectancy in men with localized PCa, which may be more accurate than life tables, are available.[7,8]

In general, age should not be an absolute contraindication for RP. The National Comprehensive Cancer Network (NCCN) Guidelines for senior adult oncology state that "irrespective of age, a person who is functionally independent and without serious

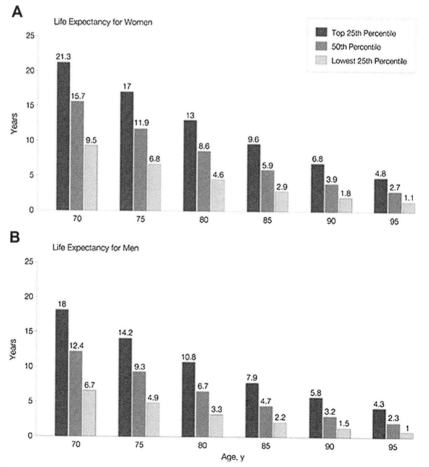

Fig. 1. Upper, middle, and lower quartiles of life expectancy for men at selected ages. (*Data from* Walter LC, Lewis CL, Barton MB. Screening for colorectal, breast, and cervical cancer in the elderly: a review of the evidence. Am J Med 2005 Oct;118(10):1079.)

comorbidity should be a good candidate for most forms of cancer treatments."[9] Furthermore, the International Society of Geriatric Oncology (ISGO) specifically addresses treatment of elderly men with localized PCa, and recommends that healthy elderly men receive standard treatment as for younger men, whereas men with vulnerable health status (reversible health problem) should be offered standard treatment exclusive of RP.[10,11] Single-institution series of elderly men undergoing RP demonstrate that in carefully selected men, RP can be beneficial.[12–15] For example, in one RP series of elderly men the 15-year PCa-specific and overall survival was 90.2% and 68.9%, much higher than in population-based series.[16]

SURGICAL TECHNIQUE

Radical removal of the prostate can be performed using open (radical retropubic or perineal) and minimally invasive (laparoscopic or robotic-assisted) techniques. The primary methods of prostate removal today are either radical retropubic or robotic-assisted, although the perineal approach and pure laparoscopic prostatectomies can provide comparable oncologic and functional outcomes in experienced hands in comparison with the more common approaches. The anatomic points of the retropubic approach were defined by Walsh in 1982, and remain the standard against which all other approaches are compared.[17] Since its first description using the Da Vinci system in 2001,[18] there has been increased adoption of robotic-assisted RP, such that 62% of RPs performed in 2009 were performed robotically.[19] A comparison of oncologic and functional outcomes between radical retropubic prostatectomy and robotic-assisted prostatectomy is beyond the scope of this article. The body of published literature that attempts to compare oncologic and functional outcomes, primarily between open and robotic-assisted approaches, is conflicting and controversial. Although it is well established that minimally invasive approaches are associated with less blood loss, decreased narcotic use, and decreased hospital stay, the primary comparative function outcomes of incontinence and erectile dysfunction are not well characterized, although multiple notable reports have addressed these issues.[20–23] Similarly, the long-term oncologic outcomes of open versus robotic-assisted methods have not been fully reported, hampering meaningful conclusions regarding the cancer-specific outcomes of open and robotic approaches.[24] A detailed analysis of the "trifecta" (continence, sexual function, and oncologic control) is beyond the scope of this article. In the authors' opinion it is the surgeon, not the approach, which is most critical to an individual's outcomes following prostatectomy, a stance that is supported by leaders in both minimally invasive and open surgical approaches.

CAVERNOSAL NERVE SPARING

The cavernosal neurovascular bundles (NVB) that are responsible for erectile function are located along the posterolateral surface of the prostate, lying directly on the prostatic capsule. Nerve-sparing techniques are frequently used whereby the NVBs are carefully dissected off the surface of the prostate, taking care not to disrupt the prostatic capsule. In the setting of organ-confined disease, the surgeon can safely spare these nerves without compromising oncologic efficacy, provided that no iatrogenic capsular incision is made. The challenge lies in accurately predicting which cancer will be organ-confined disease and which cancers may have microscopic extracapsular extension (ECE) such that nerve-sparing techniques may have an impact on surgical margin rates. Others have advocated wide-field resection of NVBs in the setting of all high-grade or high-volume disease, such as in the setting of high-risk disease.

There are several tools available for predicting the risk of ECE to guide clinicians and patients on whether or not to spare the NVB, primarily predicting the laterality of ECE. These different tools combine a varying number of several different factors: 2 factors (1 positive core with ≥7 mm of tumor and a positive base biopsy)[25]; 3 factors (Gleason score, % of core with tumor involvement, and perineural invasion[26]; Gleason score, PSA, and % of cores with cancer[27]; or Gleason score, PSA, and clinical stage[28]); and 5 factors (PSA, clinical stage, Gleason score, % of core tumor involvement, % of cores with cancer).[29,30] Individual surgeons will favor varying risk cutoffs regarding when to attempt nerve-sparing techniques.

The prostatic anatomy lends itself to various approaches of nerve-sparing versus wide resection. The detailed description of the fascial planes allows for variable depths of dissection, as shown in **Fig. 2**.[31] For example, intrafascial dissection is in close proximity to the prostatic capsule, and is more likely to be used in low-risk PCa with low probability of ECE. Conversely, an extrafascial dissection is more likely to be used in an individual for whom the risk of ECE is high.[31]

In addition, intraoperative findings can guide the decision on nerve-sparing approaches. Visual inspection or, in the case of open prostatectomy, manual palpation, can be used to help define the proximity of a tumor to the nerves.[32] Intraoperative biopsies can also assist in decisions regarding nerve sparing.[33] Others have promoted emerging technologies to identify the nerves during robotic-assisted laparoscopic prostatectomy.[34] In all cases, the decision to perform nerve sparing should not compromise the oncologic goal of complete excision of the tumor with negative surgical margins.

PELVIC LYMPH NODE DISSECTION

There are 2 major issues that surround LND for PCa. First, the boundaries of lymph node dissection are variable. Traditionally, most surgeons perform a pelvic LND (PLND) that is limited to the obturator fossa and external iliac vein. However, the extent of PLND has grown with increasing recognition that the lymphatic drainage of the prostate is linked to the external and internal iliac arteries and the presacral regions.

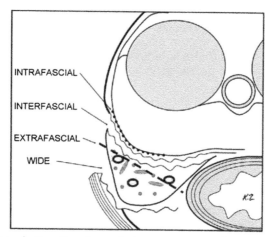

Fig. 2. The planes of dissection for radical prostatectomy. (*From* Shikanov S, Woo J, Al-Ahmadie H, et al. Extrafascial versus interfascial nerve-sparing technique for robotic-assisted laparoscopic prostatectomy: comparison of functional outcomes and positive surgical margins characteristics. Urology 2009;74(3):612; with permission.)

Several reports have found that the limited PLND will miss 20% to 40% of positive lymph nodes.[35-37] The extent of the extended PLND (ePLND) is yet to be determined. The NCCN guidelines describe the boundaries to be "external iliac vein anteriorly, the pelvic side wall laterally, the bladder wall medially, the floor of the pelvis posteriorly, Cooper's ligament distally, and the internal iliac artery proximally."[38] According to the European Association of Urology (EAU) guidelines, regions to be removed include the nodal tissue "overlying the external iliac artery and vein, the nodes within the obturator fossa located cranially and caudally to the obturator nerve, and the nodes medial and lateral to the internal iliac artery."[39] However, it should be noted that mapping studies have shown that there are additional areas of primary drainage not included in these templates (presacral, perirectal, common iliac).[40]

The therapeutic benefit of ePLND is less well defined. Whereas ePLND certainly provides more accurate staging and will detect a greater number of patients with positive lymph nodes, potentially helping identify adjuvant therapy candidates, it is not clear that it results in improved oncologic outcomes. Some patients with positive nodes experience long-term disease-free intervals, with approximately 10% to 15% of patients remaining without evidence of recurrence at up to 10 years.[41-43] Several studies have found that a greater number of lymph nodes removed is associated with improved disease-specific outcomes[44-46] or that in those with positive nodes, a lower lymph node density is associated with improved outcomes.[47,48] Along these lines, better outcomes have been observed in men with only 1 positive lymph node.[41,49-53] However, these findings must be tempered with the higher risk of complications and added operative time with ePLND.[54,55]

The second major issue surrounds the need and indication for PLND, and most have promoted LND based on probability of lymph node involvement (LNI). For example, the NCCN guidelines recommend a PLND if the probability of LNI is 2% or greater, and states that "an extended PLND will discover metastases approximately twice as often as a limited PLND."[38] Extended PLND provides more complete staging and may cure some men with microscopic metastasis; therefore, "an extended PLND is preferred when PLND is performed."[38] The EAU recommends that a PLND be performed if the risk of LNI is 5% or greater, essentially excluding a PLND for men with low-risk disease.[39] The EAU states that "extended LND should be performed in intermediate-risk, localized PCa if the estimated risk for positive lymph nodes exceeds 5%, as well as in high-risk cases. In these circumstances, the estimated risk for positive lymph nodes is 15%–40%. Limited LND should no longer be performed, because it misses at least half the nodes involved."[39] There are several nomograms available to predict the likelihood of LNI based on preoperative characteristics; these include the Partin tables,[28] the Kattan nomogram,[56] and the Briganti[57] nomogram. Older nomograms for predicting the probability of LNI were based on the more limited PLND and thus underestimate the risk of LNI. The authors suggest that an individualized risk assessment be made in each case, and when the decision is made to perform a PLND, it should be an ePLND.

SURGICAL MARGINS

Positive surgical margins (PSM) are reported to occur in 11% to 38% of cases[58] and can be influenced by the surgeon. Although PSM can result from extensive cancer for which complete resection is not possible, PSM also occur because of technical error (eg, capsular incision) or inaccurate selection of patients for nerve-sparing techniques. Nomograms are commonly used to predict the probability of extracapsular extension to assist the surgeon in determining when to perform "wide-field" cavernosal nerve resection rather than nerve sparing in an attempt to reduce PSM.[28,29] Several studies have reported PSM to be independently associated with biochemical recurrence after RP.[59–64] Furthermore, PSM are associated with PCa-specific mortality (PCSM) in some,[65,66] but not all large series.[67] In sum, it is incumbent on the surgeon to make every effort to optimize surgical technique and patient selection to achieve negative surgical margins.

Nerve grafts have been proposed as an option for men undergoing wide-field resection, using sural, genitofemoral, or ilioinguinal nerve grafts.[68–70] Several studies have suggested a beneficial effect from the grafts.[68–75] In the only randomized study performed, there was no difference in erectile dysfunction between those with and without nerve grafts, although the study was underpowered, there was poor patient compliance, and 67% of controls analyzed were potent, a number much higher than expected.[76] At present, therefore, the role of nerve grafting in PCa remains unclear.

LOW-RISK PROSTATE CANCER
Definition of Low-Risk Prostate Cancer

Risk stratification for patients with localized PCa includes PSA, Gleason, and T-stage data. The American Urological Association (AUA), the EAU, and the NCCN all define low-risk disease as PSA less than 10 AND Gleason 6 or less AND T1c/T2a. The NCCN also define a "very low risk disease" when all the following criteria are met: PSA less than 10, T1c, Gleason 6 or less, fewer than 3 biopsy cores positive, 50% or less cancer in any core, and PSA density less than 0.15 ng/mL/g.

Outcomes for Low-Risk Disease Following Radical Prostatectomy

Cancer-specific survival for men with low-risk disease is excellent, and approximately 40% of newly diagnosed PCa are thought to meet the definition of low risk. Stephenson and colleagues[77] evaluated the long-term PCSM in a cohort of 11,521 men treated with RP with the finding that only 3 of 9557 men with organ-confined, Gleason-6 PCa died of PCa, further supporting the excellent long-term outcomes of RP in the low-risk subgroups. In an observational cohort of men diagnosed in Sweden from 1997 to 2002, 2686 men younger than 70 years were diagnosed with low-risk PCa (T1c, Gleason 6, PSA<10).[78] After a median follow-up of longer than 8 years, the PCSM for those under surveillance (n = 1079) was 2.4% and was similar to those treated with RP.

RP has been shown to improve disease-specific survival in comparison with watchful waiting in randomized studies. The Scandinavian Prostate Cancer Group Study randomized 695 men to either RP or watchful waiting for localized PCa.[79] RP was associated with a 46% reduction in PCSM (hazard ratio [HR] 0.54, 95% confidence interval [CI] 0.36–0.88) with an absolute risk reduction of 5.0%. The survival difference was most significant in men younger than 65 years. However, important considerations from this study include that only 5% of the cancer was identified by screening, 70% presented with clinical T2, 40% had a PSA greater than 10, and the analysis included men with low-, intermediate-, and high-risk disease. Concerns were raised as to whether these data on men diagnosed from 1989 to 1999 were applicable to the current state of a highly screened population and men with low-risk disease.

In 2012, data from the Prostate Cancer Intervention Versus Observation Trial (PIVOT) were published, comparing RP with watchful waiting in a highly screened population.[80] The study enrolled 731 men, 296 of whom had low-risk disease (148 in each arm). After a median follow-up of 10 years, the cumulative PCSM was 2.7% in the watchful-waiting arm and 4.1% in the RP arm (HR 1.5, 95% CI 0.4–5.2). These data suggest that for men with low-risk disease, the 10-year risk of PCSM is low and not different between observation and treatment. However, longer follow-up out to 20 to 30 years may see a survival advantage for RP over active surveillance/watchful waiting. Regardless, treating physicians need to be aware of these excellent disease-specific survival numbers, and carefully select patients with low-risk disease who may benefit from active treatment and strong consideration for active surveillance given for most of these individuals.

HIGH-RISK PROSTATE CANCER
Definition of High-Risk Prostate Cancer

Unlike low-risk PCa, whereby an individual must have all 3 factors (PSA, Gleason score, and tumor stage) in the lowest categories, high-risk disease is defined by fulfilling any of the 3 factors in the highest category. The AUA, EAU, and NCCN all share the same PSA (>20) and Gleason (8–10) cutoffs, but differ slightly in the T-stage cutoff for high risk. The AUA guidelines consider T2c lesions to be high risk, whereas both the NCCN and EAU consider T3a to be high risk. Both the NCCN and EAU further define a "very high risk" subgroup with T3b to T4 disease. Although PSA screening has led to a significant decrease in those who meet high-risk criteria by either PSA level or tumor stage (ie, more tumors diagnosed as T1c with PSA at low levels), patients with high-risk disease continue to comprise approximately 25% of those with localized disease (down from >40% in the 1990s; **Fig. 3**).[81] Thus, management of these patients continues to be an active part of PCa today.

Outcomes for High-Risk Disease Following Radical Prostatectomy

Recurrence rates for high-risk PCa following any treatment, including RP, are high (approximately 50%), and **Fig. 4** shows disease-free survival curves from several different studies published in the AUA Clinical Guidelines.[82]

Although recurrence is common the outcome is excellent after RP, with multiple large series (**Table 1**) demonstrating approximately 90% 10-year disease-specific survival.

Further, RP is superior to observation in men with high-risk disease, as illustrated in the PIVOT study of RP versus observation for men with localized PCa. Men with high-risk PCa had a 60% reduction in PCSM with RP when compared with observation

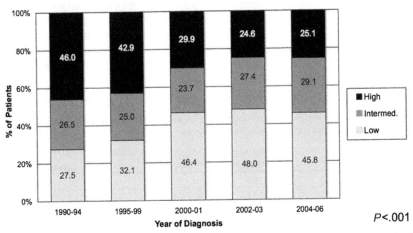

Fig. 3. Trends in prostate cancer risk categories over time. (*From* Cooperberg MR, Broering JM, Kantoff PW, et al. Contemporary trends in low risk prostate cancer: risk assessment and treatment. J Urol 2007;178(3 Pt 2):S15; with permission.)

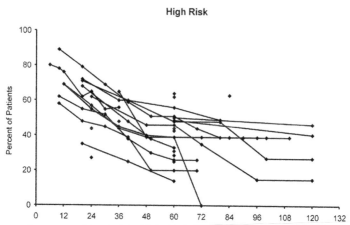

Fig. 4. Disease-free survival from various studies of radical prostatectomy. (*From* Thompson I, Thrasher JB, Aus G, et al. Guideline for the management of clinically localized prostate cancer: 2007 update. American Urological Association Education and Research, Inc. J Urol 2007;177(6):2106–31; with permission.)

(HR 0.4, 95% CI 0.2–1.0). Although any of the 3 factors can make a person "high risk," several studies have shown that having more than 1 factor is associated with worse disease-specific outcomes than having a single factor.[19,83–85] Of note, more accurate pathologic staging after RP results in both downgrading and downstaging. For example, downstaging can occur in up to 30% of cases[86–89] and downgrading in those with disease of Gleason score 8 to 10 occurs in 29% to 56% of cases.[90–93] In a recent review of 380 patients with biopsy-proven disease of Gleason 8 to 10, downgrading to Gleason 7 or less occurred in 45% of patients.[90] If tertiary pattern 5 (TP5) was considered in the pathologic grade, the downgrading occurred in only 26% of cases.

TP5 disease requires special mention, as it is not addressed in the risk strata based on biopsy. The Gleason scoring system for PCa assigns a grade to the 2 predominant patterns to yield the combined Gleason score. A third (tertiary) pattern is present in 2.3% to 48% of cases of RP specimens (by convention, a tertiary pattern is not given on biopsy specimens).[94–100] The presence of TP5 in RP specimens with Gleason-7 carcinomas is associated with an increased risk of biochemical failure compared with those carcinomas of Gleason 7 without TP5.[94,95,98,99,101] Whereas pathologic Gleason-7 disease is one criterion of the intermediate-risk group,[102] the finding of

Table 1			
Ten-year biochemical recurrence and cancer-specific survival for patients with high-risk prostate cancer in large radical prostatectomy series			
Authors,[Ref.] Year	No. of Patients	10-y Recurrence-Free Survival (%)	10-y Disease-Free Survival (%)
Briganti et al,[132] 2012	1366	54	91
Stephenson et al,[77] 2009	1962	n/a	92
Boorjian et al,[133] 2011	1238	n/a	92
Ward et al,[88] 2005	841	73	90
Yossepowitch et al,[134] 2008	1359	n/a	93

Abbreviation: n/a, no data available.

Table 2
Published large series comparing radical prostatectomy with radiation therapy for prostate cancer

Authors,[Ref.] Year	Total No. of Patients (No. with High-Risk PCa)		Notes on EBRT	10-y Prostate Cancer-Specific Mortality Rate (95% CI) in High-Risk Patients		Risk of Mortality with XRT (Compared with RP)
	RP	EBRT		RP	EBRT	
Abdollah et al,[128] 2012	20445 (7442)[a]	20445 (7442)	cGy n/a 9% ADT	6.8 (5.7–7.8)	11.5 (10.2–12.9)	1.7 (1.5–1.9)
Cooperberg et al,[125] 2010	5052 (328)	1143 (279)	cGy n/a 51% ADT	n/a	n/a	1.6 (1.1–2.5)
Kibel et al,[127] 2012	6485 (528)	2264 (676)	70–80 cGy 34% ADT	1.8 (1.6–2.1)[b]	2.9 (2.6–3.3)[b]	1.5 (1.0–2.3)
Zelefsky et al,[126] 2010	1318 (n/a)[c]	1062 (n/a)[c]	81–84.4 cGy 56% <6 mo ADT	3.8 (1.2–11.5)[d]	9.5 (4.9–17.9)[d]	2.9 (1.7–5.0)[e]

Abbreviations: ADT, androgen deprivation therapy; CI, confidence interval; EBRT, external-beam radiation therapy; n/a, no data available; PCa, prostate cancer; RP, radical prostatectomy; XRT, radiation therapy.
a Propensity-score-matched cohort analysis from Surveillance Epidemiology and End Results (SEER)-Medicare.
b PCa-specific mortality in all patients, not limited to high risk.
c Total number of patients (RP + EBRT) with high-risk disease was 409 in this study, but the number in each group was not provided.
d 8-year PCa-specific survival.
e 8-year metastasis-free survival analysis in all patients.

Table 3
Contemporary series of cryotherapy for primary treatment of localized prostate cancer

Authors,[Ref.] Year	No. of Patients	Follow-Up	Definition of Failure	Overall Recurrence-Free Survival (%)	Recurrence-Free Survival (%) in Low-Risk Patients	Recurrence-Free Survival (%) in High-Risk Patients
Levy & Jones,[135,a] 2011	2685 COLD Registry	Median = 60 mo	Nadir + 2 ng/mL	—	89 (5 y)	64 (5 y)
Ward & Jones,[136,b] 2011	1160 COLD Registry	Mean = 21.1 mo	3 consecutive PSA rises occurring 6 mo after therapy	75.7 (36 mo)	—	—
Cheetham et al,[137] 2010	25 Primary (76 total)	Median = 10.1 y	Nadir + 2 ng/mL	51.2 (of the 43 men still alive at 10 y)	—	—
Donnelly et al,[138,c] 2010	122	Median = 100 mo	Nadir + 2 ng/mL or radiologic evidence of disease or additional therapy	75 (5 y)	—	—
Ko et al,[139,d] 2010	33 high-risk	Median = 61 mo	Nadir + 2 ng/mL	97 (36 mo)	—	97 (36 mo)
Truesdale et al,[140] 2010	77	Median = 24 mo	Nadir + 2 ng/mL	72.7 (at last follow-up)	—	—
Chin et al,[141,d] 2008	33 high-risk	Mean = 37 mo	3 consecutive PSA rises	13 (4 y)	—	13 (4 y)
Cohen et al,[142] 2008	370	Median = 12. 55 y	Nadir + 2 ng/mL	62.36 (10 y)	80.56 (10 y)	45.54 (10 y)

Study	No. of Patients	Follow-up	Biochemical Recurrence Definition			
Jones et al,[143] 2008	1198 COLD Registry	Mean = 24.4 mo	Nadir + 2 ng/mL	72.9 (5 y)	91.1 (5 y)	62.2 (5 y)
Onik et al,[144,b] 2008	48	Mean = 4.5 y	3 consecutive PSA rises	94 (2 y)	—	—
Ellis et al,[145] 2007	416	Mean = 20.4 mo	3 consecutive PSA rises with a final value >1.0 ng/mL	79.6 (4 y)	83.6 (4 y)	69.1 (4 y)
Polascik et al,[146] 2007	50	Median = 18 mo	PSA ≥0.5 ng/mL	90 (at last follow-up)	—	—
Bahn et al,[147,b] 2006	31	Mean = 70 mo	3 consecutive PSA rises	92.9 (at last follow-up)	—	—
Prepelica et al,[148] 2005	65 high-risk	Median = 35 mo	3 consecutive PSA rises	81.7 (6 y)	—	81.7 (6 y)
Aus et al,[149] 2002	54	Median = 58.5 mo	PSA >1 ng/mL or positive prostate biopsy	38.9 (58.5 mo)	—	—
Bahn et al,[150] 2002	590	Mean = 5.43 y	PSA ≥0.5 ng/mL	62 (7 y)	61 (7 y)	61 (7 y)
Donnelly et al,[151] 2002	76	Median = 60.8 mo	PSA >1.0 ng/mL	—	75 (5 y)	76 (5 y)
Long et al,[152] 2001	975	Median = 24 mo	PSA <1 ng/mL	—	76 (5 y)	41 (5 y)

Abbreviation: PSA, prostate-specific antigen.
a Only reported for those patients who achieved a PSA nadir of <0.6 ng/mL.
b Limited to patients undergoing partial gland cryotherapy.
c All patients received neoadjuvant androgen deprivation therapy.
d All patients received concurrent androgen deprivation therapy.

Table 4
Contemporary series of high-intensity focused ultrasound for primary treatment of localized prostate cancer

Authors,[Ref.] Year	No. of Patients	Median Follow-Up	Definition of Failure	5-y Disease-Free Rate (Overall) (%)	5-y Disease-Free Rate (Low Risk) (%)	5-y Disease-Free Rate (High Risk) (%)
Sung et al,[153] 2012	126	Median = 61.1 mo	Nadir + 1.2 ng/mL	—	66.3 (5 y)	21.0 (5 y)
Boutier et al,[154] 2011	99	Not stated	Positive biopsy at 3–6 mo	36.4 (3–6 mo)	—	—
Ganzer et al,[155] 2011	804 from @-Registry	Median = 5.0 y	Nadir + 1.2 ng/mL	5 y BRFS PSA nadir ≤0.2 = 84 PSA nadir 0.21–0.5 = 64 PSA nadir 0.51–1 = 40 PSA nadir >1 = 30	—	—
Inoue et al,[156] 2011	137	Median = 36 mo	Nadir + 2 ng/mL or positive biopsy	77.8 (5 y)	91.3 (5 y)	61.7 (5 y)
Ripert et al,[157] 2011	53	Median = 47 mo	Nadir + 1.2 ng/mL	21.7 (5 y)	—	—
Crouzet et al,[158] 2010	803	Mean = 42 mo	Nadir + 2 ng/mL	—	83 (5 y)	68 (5 y)
Sumitomo et al,[159] 2010	115	Median = 42 mo	Nadir + 2 ng/mL or positive biopsy or salvage therapy	—	90.6 (5 y)	57.1 (5 y)
Ahmed et al,[160] 2009	172	Mean = 346 d	PSA ≤0.5 ng/mL	78.3 (1 y)	—	—

Study	No.	Follow-up	Definition of Failure			
Blana et al,[169] 2009	285	Median = 4.7 y	Positive biopsy or secondary treatment or metastatic disease or PCa death	25 (at last follow-up)	—	—
Challacombe et al,[161] 2009	31 primary (43 total)	Mean = 24.9 mo	Nadir + 2 ng/mL or PSA ≥0.5 ng/mL	At last follow-up: Nadir + 2 ng/mL = 54 PSA ≥0.5 ng/mL = 25	—	—
Mearini et al,[162] 2009	163	Median = 23.8 mo	Nadir + 2 ng/mL	—	86.1 (3 y)	56.4 (3 y)
Uchida et al,[163] 2009	517	Median = 24.0 mo	Nadir + 2 ng/mL	72 (5 y)	84 (5 y)	45 (5 y)
Blana et al,[164] 2008	163	Mean = 4.8 y	Nadir + 2 ng/mL	75 (5 y)	77 (5 y)	—
Blana et al,[165] 2008	140	Mean = 6.4 y	Nadir + 2 ng/mL	77 (5 y)	—	—
Misrai et al,[166] 2008	119	Mean = 3.9 y	Nadir + 2 ng/mL	30 (5 y)	—	—
Sumitomo et al,[167] 2008	530	Mean = 23.4 mo	Nadir + 2 ng/mL or positive biopsy or metastatic disease	64.7 (3 y)	—	—
Lee et al,[168] 2006	58	Mean = 14 mo	3 consecutive PSA rises above 1.0 ng/mL or positive biopsy	69 (at last follow-up)	85 (at last follow-up)	47 (at last follow-up)

Abbreviations: BRFS, biochemical relapse-free survival; PCa, prostate cancer; PSA, prostate-specific antigen.

TP5 disease represents substantially increased rates of recurrence, similar to rates associated with conventionally defined high-risk disease. Thus, finding TP5 has significant clinical consequences for post-RP patient management.

NEOADJUVANT THERAPY BEFORE RADICAL PROSTATECTOMY

Several studies have explored the use of neoadjuvant androgen deprivation therapy (ADT) before prostatectomy.[103–110] The initial results were encouraging, with improvements in several pathologic characteristics. In a meta-analysis, neoadjuvant ADT was associated with an increased likelihood of organ-confined disease (relative risk [RR] 1.6, 95% CI 1.4–2.0), and a reduction in risk in positive margins (RR 0.5, 95% CI 0.4–0.6) and lymph node involvement (RR 0.7, 95% CI 0.5–0.9).[111] However, there was no improvement in disease-specific outcomes with similar rates of biochemical recurrence and PCa-specific survival.

Several phase II studies of neoadjuvant chemotherapy before RP have been performed. Many of these studies have used docetaxel with or without ADT.[112–115] Additional studies have combined other agents with docetaxel (eg, estramustine, mitoxantrone).[116–120] Several phase II studies of novel agents and novel combinations of ADT are ongoing, including maximal androgen blockade with a combination of goserelin, bicalutamide, ketoconazole, and dutasteride (NCT00298155). CALGB 90203 is a phase III study of neoadjuvant docetaxel with ADT followed by RP versus RP in patients with high-risk PCa.[121] The study's primary outcome is 3-year biochemical progression-free survival, and it is anticipated to end in 2018. At present, neoadjuvant therapy before RP is not the standard of care; however, the authors encourage increased access to neoadjuvant clinical trials for patients with high-risk PCa undergoing RP.

IS RADICAL PROSTATECTOMY THE PREFERRED TREATMENT FOR HIGH-RISK PROSTATE CANCER?

Historically, many patients with high-risk disease were directed toward radiation therapy, owing in part to concerns over the risk of micrometastatic disease, along with level I data from radiation studies showing improved disease-specific survival with prolonged ADT concurrent with radiation therapy in comparison with radiation therapy alone.[122–124] Reports of excellent long-term disease-specific survival in men with high-risk PCa following RP has led increasingly to a reevaluation of the important role of RP in these men, with the argument for local control with RP serving as the first step in multimodal therapy. Although there have been no randomized studies comparing RP with radiation therapy, recent studies have suggested that RP may offer some disease-specific survival advantages over radiation (**Table 2**).[125–128] In one study with case-mix adjustment, 1318 men undergoing RP (of whom only 7% received either adjuvant radiation or ADT) were compared with 1062 men treated with 81 to 86.4 cGy with external-beam radiation therapy (EBRT) at a high-volume cancer center, including 409 total patients with high-risk disease.[126] The 8-year actuarial probability of PCSM in the high-risk group was 9.5% (95% CI 4.9–17.9) for radiation and 3.8 (95% CI 1.2–11.5) for RP. In the multivariate analysis that included all patients, the RP had a 65% reduction in risk of distant metastasis compared with the radiation group (HR 0.35, 95% CI 0.19–0.63; $P = .001$). In a second study from CaPSURE, compared with surgery, radiation treatment was associated with a 2-fold increased risk of PCSM in a multivariate model including all-risk patients (HR 2.21, 95% CI 1.50–3.24; $P<.001$).[125] A study of 6485 men undergoing RP and 2264 men treated with EBRT from 2 major PCa centers used propensity-score analysis, and found that although the 10-year PCSM rates were low in both groups, there was a 50% increased risk of PCSM with EBRT in comparison with RP (95% CI 1.0–2.3).[129] Finally, a propensity-score–matched analysis of 40,890 men using Surveillance Epidemiology and End Results (SEER)-Medicare data found similar findings with 10-year PCSM rates of 6.8% and 11.5% in the RP and EBRT groups, respectively (multivariate HR 1.7, 95% CI 1.5–1.9).[128] It should be noted, however, that these are not randomized trials, and selection bias is likely present. Furthermore, few men in the radiation group received prolonged (2–3 years) ADT for which randomized studies show an improvement in disease-specific survival. Finally, there were few salvage treatments for the radiation-failure group, and there were a limited number of events.

This potential surgical advantage is being extended to consideration in men with node-positive disease. Whereas previously it was common to send suspicious lymph nodes for frozen section with plans to abort the RP in the setting of positive lymph nodes, there are now emerging data for RP even in the face of clinically positive nodes. Two retrospective studies compared outcomes in patients based on findings on frozen section at the time of planned prostatectomy.[53,130] The decision for proceeding with RP despite positive nodes was based on physician judgment and patient preferences. In both studies, the 10-year cancer-specific survival was higher in those treated with RP (86%[130] and 76%[53]) compared with those who had RP aborted (40%[130] and 46%[53]). In both studies, aborted RP was associated with a greater than 2-fold increased risk of PCSM compared with those undergoing RP (HR 2.1, 95% CI 1.1–4.1[53]; and HR 2.0, 95% CI 1.6–2.6[130]). Although nonrandomized and unmeasured confounding in part explains the observed differences in outcome, these findings support ongoing work in the role of tumor debulking and multimodal therapy for high-risk PCa.

Alternative Surgical Therapies

Outcomes of primary high-intensity focused ultrasound and cryoablation are highly varied among published reports (**Tables 3** and **4**). Much of this variability may arise from differences in patient selection, length of follow-up, and inconsistencies in the definition used for failure. Posttreatment biopsies and PSA values have been the most common methods for determining failure after treatment. However, inconsistency in the definition of PSA failure has led to some series publishing results using multiple definitions of failure within the same published report. This inconsistency results in variable failure rates, even within the same cohort of patients, and hampers any conclusions regarding the efficacy of these ablative procedures.[131]

SUMMARY

The surgical management of PCa continues to evolve. Increased appreciation for the fascial planes surrounding the prostate along with greater knowledge of the lymphatic drainage of the prostate has led to technical modifications in surgical approaches, with several nomograms available to help guide urologists. Patients with high-risk PCa are most likely to benefit from RP; however, the rate of recurrence remains high in these patients. The current situation calls for the continued study of novel neoadjuvant therapies to improve outcomes along with better determination of those most likely to benefit from adjuvant therapies.

REFERENCES

1. American Cancer Society I. Prostate cancer: what are the key statistics about prostate cancer? Available at: http://www.cancer.org/cancer/prostatecancer/detailedguide/prostate-cancer-key-statistics. Accessed October 1, 2013.

2. Draisma G, Etzioni R, Tsodikov A, et al. Lead time and overdiagnosis in prostate-specific antigen screening: importance of methods and context. J Natl Cancer Inst 2009;101(6):374–83.

3. Cooperberg MR, Broering JM, Carroll PR. Time trends and local variation in primary treatment of localized prostate cancer. J Clin Oncol 2010;28(7):1117–23.

4. Jeldres C, Latouff JB, Saad F. Predicting life expectancy in prostate cancer patients. Curr Opin Support Palliat Care 2009;3(3):166–9.

5. Walz J, Gallina A, Perrotte P, et al. Clinicians are poor raters of life-expectancy before radical prostatectomy or definitive radiotherapy for localized prostate cancer. BJU Int 2007;100(6):1254–8.

6. Walter LC, Covinsky KE. Cancer screening in elderly patients: a framework for individualized decision making. JAMA 2001;285(21):2750–6.

7. Walz J, Gallina A, Saad F, et al. A nomogram predicting 10-year life expectancy in candidates for radical prostatectomy or radiotherapy for prostate cancer. J Clin Oncol 2007;25(24):3576–81.

8. Tewari A, Johnson CC, Divine G, et al. Long-term survival probability in men with clinically localized prostate cancer: a case-control, propensity modeling study stratified by race, age, treatment and comorbidities. J Urol 2004;171(4):1513–9.

9. Senior Adult Oncology. NCCN Clinical Practice Guidelines in Oncology. 2010;1.2010. Available at: http://www.nccn.org/professionals/physician_gls/PDF/senior.pdf. Accessed April 10, 2010.

10. Droz JP, Balducci L, Bolla M, et al. Background for the proposal of SIOG guidelines for the management of prostate cancer in senior adults. Crit Rev Oncol Hematol 2010;73(1):68–91.

11. Droz JP, Balducci L, Bolla M, et al. Management of prostate cancer in older men: recommendations of a working group of the International Society of Geriatric Oncology. BJU Int 2010;106(4):462–9.

12. Magheli A, Rais-Bahrami S, Humphreys EB, et al. Impact of patient age on biochemical recurrence rates following radical prostatectomy. J Urol 2007;178(5):1933–7 [discussion: 1937–8].

13. Malaeb BS, Rashid HH, Lotan Y, et al. Prostate cancer disease-free survival after radical retropubic prostatectomy in patients older than 70 years compared to younger cohorts. Urol Oncol 2007;25(4):291–7.

14. Siddiqui SA, Sengupta S, Slezak JM, et al. Impact of patient age at treatment on outcome following radical retropubic prostatectomy for prostate cancer. J Urol 2006;175(3 Pt 1):952–7.

15. Sun L, Caire AA, Robertson CN, et al. Men older than 70 years have higher risk prostate cancer and poorer survival in the early and late prostate specific antigen eras. J Urol 2009;182(5):2242–8.

16. Pierorazio PM, Humphreys E, Walsh PC, et al. Radical prostatectomy in older men: survival outcomes in septuagenarians and octogenarians. BJU Int 2010;106(6):791–5.

17. Walsh PC, Donker PJ. Impotence following radical prostatectomy: insight into etiology and prevention. J Urol 1982;128(3):492–7.

18. Abbou CC, Hoznek A, Salomon L, et al. Laparoscopic radical prostatectomy with a remote controlled robot. J Urol 2001;165(6 Pt 1):1964–6.

19. Pierorazio PM, Ross AE, Han M, et al. Evolution of the clinical presentation of men undergoing radical prostatectomy for high-risk prostate cancer. BJU Int 2012;109(7):988–93.

20. Trinh QD, Sammon J, Sun M, et al. Perioperative outcomes of robot-assisted radical prostatectomy compared with open radical prostatectomy: results from the nationwide inpatient sample. Eur Urol 2012;61(4):679–85.

21. Novara G, Ficarra V, Rosen RC, et al. Systematic review and meta-analysis of perioperative outcomes and complications after robot-assisted radical prostatectomy. Eur Urol 2012;62(3):431–52.

22. Ficarra V, Novara G, Ahlering TE, et al. Systematic review and meta-analysis of studies reporting potency rates after robot-assisted radical prostatectomy. Eur Urol 2012;62(3):418–30.

23. Ficarra V, Novara G, Rosen RC, et al. Systematic review and meta-analysis of studies reporting urinary continence recovery after robot-assisted radical prostatectomy. Eur Urol 2012;62(3):405–17.

24. Novara G, Ficarra V, Mocellin S, et al. Systematic review and meta-analysis of studies reporting oncologic outcome after robot-assisted radical prostatectomy. Eur Urol 2012;62(3):382–404.

25. Kamat AM, Jacobsohn KM, Troncoso P, et al. Validation of criteria used to predict extraprostatic cancer extension: a tool for use in selecting patients for nerve sparing radical prostatectomy. J Urol 2005;174(4 Pt 1):1262–5.

26. Shah O, Robbins DA, Melamed J, et al. The New York University nerve sparing algorithm decreases the rate of positive surgical margins following radical retropubic prostatectomy. J Urol 2003;169(6):2147–52.

27. Gancarczyk KJ, Wu H, McLeod DG, et al. Using the percentage of biopsy cores positive for cancer, pretreatment PSA, and highest biopsy Gleason sum to predict pathologic stage after radical prostatectomy: the Center for Prostate Disease Research nomograms. Urology 2003;61(3):589–95.

28. Makarov DV, Trock BJ, Humphreys EB, et al. Updated nomogram to predict pathologic stage of prostate cancer given prostate-specific antigen level, clinical stage, and biopsy Gleason score (Partin tables) based on cases from 2000 to 2005. Urology 2007;69(6):1095–101.

29. Ohori M, Kattan MW, Koh H, et al. Predicting the presence and side of extracapsular extension: a nomogram for staging prostate cancer. J Urol 2004;171(5): 1844–9 [discussion: 1849].

30. Tsuzuki T, Hernandez DJ, Aydin H, et al. Prediction of extraprostatic extension in the neurovascular bundle based on prostate needle biopsy pathology, serum prostate specific antigen and digital rectal examination. J Urol 2005;173(2): 450–3.

31. Shikanov S, Woo J, Al-Ahmadie H, et al. Extrafascial versus interfascial nerve-sparing technique for robotic-assisted laparoscopic prostatectomy: comparison of functional outcomes and positive surgical margins characteristics. Urology 2009;74(3):611–6.

32. Hernandez DJ, Epstein JI, Trock BJ, et al. Radical retropubic prostatectomy. How often do experienced surgeons have positive surgical margins when there is extraprostatic extension in the region of the neurovascular bundle? J Urol 2005;173(2):446–9.

33. Lepor H, Kaci L. Role of intraoperative biopsies during radical retropubic prostatectomy. Urology 2004;63(3):499–502.

34. Ponnusamy K, Sorger JM, Mohr C. Nerve mapping for prostatectomies: novel technologies under development. J Endourol 2012;26(7):769–77.

35. Bader P, Burkhard FC, Markwalder R, et al. Is a limited lymph node dissection an adequate staging procedure for prostate cancer? J Urol 2002;168(2): 514–8 [discussion: 518].

36. Heidenreich A, Varga Z, Von Knobloch R. Extended pelvic lymphadenectomy in patients undergoing radical prostatectomy: high incidence of lymph node metastasis. J Urol 2002;167(4):1681–6.

37. Weckermann D, Dorn R, Trefz M, et al. Sentinel lymph node dissection for prostate cancer: experience with more than 1,000 patients. J Urol 2007;177(3):916–20.

38. NCCN Clinical Practice Guidelines in Oncology (NCCN Guideline). Prostate cancer; version 1.2013. Available at: nccn.org. Accessed February 1, 2013.

39. Heidenreich A, Bellmunt J, Bolla M, et al. EAU guidelines on prostate cancer. Part 1: screening, diagnosis, and treatment of clinically localised disease. Eur Urol 2011;59(1):61–71.

40. Mattei A, Fuechsel FG, Bhatta Dhar N, et al. The template of the primary lymphatic landing sites of the prostate should be revisited: results of a multimodality mapping study. Eur Urol 2008;53(1):118–25.

41. Bader P, Burkhard FC, Markwalder R, et al. Disease progression and survival of patients with positive lymph nodes after radical prostatectomy. Is there a chance of cure? J Urol 2003;169(3):849–54.

42. Messing EM, Manola J, Yao J, et al. Immediate versus deferred androgen deprivation treatment in patients with node-positive prostate cancer after radical prostatectomy and pelvic lymphadenectomy. Lancet Oncol 2006;7(6):472–9.

43. Palapattu GS, Allaf ME, Trock BJ, et al. Prostate specific antigen progression in men with lymph node metastases following radical prostatectomy: results of long-term followup. J Urol 2004;172(5 Pt 1):1860–4.

44. Joslyn SA, Konety BR. Impact of extent of lymphadenectomy on survival after radical prostatectomy for prostate cancer. Urology 2006;68(1):121–5.

45. Schiavina R, Bertaccini A, Franceschelli A, et al. The impact of the extent of lymph-node dissection on biochemical relapse after radical prostatectomy in node-negative patients. Anticancer Res 2010;30(6):2297–302.

46. Masterson TA, Bianco FJ Jr, Vickers AJ, et al. The association between total and positive lymph node counts, and disease progression in clinically localized prostate cancer. J Urol 2006;175(4):1320–4 [discussion: 1324–5].

47. Allaf ME, Palapattu GS, Trock BJ, et al. Anatomical extent of lymph node dissection: impact on men with clinically localized prostate cancer. J Urol 2004; 172(5 Pt 1):1840–4.

48. Daneshmand S, Quek ML, Stein JP, et al. Prognosis of patients with lymph node positive prostate cancer following radical prostatectomy: long-term results. J Urol 2004;172(6 Pt 1):2252–5.

49. Boorjian SA, Thompson RH, Siddiqui S, et al. Long-term outcome after radical prostatectomy for patients with lymph node positive prostate cancer in the prostate specific antigen era. J Urol 2007;178(3 Pt 1):864–70 [discussion: 870–1].

50. Briganti A, Karnes JR, Da Pozzo LF, et al. Two positive nodes represent a significant cut-off value for cancer specific survival in patients with node positive prostate cancer. A new proposal based on a two-institution experience on 703 consecutive N+ patients treated with radical prostatectomy, extended pelvic lymph node dissection and adjuvant therapy. Eur Urol 2009;55(2):261–70.

51. Da Pozzo LF, Cozzarini C, Briganti A, et al. Long-term follow-up of patients with prostate cancer and nodal metastases treated by pelvic lymphadenectomy and radical prostatectomy: the positive impact of adjuvant radiotherapy. Eur Urol 2009;55(5):1003–11.

52. Schiavina R, Manferrari F, Garofalo M, et al. The extent of pelvic lymph node dissection correlates with the biochemical recurrence rate in patients with intermediate- and high-risk prostate cancer. BJU Int 2011;108(8):1262–8.

53. Steuber T, Budaus L, Walz J, et al. Radical prostatectomy improves progression-free and cancer-specific survival in men with lymph node positive prostate cancer in the prostate-specific antigen era: a confirmatory study. BJU Int 2011; 107(11):1755–61.

54. Keegan KA, Cookson MS. Complications of pelvic lymph node dissection for prostate cancer. Curr Urol Rep 2011;12(3):203–8.

55. Touijer K, Fuenzalida RP, Rabbani F, et al. Extending the indications and anatomical limits of pelvic lymph node dissection for prostate cancer: improved staging or increased morbidity? BJU Int 2011;108(3):372–7.

56. Cagiannos I, Karakiewicz P, Eastham JA, et al. A preoperative nomogram identifying decreased risk of positive pelvic lymph nodes in patients with prostate cancer. J Urol 2003;170(5):1798–803.

57. Briganti A, Larcher A, Abdollah F, et al. Updated nomogram predicting lymph node invasion in patients with prostate cancer undergoing extended pelvic lymph node dissection: the essential importance of percentage of positive cores. Eur Urol 2012;61(3):480–7.

58. Yossepowitch O, Bjartell A, Eastham JA, et al. Positive surgical margins in radical prostatectomy: outlining the problem and its long-term consequences. Eur Urol 2008;55(1):87–99.

59. Simon MA, Kim S, Soloway MS. Prostate specific antigen recurrence rates are low after radical retropubic prostatectomy and positive margins. J Urol 2006; 175(1):140–4 [discussion: 144–5].

60. Karakiewicz PI, Eastham JA, Graefen M, et al. Prognostic impact of positive surgical margins in surgically treated prostate cancer: multi-institutional assessment of 5831 patients. Urology 2005;66(6):1245–50.

61. Pettus JA, Weight CJ, Thompson CJ, et al. Biochemical failure in men following radical retropubic prostatectomy: impact of surgical margin status and location. J Urol 2004;172(1):129–32.

62. Swindle P, Eastham JA, Ohori M, et al. Do margins matter? The prognostic significance of positive surgical margins in radical prostatectomy specimens. J Urol 2005;174(3):903–7.

63. Ward JF, Zincke H, Bergstralh EJ, et al. The impact of surgical approach (nerve bundle preservation versus wide local excision) on surgical margins and biochemical recurrence following radical prostatectomy. J Urol 2004; 172(4 Pt 1):1328–32.

64. Pfitzenmaier J, Pahernik S, Tremmel T, et al. Positive surgical margins after radical prostatectomy: do they have an impact on biochemical or clinical progression? BJU Int 2008;102(10):1413–8.

65. Chalfin HJ, Dinizo M, Trock BJ, et al. Impact of surgical margin status on prostate-cancer-specific mortality. BJU Int 2012;110(11):1684–9.

66. Wright JL, Dalkin BL, True LD, et al. Positive surgical margins at radical prostatectomy predict prostate cancer specific mortality. J Urol 2010;183(6): 2213–8.

67. Boorjian SA, Karnes RJ, Crispen PL, et al. The impact of positive surgical margins on mortality following radical prostatectomy during the prostate specific antigen era. J Urol 2010;183(3):1003–9.

68. Kim ED, Nath R, Slawin KM, et al. Bilateral nerve grafting during radical retropubic prostatectomy: extended follow-up. Urology 2001;58(6):983–7.

69. Nelson BA, Chang SS, Cookson MS, et al. Morbidity and efficacy of genitofemoral nerve grafts with radical retropubic prostatectomy. Urology 2006;67(4): 789–92.

70. Srougi M, Pereira D, Dall'Oglio M. Sexual rehabilitation after radical retropubic prostatectomy: new technique using ilio-inguinal nerve graft. Int Braz J Urol 2002;28(5):446–50 [discussion: 450–1].

71. Namiki S, Saito S, Nakagawa H, et al. Impact of unilateral sural nerve graft on recovery of potency and continence following radical prostatectomy: 3-year longitudinal study. J Urol 2007;178(1):212–6 [discussion: 216].

72. Secin FP, Koppie TM, Scardino PT, et al. Bilateral cavernous nerve interposition grafting during radical retropubic prostatectomy: Memorial Sloan-Kettering Cancer Center experience. J Urol 2007;177(2):664–8.

73. Sim HG, Kliot M, Lange PH, et al. Two-year outcome of unilateral sural nerve interposition graft after radical prostatectomy. Urology 2006;68(6):1290–4.

74. Singh H, Karakiewicz P, Shariat SF, et al. Impact of unilateral interposition sural nerve grafting on recovery of urinary function after radical prostatectomy. Urology 2004;63(6):1122–7.

75. Zorn KC, Bernstein AJ, Gofrit ON, et al. Long-term functional and oncological outcomes of patients undergoing sural nerve interposition grafting during robot-assisted laparoscopic radical prostatectomy. J Endourol 2008;22(5):1005–12.

76. Davis JW, Chang DW, Chevray P, et al. Randomized phase II trial evaluation of erectile function after attempted unilateral cavernous nerve-sparing retropubic radical prostatectomy with versus without unilateral sural nerve grafting for clinically localized prostate cancer. Eur Urol 2009;55(5):1135–43.

77. Stephenson AJ, Kattan MW, Eastham JA, et al. Prostate cancer-specific mortality after radical prostatectomy for patients treated in the prostate-specific antigen era. J Clin Oncol 2009;27(26):4300–5.

78. Stattin P, Holmberg E, Johansson JE, et al. Outcomes in localized prostate cancer: National Prostate Cancer Register of Sweden follow-up study. J Natl Cancer Inst 2010;102(13):950–8.

79. Bill-Axelson A, Holmberg L, Ruutu M, et al. Radical prostatectomy versus watchful waiting in early prostate cancer. N Engl J Med 2005;352(19):1977–84.

80. Wilt TJ, Brawer MK, Jones KM, et al. Radical prostatectomy versus observation for localized prostate cancer. N Engl J Med 2012;367(3):203–13.

81. Cooperberg MR, Broering JM, Kantoff PW, et al. Contemporary trends in low risk prostate cancer: risk assessment and treatment. J Urol 2007;178(3 Pt 2):S14–9.

82. Thompson I, Thrasher JB, Aus G, et al. Guideline for the management of clinically localized prostate cancer: 2007 update. American Urological Association Education and Research, Inc. J Urol 2007;177(6):2106–31.

83. Grossfeld GD, Latini DM, Lubeck DP, et al. Predicting recurrence after radical prostatectomy for patients with high risk prostate cancer. J Urol 2003;169(1):157–63.

84. Kane CJ, Presti JC Jr, Amling CL, et al. Changing nature of high risk patients undergoing radical prostatectomy. J Urol 2007;177(1):113–7.

85. Reese AC, Pierorazio PM, Han M, et al. Contemporary evaluation of the national comprehensive cancer network prostate cancer risk classification system. Urology 2012;80(5):1075–9.

86. Mearini L, Zucchi A, Costantini E, et al. Outcomes of radical prostatectomy in clinically locally advanced N0M0 prostate cancer. Urol Int 2010;85(2):166–72.

87. Reese AC, Sadetsky N, Carroll PR, et al. Inaccuracies in assignment of clinical stage for localized prostate cancer. Cancer 2011;117(2):283–9.

88. Ward JF, Slezak JM, Blute ML, et al. Radical prostatectomy for clinically advanced (cT3) prostate cancer since the advent of prostate-specific antigen testing: 15-year outcome. BJU Int 2005;95(6):751–6.

89. Xylinas E, Drouin SJ, Comperat E, et al. Oncological control after radical prostatectomy in men with clinical T3 prostate cancer: a single-centre experience. BJU Int 2009;103(9):1173–8 [discussion: 1178].

90. Epstein JI, Feng Z, Trock BJ, et al. Upgrading and downgrading of prostate cancer from biopsy to radical prostatectomy: incidence and predictive factors using the modified Gleason grading system and factoring in tertiary grades. Eur Urol 2012;61(5):1019–24.

91. Imamoto T, Suzuki H, Utsumi T, et al. External validation of a nomogram predicting the probability of prostate cancer Gleason sum upgrading between biopsy and radical prostatectomy pathology among Japanese patients. Urology 2010; 76(2):404–10.

92. Moussa AS, Li J, Soriano M, et al. Prostate biopsy clinical and pathological variables that predict significant grading changes in patients with intermediate and high grade prostate cancer. BJU Int 2009;103(1):43–8.

93. Ruijter E, van Leenders G, Miller G, et al. Errors in histological grading by prostatic needle biopsy specimens: frequency and predisposing factors. J Pathol 2000;192(2):229–33.

94. Hattab EM, Koch MO, Eble JN, et al. Tertiary Gleason pattern 5 is a powerful predictor of biochemical relapse in patients with Gleason score 7 prostatic adenocarcinoma. J Urol 2006;175(5):1695–9 [discussion: 1699].

95. Mosse CA, Magi-Galluzzi C, Tsuzuki T, et al. The prognostic significance of tertiary Gleason pattern 5 in radical prostatectomy specimens. Am J Surg Pathol 2004;28(3):394–8.

96. Rasiah KK, Stricker PD, Haynes AM, et al. Prognostic significance of Gleason pattern in patients with Gleason score 7 prostate carcinoma. Cancer 2003; 98(12):2560–5.

97. van Oort IM, Schout BM, Kiemeney LA, et al. Does the tertiary Gleason pattern influence the PSA progression-free interval after retropubic radical prostatectomy for organ-confined prostate cancer? Eur Urol 2005;48(4):572–6.

98. Whittemore DE, Hick EJ, Carter MR, et al. Significance of tertiary Gleason pattern 5 in Gleason score 7 radical prostatectomy specimens. J Urol 2008; 179(2):516–22 [discussion: 522].

99. Pan CC, Potter SR, Partin AW, et al. The prognostic significance of tertiary Gleason patterns of higher grade in radical prostatectomy specimens: a proposal to modify the Gleason grading system. Am J Surg Pathol 2000;24(4):563–9.

100. Patel AA, Chen MH, Renshaw AA, et al. PSA failure following definitive treatment of prostate cancer having biopsy Gleason score 7 with tertiary grade 5. JAMA 2007;298(13):1533–8.

101. Sim HG, Telesca D, Culp SH, et al. Tertiary Gleason pattern 5 in Gleason 7 prostate cancer predicts pathological stage and biochemical recurrence. J Urol 2008;179(5):1775–9.

102. D'Amico AV, Whittington R, Malkowicz SB, et al. Biochemical outcome after radical prostatectomy, external beam radiation therapy, or interstitial radiation therapy for clinically localized prostate cancer. JAMA 1998;280(11):969–74.

103. Dalkin BL, Ahmann FR, Nagle R, et al. Randomized study of neoadjuvant testicular androgen ablation therapy before radical prostatectomy in men with clinically localized prostate cancer. J Urol 1996;155(4):1357–60.

104. Debruyne FM, Witjes WP, Schulman CC, et al. A multicentre trial of combined neoadjuvant androgen blockade with Zoladex and flutamide prior to radical prostatectomy in prostate cancer. The European Study Group on Neoadjuvant Treatment. European Urology 1994;26(Suppl 1):4.

105. Gleave ME, Goldenberg SL, Chin JL, et al. Randomized comparative study of 3 versus 8-month neoadjuvant hormonal therapy before radical prostatectomy: biochemical and pathological effects. J Urol 2001;166(2):500–6 [discussion: 506–7].

106. Labrie F, Cusan L, Gomez JL, et al. Neoadjuvant hormonal therapy: the Canadian experience. Urology 1997;49(Suppl 3A):56–64.

107. Prezioso D, Lotti T, Polito M, et al. Neoadjuvant hormone treatment with leuprolide acetate depot 3.75 mg and cyproterone acetate, before radical prostatectomy: a randomized study. Urol Int 2004;72(3):189–95.

108. Selli C, Montironi R, Bono A, et al. Effects of complete androgen blockade for 12 and 24 weeks on the pathological stage and resection margin status of prostate cancer. J Clin Pathol 2002;55(7):508–13.

109. Soloway MS, Pareek K, Sharifi R, et al. Neoadjuvant androgen ablation before radical prostatectomy in cT2bNxMo prostate cancer: 5-year results. J Urol 2002;167(1):112–6.

110. van der Kwast TH, Tetu B, Candas B, et al. Prolonged neoadjuvant combined androgen blockade leads to a further reduction of prostatic tumor volume: three versus six months of endocrine therapy. Urology 1999;53(3):523–9.

111. Shelley MD, Kumar S, Wilt T, et al. A systematic review and meta-analysis of randomised trials of neo-adjuvant hormone therapy for localised and locally advanced prostate carcinoma. Cancer Treat Rev 2009;35(1):9–17.

112. Chi KN, Chin JL, Winquist E, et al. Multicenter phase II study of combined neoadjuvant docetaxel and hormone therapy before radical prostatectomy for patients with high risk localized prostate cancer. J Urol 2008;180(2):565–70 [discussion: 570].

113. Dreicer R, Magi-Galluzzi C, Zhou M, et al. Phase II trial of neoadjuvant docetaxel before radical prostatectomy for locally advanced prostate cancer. Urology 2004;63(6):1138–42.

114. Febbo PG, Richie JP, George DJ, et al. Neoadjuvant docetaxel before radical prostatectomy in patients with high-risk localized prostate cancer. Clin Cancer Res 2005;11(14):5233–40.

115. Oh WK, George DJ, Kaufman DS, et al. Neoadjuvant docetaxel followed by radical prostatectomy in patients with high-risk localized prostate cancer: a preliminary report. Semin Oncol 2001;28(4 Suppl 15):40–4.

116. Prayer-Galetti T, Sacco E, Pagano F, et al. Long-term follow-up of a neoadjuvant chemohormonal taxane-based phase II trial before radical prostatectomy in patients with non-metastatic high-risk prostate cancer. BJU Int 2007;100(2):274–80.

117. Ross RW, Galsky MD, Febbo P, et al. Phase 2 study of neoadjuvant docetaxel plus bevacizumab in patients with high-risk localized prostate cancer: a Prostate Cancer Clinical Trials Consortium trial. Cancer 2012;118(19):4777–84.

118. Vuky J, Porter C, Isacson C, et al. Phase II trial of neoadjuvant docetaxel and gefitinib followed by radical prostatectomy in patients with high-risk, locally advanced prostate cancer. Cancer 2009;115(4):784–91.

119. Garzotto M, Higano CS, O'Brien C, et al. Phase 1/2 study of preoperative docetaxel and mitoxantrone for high-risk prostate cancer. Cancer 2010;116(7):1699–708.

120. Hussain M, Smith DC, El-Rayes BF, et al. Neoadjuvant docetaxel and estramustine chemotherapy in high-risk/locallyadvanced prostate cancer. Urology 2003;61(4):774–80.

121. Eastham JA, Kelly WK, Grossfeld GD, et al, Cancer, Leukemia Group B. Cancer and Leukemia Group B (CALGB) 90203: a randomized phase 3 study of radical

prostatectomy alone versus estramustine and docetaxel before radical prostatectomy for patients with high-risk localized disease. Urology 2003;62(Suppl 1): 55–62.

122. Bolla M, Gonzalez D, Warde P, et al. Improved survival in patients with locally advanced prostate cancer treated with radiotherapy and goserelin. N Engl J Med 1997;337(5):295–300.

123. D'Amico AV, Manola J, Loffredo M, et al. 6-month androgen suppression plus radiation therapy vs radiation therapy alone for patients with clinically localized prostate cancer: a randomized controlled trial. JAMA 2004;292(7):821–7.

124. Warde P, Mason M, Ding K, et al. Combined androgen deprivation therapy and radiation therapy for locally advanced prostate cancer: a randomised, phase 3 trial. Lancet 2011;378(9809):2104–11.

125. Cooperberg MR, Vickers AJ, Broering JM, et al. Comparative risk-adjusted mortality outcomes after primary surgery, radiotherapy, or androgen-deprivation therapy for localized prostate cancer. Cancer 2010;116(22):5226–34.

126. Zelefsky MJ, Eastham JA, Cronin AM, et al. Metastasis after radical prostatectomy or external beam radiotherapy for patients with clinically localized prostate cancer: a comparison of clinical cohorts adjusted for case mix. J Clin Oncol 2010;28(9):1508–13.

127. Kibel AS, Ciezki JP, Klein EA, et al. Survival among men with clinically localized prostate cancer treated with radical prostatectomy or radiation therapy in the prostate specific antigen era. J Urol 2012;187(4):1259–65.

128. Abdollah F, Schmitges J, Sun M, et al. Comparison of mortality outcomes after radical prostatectomy versus radiotherapy in patients with localized prostate cancer: a population-based analysis. Int J Urol 2012;19(9):836–44 [author reply: 844–5].

129. Freedland SJ, Partin AW, Humphreys EB, et al. Radical prostatectomy for clinical stage T3a disease. Cancer 2007;109(7):1273–8.

130. Engel J, Bastian PJ, Baur H, et al. Survival benefit of radical prostatectomy in lymph node-positive patients with prostate cancer. European Urology 2010; 57(5):754–61.

131. Babaian RJ, Donnelly B, Bahn D, et al. Best practice statement on cryosurgery for the treatment of localized prostate cancer. J Urol 2008;180(5):1993–2004.

132. Briganti A, Joniau S, Gontero P, et al. Identifying the best candidate for radical prostatectomy among patients with high-risk prostate cancer. Eur Urol 2012; 61(3):584–92.

133. Boorjian SA, Karnes RJ, Viterbo R, et al. Long-term survival after radical prostatectomy versus external-beam radiotherapy for patients with high-risk prostate cancer. Cancer 2011;117(13):2883–91.

134. Yossepowitch O, Eggener SE, Serio AM, et al. Secondary therapy, metastatic progression, and cancer-specific mortality in men with clinically high-risk prostate cancer treated with radical prostatectomy. European Urology 2008;53(5): 950–9.

135. Levy DA, Jones JS. Impact of prostate gland volume on cryoablation prostate-specific antigen outcomes. Urology 2011;77(4):994–8.

136. Ward JF, Jones JS. Focal cryotherapy for localized prostate cancer: a report from the national Cryo On-Line Database (COLD) Registry. BJU Int 2012; 109(11):1648–54.

137. Cheetham P, Truesdale M, Chaudhury S, et al. Long-term cancer-specific and overall survival for men followed more than 10 years after primary and salvage cryoablation of the prostate. J Endourol 2010;24(7):1123–9.

138. Donnelly BJ, Saliken JC, Brasher PM, et al. A randomized trial of external beam radiotherapy versus cryoablation in patients with localized prostate cancer. Cancer 2010;116(2):323–30.

139. Ko YH, Kang SH, Park YJ, et al. The biochemical efficacy of primary cryoablation combined with prolonged total androgen suppression compared with radiotherapy on high-risk prostate cancer: a 3-year pilot study. Asian J Androl 2010; 12(6):827–34.

140. Truesdale MD, Cheetham PJ, Hruby GW, et al. An evaluation of patient selection criteria on predicting progression-free survival after primary focal unilateral nerve-sparing cryoablation for prostate cancer: recommendations for follow up. Cancer J 2010;16(5):544–9.

141. Chin JL, Ng CK, Touma NJ, et al. Randomized trial comparing cryoablation and external beam radiotherapy for T2C-T3B prostate cancer. Prostate Cancer Prostatic Dis 2008;11(1):40–5.

142. Cohen JK, Miller RJ Jr, Ahmed S, et al. Ten-year biochemical disease control for patients with prostate cancer treated with cryosurgery as primary therapy. Urology 2008;71(3):515–8.

143. Jones JS, Rewcastle JC, Donnelly BJ, et al. Whole gland primary prostate cryoablation: initial results from the cryo on-line data registry. J Urol 2008;180(2): 554–8.

144. Onik G, Vaughan D, Lotenfoe R, et al. The "male lumpectomy": focal therapy for prostate cancer using cryoablation results in 48 patients with at least 2-year follow-up. Urol Oncol 2008;26(5):500–5.

145. Ellis DS, Manny TB Jr, Rewcastle JC. Cryoablation as primary treatment for localized prostate cancer followed by penile rehabilitation. Urology 2007; 69(2):306–10.

146. Polascik TJ, Nosnik I, Mayes JM, et al. Short-term cancer control after primary cryosurgical ablation for clinically localized prostate cancer using third-generation cryotechnology. Urology 2007;70(1):117–21.

147. Bahn DK, Silverman P, Lee F Sr, et al. Focal prostate cryoablation: initial results show cancer control and potency preservation. J Endourol 2006;20(9):688–92.

148. Prepelica KL, Okeke Z, Murphy A, et al. Cryosurgical ablation of the prostate: high risk patient outcomes. Cancer 2005;103(8):1625–30.

149. Aus G, Pileblad E, Hugosson J. Cryosurgical ablation of the prostate: 5-year follow-up of a prospective study. European Urology 2002;42(2):133–8.

150. Bahn DK, Lee F, Badalament R, et al. Targeted cryoablation of the prostate: 7-year outcomes in the primary treatment of prostate cancer. Urology 2002; 60(2 Suppl 1):3–11.

151. Donnelly BJ, Saliken JC, Ernst DS, et al. Prospective trial of cryosurgical ablation of the prostate: five-year results. Urology 2002;60(4):645–9.

152. Long JP, Bahn D, Lee F, et al. Five-year retrospective, multi-institutional pooled analysis of cancer-related outcomes after cryosurgical ablation of the prostate. Urology 2001;57(3):518–23.

153. Sung HH, Jeong BC, Seo SI, et al. Seven years of experience with high-intensity focused ultrasound for prostate cancer: advantages and limitations. Prostate 2012;72(13):1399–406.

154. Boutier R, Girouin N, Cheikh AB, et al. Location of residual cancer after transrectal high-intensity focused ultrasound ablation for clinically localized prostate cancer. BJU Int 2011;108(11):1776–81.

155. Ganzer R, Robertson CN, Ward JF, et al. Correlation of prostate-specific antigen nadir and biochemical failure after high-intensity focused ultrasound of localized

prostate cancer based on the Stuttgart failure criteria—analysis from the @-Registry. BJU Int 2011;108(8 Pt 2):E196–201.

156. Inoue Y, Goto K, Hayashi T, et al. Transrectal high-intensity focused ultrasound for treatment of localized prostate cancer. Int J Urol 2011;18(5):358–62.

157. Ripert T, Azemar MD, Menard J, et al. Six years' experience with high-intensity focused ultrasonography for prostate cancer: oncological outcomes using the new 'Stuttgart' definition for biochemical failure. BJU Int 2011;107(12):1899–905.

158. Crouzet S, Rebillard X, Chevallier D, et al. Multicentric oncologic outcomes of high-intensity focused ultrasound for localized prostate cancer in 803 patients. European Urology 2010;58(4):559–66.

159. Sumitomo M, Asakuma J, Yoshii H, et al. Anterior perirectal fat tissue thickness is a strong predictor of recurrence after high-intensity focused ultrasound for prostate cancer. Int J Urol 2010;17(9):776–82.

160. Ahmed HU, Zacharakis E, Dudderidge T, et al. High-intensity-focused ultrasound in the treatment of primary prostate cancer: the first UK series. Br J Cancer 2009;101(1):19–26.

161. Challacombe BJ, Murphy DG, Zakri R, et al. High-intensity focused ultrasound for localized prostate cancer: initial experience with a 2-year follow-up. BJU Int 2009;104(2):200–4.

162. Mearini L, D'Urso L, Collura D, et al. Visually directed transrectal high intensity focused ultrasound for the treatment of prostate cancer: a preliminary report on the Italian experience. J Urol 2009;181(1):105–11 [discussion: 111–2].

163. Uchida T, Shoji S, Nakano M, et al. Transrectal high-intensity focused ultrasound for the treatment of localized prostate cancer: eight-year experience. Int J Urol 2009;16(11):881–6.

164. Blana A, Rogenhofer S, Ganzer R, et al. Eight years' experience with high-intensity focused ultrasonography for treatment of localized prostate cancer. Urology 2008;72(6):1329–33 [discussion: 1333–4].

165. Blana A, Murat FJ, Walter B, et al. First analysis of the long-term results with transrectal HIFU in patients with localised prostate cancer. European Urology 2008;53(6):1194–201.

166. Misrai V, Roupret M, Chartier-Kastler E, et al. Oncologic control provided by HIFU therapy as single treatment in men with clinically localized prostate cancer. World J Urol 2008;26(5):481–5.

167. Sumitomo M, Hayashi M, Watanabe T, et al. Efficacy of short-term androgen deprivation with high-intensity focused ultrasound in the treatment of prostate cancer in Japan. Urology 2008;72(6):1335–40.

168. Lee HM, Hong JH, Choi HY. High-intensity focused ultrasound therapy for clinically localized prostate cancer. Prostate Cancer Prostatic Dis 2006;9(4):439–43.

169. Blana A, Brown SC, Chaussy C, et al. High-intensity focused ultrasound for prostate cancer: comparative definitions of biochemical failure. BJU Int 2009;104(8):1058–62.

Contemporary Issues in Radiotherapy for Clinically Localized Prostate Cancer

Richard Khor, MBBS, FRANZCR*, Scott Williams, MD, FRANZCR

KEYWORDS

- Prostate carcinoma • Radiotherapy • Image-guided radiotherapy • Brachytherapy
- Stereotactic body radiotherapy

KEY POINTS

- Radiation is a potent genotoxic agent that induces clonogenic cell death through apoptosis and terminal senescence.
- Increasing radiation dose is associated with improved biochemical outcomes, and is facilitated by improvements in image guidance and better target delineation.
- Neoadjuvant or adjuvant androgen deprivation improves biochemical and survival outcomes in intermediate-risk and high-risk patients, but the benefits must be measured against potential toxicity.
- Prostate cancer may respond to higher doses per fraction than other tumors, which has led to the current interest in brachytherapy and stereotactic body radiotherapy.
- There is level 1 evidence regarding the improved outcomes achieved with adjuvant postprostatectomy radiotherapy, with current trials investigating the role of early salvage postprostatectomy radiotherapy.
- Future improvement in outcomes may be derived from improved adjuvant therapies or technological advancements in radiotherapy delivery techniques.

INTRODUCTION

Radiation therapy remains a valid curative approach to prostate cancer therapy. Significant technological advances over the past 2 decades have facilitated the safe delivery of increasingly higher doses of radiation therapy to the prostate while avoiding relevant adjacent tissues. In turn, short-term and medium-term outcomes have improved, and the addition of endocrine manipulation either before (neoadjuvant) or

Disclosure: Nothing to disclose.
Division of Radiation Oncology and Cancer Imaging, Peter MacCallum Cancer Centre, Locked Bag 1, A'Beckett Street, Victoria 8006, Australia
* Corresponding author.
E-mail address: richard.khor@petermac.org

after (adjuvant) curative therapy has shown a substantial impact. Furthermore, radiotherapy in the postprostatectomy setting has gained prominence in recent years.

PRINCIPLES OF RADIATION THERAPY

Therapeutic radiation can be delivered with multiple techniques. For most patients, this involves external beam radiotherapy (EBRT) using a linear accelerator to deliver high-energy photons. Alternatively, brachytherapy uses temporary high-dose-rate (HDR) or permanent low-dose-rate (LDR) radioactive sources to deliver the prescribed dose to the target.

Ionizing radiation is a potent genotoxic agent that predominately interacts with biological matter by inducing double-stranded deoxyribonucleic acid (DNA) breaks. Tumor growth is halted by either induction of tumor cell death by necrosis or loss of cell reproductive integrity; together termed clonogenic cell death. It seems that clonogenic inactivation through instigation of terminal differentiation (senescence) may also be central in the response of prostate cancer to radiation.[1,2]

The aim of traditional fractionated radiation therapy is to exploit potentially defective DNA repair mechanisms through delivery of daily doses, nominally 1.8–2 Gy per day. This allows for normal tissues with ostensibly intact DNA damage repair mechanisms to repair a substantial portion of the DNA damage between fractions. Tumors are usually unable to mount a similar DNA repair response, and thus sustain more damage over multiple fractions than normal tissues.[3] As the total delivered dose accumulates, so does the DNA damage, and more tumor control is achieved.

Different tissues have different patterns of response depending on the dose and dose per fraction given. As a generalization, the model of dose-response shows an initial linear component and subsequent quadratic components to this relationship. In general, normal tissues are more damaged by higher doses of radiation per fraction, whereas most malignancies show a much more linear response to increasing dose per fraction, meaning there is an advantage to delivering high total radiation doses. Recent data suggest that prostate cancer may behave differently, and exhibit a similar fraction size sensitivity to that of normal tissues, suggesting that larger fraction sizes rather than total dose are optimal.[4–7] With approaches such as HDR brachytherapy, impressive biochemical outcomes have been reported with lower doses of radiotherapy delivered in large fractions.[8,9]

PATIENT SELECTION FOR RADIATION THERAPY WITH CURATIVE INTENT
Risk Stratification

There is significant heterogeneity in the biological behavior observed in prostate cancer. The risk of biochemical failure after local therapy has been explored in detail. Increasing stage at presentation, prostate specific antigen (PSA) level, and grade of tumor all predict for PSA recurrence after therapy with curative intent.[10,11]

The National Comprehensive Cancer Network (NCCN) risk stratification (**Table 1**)[11] can be used to stratify patients by risk of biochemical failure after curative therapy

Table 1			
NCCN risk stratification and PSA control			
NCCN Risk Stratification	**AJCC Clinical Stage**	**Presenting PSA (ng/mL)**	**Gleason Grade**
Low	T1 to T2a, N0	≤10	6 or less
Intermediate	T2b to T2c, N0	>10–20	7
High	T3 or T4, N0–1	>20	8 or greater

(eg, low, intermediate, or high risk). It should also be realized that many men with low-risk disease have a low chance of prostate cancer death and may be candidates for active surveillance, and if more than 60 years of age are unlikely to die of prostate cancer irrespective of local treatment.[12,13] Some patients with Gleason 7 disease more than 70 years of age may even be able to avoid treatment all together without a mortality penalty.[14,15] In intermediate-risk disease, the benefits of therapy must be carefully weighed against the potential side effects of therapy and associated costs.

Conversely, the risk of prostate cancer death in patients with high-risk disease increases considerably.[16] Despite a high baseline risk of micrometastatic disease, local therapy has an impact on long-term outcomes in this group. An absolute survival benefit of 10% at 7 years was demonstrated in the SPCG-7 randomized trial of androgen deprivation therapy with or without local radiation therapy.[17] A comparable benefit was confirmed in a similarly structured Canadian study, further reinforcing the use of radiation in this setting.[18]

Assessment, Comorbidities, and Contraindications

A thorough history and examination should be performed to assess the patient's suitability for radiation therapy, especially given that the avoidance of therapy is intrinsically linked with anticipated life expectancy. Thus, patients with a low life expectancy because of either medical comorbidities or a life expectancy less than 10 years are less likely to benefit from therapy.[11] The presence of comorbidities can significantly affect the choice of recommended therapy and treatment modality; for example, in the avoidance of anesthetic and postoperative risks in men with significant comorbidities. However, certain comorbidities may interact with radiotherapy, such as the presence of type 2 diabetes, or increase risk of rectal toxicity (especially with concurrent inflammatory bowel disease) after radiotherapy.[19]

Assessment of urinary symptoms is central as symptomatic benign prostatic hypertrophy (BPH) often coexists with carcinoma. Qualitative as well as quantitative validated assessments, such as the American Urologic Association (AUA) Prostate Symptom Score or the identical International Prostate Symptom Score (IPSS),[20] should be attained. Men with significant lower urinary tract obstructive symptoms are at higher risk of late genitourinary toxicity such as incontinence from both external beam[21–23] and brachytherapy.[24,25] Men with a higher IPSS are also more likely to experience urinary obstructive symptoms during external beam radiotherapy.[26] These may also be mitigated with cytoreductive androgen suppression therapy before commencement of treatment.[27] A transurethral resection of prostate (TURP) before radiation may be required in some to alleviate obstruction, but conflicting nonrandomized studies have been published regarding whether it is has a long-term deleterious effect on urinary continence.[21,22,24]

Potency after local therapy for prostate cancer is an important end point. A sexual history should be taken, in terms of sexual activity, erectile function, and libido. Validated surveys such as the International Index of Erectile Function (IIEF)[28] provide an objective measure of sexual function and health.

If testosterone manipulation is being considered, cardiovascular risk factors must be carefully assessed and aggressively managed, because of the potential for increased cardiovascular events in patients with significant underlying cardiac dysfunction.[29] This could influence the decision about the prescription of endocrine therapy and its duration.

Radiation should be avoided in patients with active inflammatory bowel disease, which can increase the severity of gastrointestinal (GI) symptoms significantly.[30,31] Previous pelvic surgery, particularly for rectal cancer, can result in loops of radiosensitive small bowel entering the pelvis and possibly being tethered by postoperative adhesions, which may limit the ability to administer a full therapeutic dose. Previous high-dose pelvic radiotherapy is a contraindication to further EBRT to respect the radiotolerance of normal tissues. In this case, other modalities such as surgery or brachytherapy should be considered.[32,33]

In broad terms, patients with an increased risk of radiographic evidence of metastatic disease at presentation (eg, men with high-risk disease) should be staged with nuclear medicine bone scan and computed tomography (CT) of the abdomen and pelvis.[11] Magnetic resonance imaging (MRI) of the pelvis is useful for detecting extraprostatic extension of tumor and defining the prostatic anatomy.

A full PSA history should be obtained. Apart from the impact of the current absolute PSA level, there may be prognostic significance to the pretreatment PSA dynamics.[34,35] Similarly, the histopathology report may contain information of relevance beyond the Gleason score, with much attention focused on whether the burden of disease can be better captured using biopsy core volumetrics. The general consensus is that the metrics of a heavier cancer burden, such as an increasing number of cores involved, a higher percentage of biopsy cores positive for cancer, and increased core length, are all associated with poorer outcome and should be considered in the selection of treatment intensity.[36,37]

DEFINING THE RADIATION TARGET
Prostate and Seminal Vesicles

The extent of radiation fields is based on understanding the natural history and potential routes of spread. The multifocal nature of prostate cancer[38] has typically suggested that a uniform radiation dose to the whole prostate is required. Tumors may also breach the capsule of the prostate and be found in the periprostatic fat, or involve the adjacent seminal vesicles. The risk of extraprostatic extension and seminal vesicle invasion (SVI) increases significantly in higher-risk groups, as reflected in published nomograms.[39,40] In cases where extraprostatic extension is detected, the mean length of extension is 1.1 mm, and 90% of cases were within 3.8 mm in 1 series.[41] This information affects treatment planning.

There are conflicting data regarding the distribution of SVI, which has resulted in variation in the amount of seminal vesicle (SV) included in the prophylactic volume. Davis and colleagues[42] reported a cohort of patients in whom SVI was identified on prostatectomy, and 40% of specimens had tumor less than 0.5 cm from the SV tip. Conversely, Kestin and colleagues[43] reported that a cohort of patients with low-risk disease had a 1% incidence of SVI, compared with 27% SVI incidence in those with high-risk disease. In those with SVI, only 7% were observed to have tumor extending beyond 1 cm of the base of the SV and 1% beyond 2 cm.

Taking these basic biological underpinnings into account, the whole prostate is generally defined as an area of clinical risk, and included in the clinical target volume (CTV). Gross tumor seen on correlative imaging is included in the CTV, and any visible extracapsular extension may entail using a small volume expansion to ensure coverage of regions of apparent disease as well as incorporate areas of subclinical spread. In the event of confirmed SVI, the whole seminal vesicle is typically incorporated into the high-dose volume. Similarly, with a high risk of subclinical SVI, a prophylactic dose is generally prescribed to either the proximal or whole SVs. SVs lie immediately adjacent to the anterior fascial plane of the mesorectum, and most treatment including the SV can entail a compromise between coverage of the SV and dose constraints of the rectum.

Whole Pelvic Irradiation

Prostate cancer dissemination is commonly ascribed to lymphovascular permeation, via largely stepwise spread through the pelvic nodes. Despite this, the prophylactic treatment of pelvic nodes is controversial, with no clear consensus on the subgroup of patients who derive benefit from treatment. Several randomized trials of whole pelvis radiotherapy (WPRT) have been conducted, and all concluded that there was no clear biochemical or clinical control improvement with the addition of whole pelvic therapy to prostate only radiotherapy.[44–46] The major criticisms of these studies were that patients may have been either too low risk or too high risk to benefit from pelvic therapy. However, pelvic nodes may represent an important source of treatment failures if only the prostate is treated, especially in high-risk patients. New highly conformal therapy such as intensity-modulated radiotherapy (IMRT) has allowed adjuvant radiation to be delivered with acceptable toxicity. These observations infer that, in the right patient population, pelvic prophylaxis may be feasible with low toxicity and possible clinical benefit nomograms have been developed and refined, with the aim of identifying men most likely to benefit from WPRT.[47–50] For those believed to potentially benefit from WPRT, consensus guidelines have been published and can guide treatment volume definition; further definitive trials are ongoing.[51] The most commonly involved first echelon nodal regions are fully included in the target volume. These have been defined by MRI imaging studies, as well as sentinel node imaging.[52,53] One study using sentinel node imaging found these to be the external iliac (34.3%), internal iliac (17.9%), common iliac (12.7%), sacral (8.6%), and perirectal (6.2%) regions. The paraaortic nodes were less commonly involved[53] and are generally not included. Studies to define the role of nodal irradiation are ongoing, such as RTOG 09-24.

EXTERNAL BEAM RADIOTHERAPY
IMRT

IMRT is based on 2 principles: (1) dynamically changing the open area of each field during each fraction and (2) computer software to divide the planning CT into spatial units (voxels) and then determine the optimal solution to deliver the dose to each voxel for a given beam arrangement. This differs from conventional radiotherapy because target dose characteristics and normal tissue tolerances are specified before plan construction (inverse planning). IMRT prescriptions are highly proscriptive to adequately direct the resultant computer-generated dosimetry. Compared with three-dimensional conformal radiation therapy, prostate IMRT allows optimization of the therapeutic ratio through limiting areas of high dose outside the target volume while preserving tumor coverage. IMRT can be delivered using 7 to 9 static fields, or a single beam treating in an arc about the patient (volume-modulated arc therapy). Variants of IMRT include the Cyberknife (Accuray, Inc, Sunnyvale, CA), which uses a small 6 MV linear accelerator mounted on an articulated mechanical gantry and tomotherapy, using a therapy source moving in an arc that delivers treatment a slice at a time.

Image-Guided Radiation Therapy

One of the major technical hurdles in treating prostate cancer is target localization. The prostate is a deformable gland that is influenced by both bowel and bladder filling, and thus mobile within the pelvis.[54] Traditional bony matching techniques do not account for day-to-day variation of prostate motion, which is independent of pelvic position. Failure to account for prostatic motion could result in underdosing of the target and overdosing of surrounding normal tissues. This uncertainly is translated into a larger planning target volume (PTV) margin.

Common methods of image guidance are implanted fiducial markers and cone-beam CT scan. Fiducial markers, usually implanted via the transrectal route, can account for prostate motion when used in conjunction with kilovoltage or orthovoltage daily imaging. The patient is set up on the treatment couch, a set of verification images taken, and then the three-dimensional shift required to account for prostatic motion is applied. This approach minimizes the systematic error in patient positioning, allowing for both dose escalation with isotoxic therapy and minimization of PTV margins.[55] Clinical results indicate that such an approach can reduce toxicity significantly, including doses of up to 86.4 Gy.[56]

An alternative to implanted fiducial markers is volumetric imaging such as cone-beam CT. The imaging apparatus on the linear accelerator is rotated about the patient while imaging to obtain a three-dimensional image.[57,58] These systems can be used in patients who have a contraindication to implanted fiducial markers; acceptable levels of systematic error are maintained even when matching to prostate rather than implanted fiducials.[59,60] Furthermore, direct monitoring of intrafraction motion is possible using sophisticated electronic transponders implanted into the prostate.[61]

Dose-Escalated Radiotherapy

The ability to deliver higher doses of radiotherapy in contemporary practice is based on minimizing tumor localization uncertainties and minimizing the high-dose irradiated volume.

There is level 1 evidence that increasing radiation dose has a substantial positive effect on biochemical control.[62–66] Increasing the prescribed dose of radiation from 68 to 70 Gy to more than 78 Gy can result in impressive PSA control rates. For example, the MD Anderson Cancer Center dose escalation trial reported that increasing the radiation dose from 70 Gy to 78 Gy improved biochemical control outcomes from 59% to 78% ($P = .004$). This effect was more pronounced in intermediate and high-risk tumors, although other studies have also documented a response in all risk groups.[67,68] Similar dose escalation trials were conducted in the United Kingdom and the Netherlands (**Table 2**).

Table 2					
Randomized trials of radiation dose escalation in prostate cancer					
Study	**Number**	**Risk Groups**	**Dose**	**Outcome**	**P Value**
MDACC (Kuban et al,[65] 2008)	301	Low: 61 Intermediate: 139 High: 101	70 Gy 78 Gy	8-y bNED 59% 8-y bNED 78%	.004
PROG (Zietman et al,[63] 2005)	392	Low: 227 Intermediate: 129 High: 33	70 GyE 79.2 GyE	5-y bNED 61% 5-y bNED 80%	<.001
Dutch (Peeters et al,[62] 2006)	664	Low: 120 Intermediate: 182 High: 362	68 Gy 78 Gy	5-y FFF 54% 5-y FFF 64%	.01
MRC (Dearnaley et al,[64] 2007)	843	Low: 204 Intermediate: 264 High: 362	NADT-64 Gy NADT-74 Gy	5-y bPFS 60% 5-y bPFS 71%	.0007

Abbreviations: bNED, biochemically no evidence of disease; bPFS, biochemical progression-free survival; FFF, freedom from failure; GyE, Gray equivalent; MDACC, MD Anderson Cancer Center; MRC, Medical Research Council; NADT, neoadjuvant androgen deprivation therapy; PROG, Proton Radiation Oncology Group.

Although the biochemical outcome may be an indicator of clinical benefit, it is yet to be shown to be a potential surrogate for overall survival, and no overall survival benefit has ever been demonstrated with dose-escalated radiotherapy. Given that in many trials the risk of noncancer mortality is often double that of prostate cancer mortality,[65] these studies are underpowered to show a relatively modest decrease in mortality brought about by the biochemical failure improvements.

Although photon-based EBRT is the most common method for delivering high biological doses to the prostate, other modalities, such as proton beam therapy[63] and HDR brachytherapy,[8] can also produce similar results. Particle beam therapy uses a large particle accelerator to produce a therapeutic beam of heavy ions such as protons or carbon nuclei. The major advantage in using protons as opposed to conventional high-energy photons is the ability of a proton beam to deposit a greater proportion of energy at depth, thus potentially protecting normal tissues.

One randomized trial has used proton beams to boost an EBRT dose of 50.4 Gy to a total of either 70.2 or 79.2 Gy (photon equivalent dose).[63] The higher boost dose gave better 10-year freedom from biochemical relapse (83% v 68%) but also a somewhat higher grade 2 or more GI toxicity rate (24% vs 13%), analogous to the EBRT dose escalation experience.[69] However, no direct comparisons have been conducted between proton beam and modern IMRT techniques, and nonrandomized comparisons are conflicting. Although planning studies suggest that dose distributions and subsequent toxicity are likely to be similar,[70] larger observational studies have found higher rates of hip fractures and GI toxicity with proton therapy.[71] Perhaps the most significant drawback of proton therapy is the substantial capital and running costs of proton facilities.[72]

Toxicity

Increasing GI and genitourinary (GU) toxicity has been reported with dose-escalated regimens. The MD Anderson Cancer Center dose escalation trial reported a 10-year actuarial incidence of GI toxicity of grade 2 severity or greater as 26% for those who received 78 Gy compared with 13% for those who received 70 Gy ($P = .013$). Likewise, there was a trend toward higher grade 2 GU toxicity in the high-dose arm, which was observed in 13% and 8% of those in the high-dose and low-dose arms, respectively. This trial did not have universal use of CT to delineate normal tissues or image-guided radiation therapy (IGRT) to minimize set up uncertainty. Modern approaches using these measures are likely to result in decreased toxicity.[56]

Erectile dysfunction (ED) is the other major toxicity experienced by those treated with EBRT. The prostate lies just superior to the penile bulb, and sensitive neurovascular bundles controlling erectile function course posterolateral to the prostate. These structures can often be included in the high-dose irradiated volume and thus ED is likely to become an increasingly common issue with any form of dose-escalated therapy. The average time to ED after EBRT is 12 to 18 months, with institutional reports of 40% to 50% potency rates after 2 years[73,74]; a meta-analysis of EBRT data confirmed a potency rate of 55% at 1 year (95% confidence interval [CI] 52%–58%).[75] Prospective quality-of-life surveys reported that 50% to 60% of irradiated men (including EBRT and brachytherapy) reported distress about perceived sexual health, which may peak after 2 to 6 months, stabilizing thereafter. This implies that other factors such as acute toxicity from radiotherapy and hormone therapy are likely to adversely affect quality of life before the onset of ED from radiotherapy alone.[76] ED management with phosphodiesterase inhibitors has been shown to be effective after EBRT in randomized trials.[77,78]

Role of Androgen Deprivation Therapy

Androgens are an important mitogen in prostate cancer in all phases of disease.[79] There is level 1 evidence that the addition of androgen deprivation therapy (ADT) to radiotherapy improves biochemical and survival outcomes in patients with locally advanced disease or with poor risk factors.[80–83] There seems to be a stepwise improvement in outcome with increasing length of adjuvant androgen deprivation. RTOG 86-10 randomized patients in all risk groups between 66.6 Gy EBRT with and without 2 months of neoadjuvant goserelin. Most impressively, statistically significant improvements in biochemical progression-free survival, distant metastasis rate, local control, and cause-specific survival were found.[81] The Australian Trans-Tasman Radiation Oncology Group (TROG) 96.01 randomized study treated patients with 66 Gy of EBRT with and without neoadjuvant goserelin and flutamide (3 or 6 months) in a high-risk population. The addition of 6 months of neoadjuvant ADT to radiation resulted in improved distant progression (adjusted hazard ratio [aHR] 0.49, 95% CI 0.31–0.76; $P = .001$), prostate cancer-specific mortality (aHR 0.49, 95% CI 0.32–0.74; $P = .0008$), and all-cause mortality (aHR 0.63, 95% CI 0.48–0.83; $P = .0008$), a finding that was not reproduced in those who received 3 months of ADT.[80]

Compared with 66 to 70 Gy of radiation alone, multiple trials demonstrate survival benefits for the addition of long-term adjuvant ADT,[82,84] with 1 trial demonstrating an improvement in distant metastasis-free survival as well.[82] However, the benefit for the incremental benefit of 2 or 3 years of ADT after neoadjuvant ADT is more modest. The European Organisation for the Research and Treatment of Cancer (EORTC) 22961 trial treated patients with 6 months of ADT and 70 Gy EBRT, with or without an additional 2.5 years of ADT. A small statistically significant difference in prostate cancer–specific survival was noted, but no additional overall survival benefit was found, consistent with ADT duration effect modeling.[85] Likewise, the RTOG 92-02 trial treated patients with 2 months of goserelin, flutamide, and 65 to 70 Gy EBRT, randomizing patients between 24 months of goserelin versus no adjuvant therapy. Only a trend toward an overall survival benefit was found (80.0% vs 78.5% at 5 years, $P = .73$), although improvements in other end point surrogates such as disease-free survival and biochemical progression-free survival were found.[86]

In addition to disease control benefits, a period of neoadjuvant ADT may also confer the added benefit of modulating lower urinary tract symptoms[87] and decreasing prostate size,[88] which has the potential to translate into improved long-term toxicity rates.

All these data have predated modern dose-escalated radiotherapy, IGRT, as well as the widespread use of PSA screening. It is postulated that the effect of neoadjuvant or adjuvant ADT may not be as large when combined with dose-escalated radiotherapy.[85] However, it must be noted that no trial assessing increased radiation dose has ever demonstrated a survival advantage, in contradistinction to trials with ADT and radiotherapy. Randomized trials have been activated to address this issue in the intermediate-risk group (RTOG 08-15).

BRACHYTHERAPY

Brachytherapy (short distance therapy) involves the temporary or permanent implantation of radioactive sources to deliver tumoricidal radiation doses within the proposed target volume. Radioactive material exists as an unstable isotope of a base element. The decay of these isotopes into inert substances produces secondary particles and photons. These secondary particles are identical to those emitted by linear accelerators, with 2 chief advantages of being lower in energy and being created within the target volume. Thus, the radiation produced is less penetrating and is not required to traverse normal tissue before the target volume. Furthermore, the high dose fall off inherent to radioactive sources (inverse-square law) results in decreased doses to the rectum, but at the cost of potentially underdosing occult extraprostatic extension. Thus, supplemental EBRT is often recommended in patients with intermediate-risk or high-risk features.[89] Sources are classified by the dose rate at which they decay to produce therapeutic ionizing radiation (typically X-rays). In general, LDR implants for prostate cancer are achieved through the permanent implantation of many radioactive sources into and surrounding the prostate. HDR implants can deliver clinical dose rates similar to that of EBRT and are temporary.

LDR Brachytherapy

LDR brachytherapy involves the permanent implantation of radioactive sources into the prostate to achieve high intraprostatic doses of radiation. The availability of real-time ultrasonography or MRI feedback to place seeds accurately, along with short-range radioisotopes that decay into inert substances form the basis for LDR brachytherapy. Isotopes such as iodine 125 (^{125}I) and palladium 103 (^{103}Pd) are commonly used in clinical practice. These seeds are placed under direct image guidance, following a predefined customized plan (done in real time, or via a previous volume study) that peripherally loads the prostate gland to deliver maximum radiation dose to the prostate while sparing the urethra. Seeds are implanted via the transperineal route by means of a template affixed to the perineum. Typical delivered doses prescribed to a minimum peripheral dose (MPD) are 145 Gy and 125 Gy for ^{125}I and ^{103}Pd, respectively.[89] In patients at risk of nodal disease or extraprostatic extension, LDR brachytherapy may be combined with EBRT to the whole pelvis or limited fields to cover periprostatic tissues and SVs.

Patient selection for brachytherapy

Because of the transperineal route of application, additional care must be exercised when selecting patients suitable for brachytherapy. For this reason, patients with a large or poorly healed TURP defect, large prostatic size, or large median lobe are less suitable for an LDR approach. Low-risk patients, who are unlikely to harbor occult extraprostatic disease or SVI, are candidates for an LDR implant alone. Current American College of Radiology/American Society for Radiation Oncology guidelines recommend supplemental external beam radiotherapy in higher-risk patients for prophylaxis against extraprostatic extension or unrecognized SVI.[89]

Outcomes

LDR brachytherapy can achieve excellent outcomes, as demonstrated in multiple prospective trials with adequate follow-up.[90–94] Increasing prostate cancer grade is associated with higher biochemical failure rates. In 1 study, the biochemical control rate at 5 years was 98% for those with Gleason 6 cancer, compared with 91% to 92% for those with higher-grade cancers.[95] Implant quality significantly affects the chance of treatment success. For example, Zelefsky and colleagues[93] reported that the dose to 90% of the target volume (D90%) of less than 130 Gy using ^{125}I seeds was 75% at 8 years, compared with 93% if the D90% was greater than 130 Gy.

Combination LDR-EBRT has been shown in large series to provide outcomes comparable with EBRT alone. Critz and colleagues[96] reported the outcomes of 3546 men treated without ADT in all risk groups with up to 25 years of follow-up. The 5-year disease-free survival rates were 95%, 81%, and 55% for low-risk, intermediate-risk and high-risk men, respectively. Similar outcomes have been published in other series.[97,98] The addition of EBRT to LDR may come at the risk of increased rectal morbidity.[99] Outcomes from the RTOG 0232 (NCT00063882) and the Canadian ASCENDE-RT randomized studies comparing EBRT monotherapy to combination LDR-EBRT are awaited.

Toxicity

An increase in urinary symptoms is often observed after LDR brachytherapy. In the acute phase immediately after treatment, postoperative swelling and acute urinary retention occurs in 5% to 10% of men.[100] In the subacute phase, when the bulk of radiation dose deposition occurs, radiation urethritis is common. This may persist for several months with 75% or more returning to normal within 1 year,[100–104] with slow subsequent improvements.[105] Long-term data suggest that urinary symptoms are stable even 9 years after LDR brachytherapy.[101] Alpha-adrenergic blockade can be helpful in reducing symptoms until urinary function normalizes. Studies have found that baseline obstructive symptoms,[100] low peak urinary flow rate,[100,106] previous TURP, or a large prostate volume[106] can all predispose patients to toxicity. After LDR brachytherapy, treatment of future obstructive symptoms with TURP should best be avoided for at least 2 years, as it may be associated with urinary incontinence.[107] Early maintenance of erectile function with LDR exceeds that achieved with EBRT. A meta-analysis of ED at 1 year found that erectile preservation rates were 76% (95% CI 69%–82%), which compares favorably with EBRT outcomes.[75] However, quality-of-life data suggest that patient-reported sexual health scores decrease initially, then gradually improve, but have not normalized 2 years after implant.[101] Long-term maintenance of erectile function in patients after LDR brachytherapy has been reported as 39% at 6 years.[108]

HDR Brachytherapy

HDR brachytherapy temporary implants are another method of delivering radiation via a radioactive source. In this case, the dose rate is high and can exceed 6 Gy per minute at calibration distances, with doses increasing exponentially closer to the source. These dose rates are similar to that deliverable via linear accelerator, and allow for the delivery of large radiation fractions, which may exploit the proposed sensitivity of prostate cancer to high fractional doses. The most common isotope used is iridium 192 (^{192}Ir). A series of hollow transfer catheters are inserted into the prostate facilitated by a perineal template similar to that of LDR brachytherapy, with transrectal ultrasonographic guidance to visualize the catheter track. During treatment, the ^{192}Ir source is sequentially introduced into each transfer catheter to deliver a composite dose to the prostate with high conformity while sparing surrounding critical structures.

Hoskin and colleagues[8] reported the results of a randomized trial demonstrating increased biochemical control outcomes when an HDR boost to EBRT was compared with EBRT alone. The control arm received 55 Gy in 20 fractions of EBRT, and the experimental arm received 35.75 Gy in 13 fractions with an HDR boost of 17 Gy in 2 fractions. The 5-year freedom from biochemical failure estimates were 75% for HDR and 61% for the control arm, which was a statistically significant result. Although the radiation doses used in this study would no longer be considered optimal, well-controlled retrospective studies have also reproduced these findings with more contemporary dose fractionation schedules.[109]

Given the improvement in outcomes and brevity of treatment, HDR monotherapy trials have been conducted to establish its efficacy in patients in all risk groups with encouraging results.[110–112] For example, Demanes and colleagues[110] reported the results of a cohort of 298 patients treated with HDR monotherapy (42 Gy in 6 fractions or

38 Gy in 4 fractions). With a median follow-up time of 5.2 years, the 8-year biochemical control rate was 97% and overall survival was 95% with acceptable toxicity.

Toxicity

HDR brachytherapy results in posttreatment side effects of urinary irritation, which is found at 3 months in 15% of men.[5] In the only randomized trial of brachytherapy, HDR was found to have a similar late GI and GU toxicity incidence to hypofractionated radiotherapy. However, late GU toxicity mainly manifested as urethral strictures, with an actuarial rate of 8% at 7 years,[8] reflecting the high biological doses delivered to the urethra compared with other techniques. The risk of urethral strictures ranges from as low as 4% to as high as 30% in some series,[109,113–116] with previous TURP a likely predisposing factor to stricture formation.[117] These studies were conducted before a true appreciation of robust image guidance was widespread, and analyzing the interaction between fraction size, number of fractions, and dosimetric comparisons is complex. This has been demonstrated in a randomized trial of brachytherapy, in which quality-of-life data revealed that ED was a major component of additional toxicity from a combined EBRT-HDR approach compared with EBRT alone.[118]

POSTPROSTATECTOMY RADIOTHERAPY

Planned postprostatectomy radiotherapy (PPRT) after prostatectomy is a controversial issue in uro-oncology. Although radical prostatectomy (RP) provides excellent local control for organ-confined disease, when the tumor extends beyond the prostatic capsule, the risk of local relapse is between 10% and 50%.[119–123] This population of patients may benefit from further local therapy to secure long-term disease control. However, patient selection is likely to play an important role in the successful application of adjuvant therapy because not all patients who develop biochemical failure will die of disease. Surgical data suggest that the median time from biochemical progression to clinically apparent distant metastasis is 8 years, and the time to death from distant metastases is 5 years.[124] The median survival had not been reached after 16 years of follow-up after biochemical relapse.[125] There are 2 broad approaches to further local therapy with radiation: immediate adjuvant therapy and early initiation of salvage therapy at the time of biochemical relapse.

PPRT Volume Delineation

Patterns of failure studies have identified that the most common area for local recurrence after surgery is the vesicourethral anastomosis (VUA), found in up to two-thirds of cases.[126] The bladder trigone and bladder neck are also at risk. However, despite an intact prostatic capsule, surface secretions from prostatectomy specimens often contain detectable levels of PSA, implying that the whole surgical bed is at risk of recurrence.[127] Several consensus guidelines exist detailing the subsequent volume at risk, but commonly include the VUA, SV remnant, and posterior wall of the bladder, encompassing any surgical clips.[59,128,129] Irradiation of the pelvic nodes in this case is a controversial issue, as in definitive radiotherapy, and may be considered in those with high-risk disease.[130]

Adjuvant Therapy

Immediate adjuvant therapy aims to identify patients at risk of local recurrence after RP, and offer treatment to this population based on their high propensity for recurrence. The theoretic advantage of immediate therapy is that if disease is present, it will be treated at the lowest possible levels. The disadvantage is that all at-risk patients receive treatment and are thus exposed to treatment side effects, although only a proportion of them will benefit.

Early salvage therapy foregoes the opportunity of immediate PPRT if the PSA decreases to undetectable levels, limiting treatment to those patients who subsequently develop a detectable level of PSA. The major theoretic advantage of this approach is in minimizing the number of patients subjected to the potential side effects of radiation. Practically, delaying radiation may also decrease the potential impact on continence recovery. One large multiinstitutional retrospective study demonstrated grade 3 GU toxicity rates at less than 1%, and grade 3 GI side effects of 0.4%, based on the practice of awaiting return of continence before commencing therapy.[131]

Three randomized studies have compared immediate adjuvant therapy to a watchful waiting approach in men with T3N0 or pathology with a positive surgical margin (SM) (Table 3). These studies were conducted by the Southwest Oncology Group (SWOG), Arbeitsgemeinschaft Radiologischer Onkologie (ARO), and EORTC cooperative trials groups.[132–134] The SWOG trial demonstrated an improvement of metastasis-free survival at 10 years favoring immediate therapy from 61% to 71%, which was statistically significant. There was a corresponding improvement in overall survival with a hazard ratio of 0.72 (95% CI 0.55, 0.96; $P = .023$). However, the number needed to treat to prevent 1 case of metastatic disease at a median of 12.6 years was 12.2, underscoring the long-term nature of outcomes. The magnitude of the survival benefit was 1.7 years.

In contrast, the EORTC trial demonstrated an improvement in biochemical progression-free survival from 41.1% to 60.6% at 10 years, but no corresponding difference in clinical progression-free survival or overall survival. The benefit was strongest in those with SM positivity and those aged less than 70 years. The investigators reflected that this could be due to poorer long-term survival in the EORTC study, which could overpower any treatment effect, or the increased use of salvage radiotherapy in the EORTC study. The German ARO trial reported likewise, demonstrating improvements in early biochemical progression-free survival with adjuvant therapy of 71% versus 54% at 5 years. However, the short follow-up time (4.5 years) meant that only 3.1% had experienced clinical distant metastasis in the wait-and-see arm compared with 2% in the adjuvant arm. A meta-analysis performed by the Cochrane group examining these 3 trials demonstrated improved biochemical progression-free survival at 5 years, and improved distant metastasis-free survival and overall survival at 10 years,[135] providing level 1 evidence for adjuvant PPRT. The incidence of reported strictures increased at 10 years, but there was no difference in incontinence at any time point.

Table 3
Randomized trials of postprostatectomy radiotherapy and watchful waiting

Study/Publication	Enrolled	Median Follow-Up (y)	Primary End Point	Results	% PSA >0.2 ng/mL Adjuvant Arm
EORTC (Bolla et al,[132] 2012)	1992–2001	10.6	bPFS10	ADJ: 60.6% WW: 41.1%	28.7%
SWOG (Thompson et al,[134] 2009)	1988–1997	12.5–12.7	DMFS10	ADJ: 71% WW: 61%	35%
ARO (Wiegel et al,[133] 2009)	1997–2004	4.5	bPFS5	ADJ: 72% WW: 54%	20%[a]

Abbreviations: ADJ, adjuvant; ARO, Arbeitsgemeinschaft Radiologischer Onkologie; EORTC, European Organisation for the Research and Treatment of Cancer; SWOG, Southwest Oncology Group; WW, watchful waiting.
[a] PSA cut-off was 0.1ng/mL.

One criticism of these trials was that men with detectable PSA tests were allowed into the trial, thus the adjuvant arms were not truly adjuvant in nature. Consequently, the immediate postoperative arms of these trials included immediate adjuvant and early salvage patients, and the wait-and-see approach included delayed salvage patients. Opponents of immediate adjuvant therapy argue that these trials merely justify that an immediately detectable PSA after surgery is a strong indication for radiotherapy. However, subgroup analyses of these trials indicate that although men with detectable PSA before adjuvant radiotherapy are at higher risk of metastasis, they still derive a benefit from adjuvant therapy.[134]

Salvage Therapy

The usefulness of salvage radiation is based on large retrospective series demonstrating durable PSA control outcomes after therapy.[136,137] With detectable levels of PSA, differentiating whether the recurrence is distant or local is paramount in selecting patients who stand to benefit from salvage radiotherapy. Factors correlating with a low probability of benefiting from salvage radiation mirror the risk factors for distant recurrence: a higher PSA level at the time of salvage, specimen-confined disease at RP, Gleason 8+ tumors, a PSA doubling time of less than 10 months, and SV involvement or node-positive disease. Because of heterogeneity in terms of pathologic and biochemical parameters, the likelihood of treatment success varies accordingly. In the largest salvage series, the probability of biochemical control at 4 years ranged from 18% to 69%.[136] The PSA threshold at which to offer salvage therapy seems to have no lower bound,[138] reflecting the fact that even men without a detectable PSA can potentially harbor residual disease in higher-risk patients. King and colleagues[138] demonstrated a loss of 2.6% in biochemical progression-free survival for each increment in PSA of 0.2 ng/mL above 0.1 ng/mL, demonstrating the importance of initiating salvage therapy at low levels. Ideally, salvage therapy should be offered when isolated local recurrence is suspected, such as those with a positive resection margin, extracapsular invasion, Gleason grade less than 8, and PSA kinetics and absolute levels suggestive of residual local disease.

PPRT Toxicity (Adjuvant and Salvage)

The acute side effects of radiotherapy are usually tolerable to patients in the GU and GI domains. Quality-of-life data from the SWOG study demonstrated that 47% of men had GI tenderness or bowel urgency at 6 weeks, compared with only 5% of men in the observation arm. Severe acute reactions are uncommon; in the EORTC trial, 5.3% of men experienced grade 3 diarrhea.

Late GU toxicity consists mainly of urethral strictures, ED, and urinary frequency or dysuria. In the SWOG trial, the rate of urethral strictures in the adjuvant group was reported as 17.8% in the immediate postoperative arm compared with 9.5% in the wait-and-see arm, illustrating the interaction between surgery and radiation. In 1 meta-analysis, the pooled data from the ARO and SWOG trials demonstrated a 10% stricture rate with adjuvant radiotherapy compared with 5.8% in the wait-and-see arm at 10 years, which was statistically significant.[135] Incontinence was observed in 6.5% versus 2.8% in the adjuvant radiotherapy versus observation arm, respectively. In the EORTC trial, any grade 3 toxicity was seen in only 4.2% of men in the postoperative radiotherapy arm, compared with 2.6% in the wait-and-see arm. In terms of potency rates, the SWOG trial reported that the proportion of men with ED significantly decreased over time ($P = .02$), but did not vary significantly according to treatment arm ($P = .16$). Overall quality-of-life data from this trial demonstrated that the number of men with normal Global Health Related Quality of Life scores did not differ at 5 years.

Ongoing Trials

Current clinical trials comparing a true adjuvant approach with early salvage are under way. The TROG Radiotherapy - Adjuvant Versus Early Salvage (RAVES) trial is randomizing high-risk patients to either immediate adjuvant therapy or early salvage therapy (action point PSA 0.2 ng/mL) with a dose of 64 Gy. The multinational RADI-CALS trial has a similar design, but patients who receive radiotherapy are also eligible to be randomized to radiotherapy alone or with concurrent/adjuvant hormone therapy. The dose of radiation is either 66 Gy in 33 fractions or 52.5 Gy in 20 fractions. The hypothesis that ADT may improve outcomes is based on surgical trials suggesting that ADT improves biochemical outcomes in men with node-positive disease detected at prostatectomy,[139] and extrapolated from radiotherapy data on intact prostate.[29,84,140]

SECOND MALIGNANCY RISKS FROM RADIOTHERAPY

There is a risk of second primary malignancy after radiation; patients who have had prostate cancer are most likely to get these lesions in the rectum and bladder.[141,142] Estimates suggests that when compared with surgical therapy, prostate radiotherapy increases the relative risk of developing a second solid tumor by approximately 6% (equating to a risk increase of around 1 in 300 compared with surgery) in a study by Brenner and colleagues.[142] However, the relative risk seems to increase with increasing follow-up, to more than 27% at 10 years. When the number of radiation portals is increased as in rotational or intensity-modulated techniques, the overall amount of normal tissue exposed to low doses of radiotherapy and increased beam-on time may also theoretically increase the risk of second malignancies.[143] Although this risk is low, less discriminating patient selection and overall population longevity improvements could result in a larger population of patients exposed to the risk. As men are diagnosed and often treated earlier, this risk needs to be added into the counseling process.

FUTURE DIRECTIONS IN PROSTATE RADIOTHERAPY
Anatomic and Molecular Imaging

Imaging is likely to have a significant effect on the way radiotherapy is delivered to the prostate in the future. Multiparametric MRI, which adds capabilities such as diffusion maps, dynamic contrast sequences, and spectroscopy,[144,145] can often identify a dominant intraprostatic tumor lesion (DIL), which are regions that often correlate with sites of postradiation treatment failure.[146,147] The usefulness of boosting the DIL is being tested in a randomized trial (FLAME/NCT01168479).[148]

Positron emission tomography (PET) goes beyond anatomic definition of the cancer to also offer noninvasive biological characterization of the cancer phenotype, and holds promise in identification of parameters relevant to radiobiology such as cellular doubling time, hypoxia, and cell density. Although most PET research has focused on the improvement of sensitivity as a staging test, similar sensitivities have been noted between scans based on conventional glucose and those of acetate or choline.[149,150] As these agents rely on different metabolic pathways to accumulate tracer, opportunities exist to understand how differences in uptake, or combinations of parameters,[151] act as biomarkers for radiation response and outcome.

Hypofractionation

Extensive clinical data suggest that prostate cancer may exhibit a similar fraction size sensitivity to that of normal tissues, and thus be more sensitive to larger fraction sizes.[4–7] Thus, the fraction size could potentially be increased, which could facilitate shortening of radiation schedules with equal toxicity, while maintaining a very high biological dose effect to the prostate. Modern intensity-modulated techniques and the addition of image guidance can further augment this biological phenomenon by reducing the dose to normal tissues outside the target volume, thus preferentially sparing normal tissues.[56,152]

Several randomized trials have been conducted that support this hypothesis. Arcangeli and colleagues[153] randomized patients between standard fractionation (80 Gy in 40 fractions) and hypofractionated radiotherapy (62 Gy in 20 fractions). The population under study consisted largely of high-risk patients. There was a statistically significant biochemical control advantage observed in the hypofractionated arm of 87% versus 79% ($P<.035$) with a median follow-up of 3 years. Toxicity was comparable between the 2 arms,[154] which has been reproduced in other randomized data.[155,156] Two other randomized trials have been reported, but with lower doses of radiation. Lukka and colleagues[157] reported a randomized trial comparing 66 Gy in 33 fractions against 52.5 Gy in 20 fractions. The biochemical control rates favored the standard fractionation arm, with 59.95% of patients free from progression versus 52.95% of those in the hypofractionated arm. Yeoh and colleagues[158] reported the results of a randomized trial comparing 64 Gy in 32 fractions against 55 Gy in 20 fractions with no difference in PSA outcomes or toxicity.

The results of several trials are awaited. Two trials are comparing dose fractionation of 78 Gy in 39 fractions with 60 Gy in 20 fractions (ISRCTN 43853433). Data from RTOG 04-15, which compared 73.8 Gy in 41 fractions against 70 Gy in 28 fractions, are also maturing.

Stereotactic Body Radiotherapy

Stereotactic body radiotherapy (SBRT) is the practice of giving a small number of large fractional radiation doses with the intent of ablating the tumor and supporting host processes. Interest in this technique has been paralleled in other tumor types such as early non–small cell lung cancer, in which nonrandomized studies have demonstrated similar results to surgical techniques.[159,160] This relies on high-precision immobilization of the patient, high conformity delivery methods, and intrafraction motion management to minimize margin uncertainty.

Early clinical results in prostate cancer have demonstrated promising outcomes. With dose fractionations in the order of 37.25 Gy in 5 fractions delivered by Cyberknife or linac-based SBRT, the biochemical control rates in low-risk prostate cancer approximate 92% to 93%.[9,161] There are multiple trials assessing the usefulness of SBRT, including the usefulness of attempting to reproduce HDR brachytherapy dose distributions with SBRT or MRI-guided dominant nodule boosting with SBRT.

New Endocrine Therapies

New endocrine agents such as abiraterone and enzalutamide may be effective as either neoadjuvant or adjuvant therapy for men with high-risk prostate cancer. Both agents have been shown to improve overall survival in randomized trials consisting of castrate-resistant patients following docetaxel chemotherapy.[162–164] Abiraterone is currently being assessed in at least 2 recruiting clinical trials (NCT01717053 and NCT01023061), in which it is used along with luteinizing hormone-releasing hormone analogues as neoadjuvant and adjuvant therapy. The benefit of neoadjuvant enzaluta-mide before prostatectomy is currently under study, and neoadjuvant trials in the context of radiotherapy are sure to follow. Other agents, such as TAK-700 (Ortonel), an inhibitor of hormone synthesis (CYP17A), are being tested in addition to radiation therapy (RTOG 1115/NCT01546987).

SUMMARY

Our understanding of the radiation biology of prostate cancer continues to improve. It is well accepted that higher radiation doses are beneficial in prostate cancer, but the strength of the interaction between higher doses of radiation and androgen depriva-tion is still a compelling question. Newer approaches exploiting the proposed fraction size sensitivity of prostate cancer may lead to a reduction in treatment duration with equivalent toxicity in selected patients. Technological advances have improved target delineation and localization and have translated into improved toxicity outcomes for patients. These advances have also facilitated extreme hypofractionation techniques such as HDR brachytherapy and stereotactic body radiotherapy, which have the po-tential to transform the way modern prostate cancer therapy is delivered. Radiation also has a place in the management of men with suspected or confirmed local recur-rence after surgery, with current clinical trials seeking to optimize the timing of PPRT.

REFERENCES

1. Lehmann BD, McCubrey JA, Jefferson HS, et al. A dominant role for p53-dependent cellular senescence in radiosensitization of human prostate cancer cells. Cell Cycle 2007;6(5):595–605.
2. Bromfield GP, Meng A, Warde P, et al. Cell death in irradiated prostate epithelial cells: role of apoptotic and clonogenic cell kill. Prostate Cancer Prostatic Dis 2003;6(1):73–85.
3. Thames HD. An 'incomplete-repair' model for survival after fractionated and continuous irradiations. Int J Radiat Biol Relat Stud Phys Chem Med 1985; 47(3):319–39.
4. Proust-Lima C, Taylor JM, Secher S, et al. Confirmation of a low alpha/beta ratio for prostate cancer treated by external beam radiation therapy alone using a post-treatment repeated-measures model for PSA dynamics. Int J Radiat Oncol Biol Phys 2011;79(1):195–201.
5. Williams SG, Taylor JM, Liu N, et al. Use of individual fraction size data from 3756 patients to directly determine the alpha/beta ratio of prostate cancer. Int J Radiat Oncol Biol Phys 2007;68(1):24–33.
6. Fowler J, Chappell R, Ritter M. Is alpha/beta for prostate tumors really low? Int J Radiat Oncol Biol Phys 2001;50(4):1021–31.
7. Brenner DJ, Hall EJ. Fractionation and protraction for radiotherapy of prostate carcinoma. Int J Radiat Oncol Biol Phys 1999;43(5):1095–101.
8. Hoskin PJ, Rojas AM, Bownes PJ, et al. Randomised trial of external beam radiotherapy alone or combined with high-dose-rate brachytherapy boost for lo-calised prostate cancer. Radiother Oncol 2012;103(2):217–22.
9. King CR, Rojas AM, Bownes PJ, et al. Long-term outcomes from a prospective trial of stereotactic body radiotherapy for low-risk prostate cancer. Int J Radiat Oncol Biol Phys 2012;82(2):877–82.
10. D'Amico AV, Whittington R, Malkowicz SB, et al. Biochemical outcome after radical prostatectomy, external beam radiation therapy, or interstitial radiation therapy for clinically localized prostate cancer. JAMA 1998;280(11):969–74.

11. National Comprehensive Cancer Network. NCCN clinical practice guidelines in oncology: prostate cancer. J Natl Compr Canc Netw 2004;2:224–48.
12. Albertsen PC, Hanley JA, Fine J. 20-year outcomes following conservative management of clinically localized prostate cancer. JAMA 2005;293(17): 2095–101.
13. Wilt TJ, Brawer MK, Jones KM, et al. Radical prostatectomy versus observation for localized prostate cancer. N Engl J Med 2012;367(3):203–13.
14. Klotz L, Zhang L, Lam A, et al. Clinical results of long-term follow-up of a large, active surveillance cohort with localized prostate cancer. J Clin Oncol 2010; 28(1):126–31.
15. Bill-Axelson A, Holmberg L, Filén F, et al. Radical prostatectomy versus watchful waiting in localized prostate cancer: the Scandinavian prostate cancer group-4 randomized trial. J Natl Cancer Inst 2008;100(16):1144–54.
16. Bill-Axelson A, Holmberg L, Ruutu M, et al. Radical prostatectomy versus watchful waiting in early prostate cancer. N Engl J Med 2011;364(18):1708–17.
17. Widmark A, Klepp O, Solberg A, et al. Endocrine treatment, with or without radiotherapy, in locally advanced prostate cancer (SPCG-7/SFUO-3): an open randomised phase III trial. Lancet 2009;373(9660):301–8.
18. Warde P, Mason M, Ding K, et al. Combined androgen deprivation therapy and radiation therapy for locally advanced prostate cancer: a randomised, phase 3 trial. Lancet 2011;378(9809):2104–11.
19. Skwarchuk MW, Jackson A, Zelefsky MJ, et al. Late rectal toxicity after conformal radiotherapy of prostate cancer (I): multivariate analysis and dose–response. Int J Radiat Oncol Biol Phys 2000;47(1):103–13.
20. Barry MJ, Fowler F Jr, O'Leary MP, et al. The American Urological Association symptom index for benign prostatic hyperplasia. the measurement committee of the American Urological Association. J Urol 1992;148(5):1549.
21. Sandhu AS, Zelefsky MJ, Lee HJ, et al. Long-term urinary toxicity after 3-dimensional conformal radiotherapy for prostate cancer in patients with prior history of transurethral resection. Int J Radiat Oncol Biol Phys 2000;48(3):643–7.
22. Lee WR, Schultheiss TE, Hanlon AL, et al. Urinary incontinence following external-beam radiotherapy for clinically localized prostate cancer. Urology 1996;48(1):95–9.
23. Perez CA, Lee HK, Georgiou A, et al. Technical factors affecting morbidity in definitive irradiation for localized carcinoma of the prostate. Int J Radiat Oncol Biol Phys 1994;28(4):811–9.
24. Ishiyama H, Hirayama T, Jhaveri P, et al. Is there an increase in genitourinary toxicity in patients treated with transurethral resection of the prostate and radiotherapy?: a systematic review. Am J Clin Oncol 2012. [Epub ahead of print].
25. Blasko JC, Ragde H, Grimm PD. Transperineal ultrasound-guided implantation of the prostate: morbidity and complications. Scand J Urol Nephrol Suppl 1991; 137:113–8.
26. Malik R, Jani AB, Liauw SL. External beam radiotherapy for prostate cancer: urinary outcomes for men with high International Prostate Symptom Scores (IPSS). Int J Radiat Oncol Biol Phys 2011;80(4):1080–6.
27. Bosch R, Griffiths D, Blom J, et al. Treatment of benign prostatic hyperplasia by androgen deprivation: effects on prostate size and urodynamic parameters. J Urol 1989;141(1):68.
28. Rosen RC, Riley A, Wagner G, et al. The international index of erectile function (IIEF): a multidimensional scale for assessment of erectile dysfunction. Urology 1997;49(6):822.

29. D'Amico AV, Chen MH, Renshaw AA, et al. Androgen suppression and radiation vs radiation alone for prostate cancer: a randomized trial. JAMA 2008;299(3):289–95.

30. Song DY, Lawrie WT, Abrams RA, et al. Acute and late radiotherapy toxicity in patients with inflammatory bowel disease. Int J Radiat Oncol Biol Phys 2001; 51(2):455–9.

31. Willett CG, Ooi CJ, Zietman AL, et al. Acute and late toxicity of patients with inflammatory bowel disease undergoing irradiation for abdominal and pelvic neoplasms. Int J Radiat Oncol Biol Phys 2000;46(4):995–8.

32. Grann A, Wallner K. Prostate brachytherapy in patients with inflammatory bowel disease. Int J Radiat Oncol Biol Phys 1998;40(1):135–8.

33. Peters CA, Cesaretti JA, Stone NN, et al. Low-dose rate prostate brachytherapy is well tolerated in patients with a history of inflammatory bowel disease. Int J Radiat Oncol Biol Phys 2006;66(2):424–9.

34. Soto DE, Andridge RR, Pan CC, et al. In patients experiencing biochemical failure after radiotherapy, pretreatment risk group and PSA velocity predict differences in overall survival and biochemical failure-free interval. Int J Radiat Oncol Biol Phys 2008;71(5):1295–301.

35. Soto DE, Andridge RR, Pan CC, et al. Determining if pretreatment PSA doubling time predicts PSA trajectories after radiation therapy for localized prostate cancer. Radiother Oncol 2009;90(3):389–94.

36. Huang J, Vicini FA, Williams SG, et al. Percentage of positive biopsy cores: a better risk stratification model for prostate cancer? Int J Radiat Oncol Biol Phys 2012;83(4):1141–8.

37. Williams SG, Buyyounouski MK, Pickles T, et al. Percentage of biopsy cores positive for malignancy and biochemical failure following prostate cancer radiotherapy in 3,264 men: statistical significance without predictive performance. Int J Radiat Oncol Biol Phys 2008;70(4):1169–75.

38. Andreoiu M, Cheng L. Multifocal prostate cancer: biologic, prognostic, and therapeutic implications. Hum Pathol 2010;41(6):781–93.

39. Gallina A, Chun FK, Briganti A, et al. Development and split-sample validation of a nomogram predicting the probability of seminal vesicle invasion at radical prostatectomy. Eur Urol 2007;52(1):98–105.

40. Koh H, Kattan MW, Scardino PT, et al. A nomogram to predict seminal vesicle invasion by the extent and location of cancer in systematic biopsy results. J Urol 2003;170(4 Pt 1):1203–8.

41. Sohayda C, Kupelian PA, Levin HS, et al. Extent of extracapsular extension in localized prostate cancer. Urology 2000;55(3):382–6.

42. Davis BJ, Cheville JC, Wilson TM, et al. Histopathologic characterization of seminal vesicle invasion in prostate cancer: implications for radiotherapeutic management. Int J Radiat Oncol Biol Phys 2001;51(3 Supplement 1):140–1.

43. Kestin LL, Goldstein NS, Vicini FA, et al. Treatment of prostate cancer with radiotherapy: should the entire seminal vesicles be included in the clinical target volume? Int J Radiat Oncol Biol Phys 2002;54(3):686–97.

44. Pommier P, Chabaud S, Lagrange JL, et al. Is there a role for pelvic irradiation in localized prostate adenocarcinoma? Preliminary results of GETUG-01. J Clin Oncol 2007;25(34):5366–73.

45. Lawton CA, DeSilvio M, Roach M III, et al. An update of the phase III trial comparing whole pelvic to prostate only radiotherapy and neoadjuvant to adjuvant total androgen suppression: updated analysis of RTOG 94-13, with emphasis on unexpected hormone/radiation interactions. Int J Radiat Oncol Biol Phys 2007;69(3):646–55.

46. Hanks GE, Asbell S, Krall JM, et al. Outcome for lymph node dissection negative T-1b, T-2 (A-2, B) prostate cancer treated with external beam radiation therapy in RTOG 77-06. Int J Radiat Oncol Biol Phys 1991;21(4):1099–103.

47. Makarov DV, Trock BJ, Humphreys EB, et al. Updated nomogram to predict pathologic stage of prostate cancer given prostate-specific antigen level, clinical stage, and biopsy Gleason score (Partin tables) based on cases from 2000 to 2005. Urology 2007;69(6):1095–101.

48. Roach M 3rd, Chen A, Song J, et al. Pretreatment prostate-specific antigen and Gleason score predict the risk of extracapsular extension and the risk of failure following radiotherapy in patients with clinically localized prostate cancer. Semin Urol Oncol 2000;18(2):108–14.

49. Diaz A, Roach M 3rd, Marquez C, et al. Indications for and the significance of seminal vesicle irradiation during 3D conformal radiotherapy for localized prostate cancer. Int J Radiat Oncol Biol Phys 1994;30(2):323–9.

50. Briganti A, Larcher A, Abdollah F, et al. Updated nomogram predicting lymph node invasion in patients with prostate cancer undergoing extended pelvic lymph node dissection: the essential importance of percentage of positive cores. Eur Urol 2012;61(3):480–7.

51. Lawton CA, Michalski J, El-Naqa I, et al. RTOG GU radiation oncology specialists reach consensus on pelvic lymph node volumes for high-risk prostate cancer. Int J Radiat Oncol Biol Phys 2009;74(2):383.

52. Shih HA, Harisinghani M, Zietman AL, et al. Mapping of nodal disease in locally advanced prostate cancer: rethinking the clinical target volume for pelvic nodal irradiation based on vascular rather than bony anatomy. Int J Radiat Oncol Biol Phys 2005;63(4):1262–9.

53. Ganswindt U, Schilling D, Müller A-C, et al. Distribution of prostate sentinel nodes: a SPECT-derived anatomic atlas. Int J Radiat Oncol Biol Phys 2011;79(5): 1364–72.

54. Crook JM, Raymond Y, Salhani D, et al. Prostate motion during standard radiotherapy as assessed by fiducial markers. Radiother Oncol 1995;37(1):35–42.

55. Litzenberg D, Dawson LA, Sandler H, et al. Daily prostate targeting using implanted radiopaque markers. Int J Radiat Oncol Biol Phys 2002;52(3):699–703.

56. Zelefsky MJ, Kollmeier M, Cox B, et al. Improved clinical outcomes with high–dose image guided radiotherapy compared with non-IGRT for the treatment of clinically localized prostate cancer. Int J Radiat Oncol Biol Phys 2012;84:125–9.

57. Pouliot J, Bani-Hashemi A, Chen J, et al. Low-dose megavoltage cone-beam CT for radiation therapy. Int J Radiat Oncol Biol Phys 2005;61(2):552–60.

58. Jaffray DA, Siewerdsen JH, Wong JW, et al. Flat-panel cone-beam computed tomography for image-guided radiation therapy. Int J Radiat Oncol Biol Phys 2002;53(5):1337–49.

59. Wiltshire K, Brock K, Haider M, et al. Anatomic boundaries of the clinical target volume (prostate bed) after radical prostatectomy. Int J Radiat Oncol Biol Phys 2007;69(4):1090–9.

60. Oldham M, Letourneau D, Watt L, et al. Cone-beam-CT guided radiation therapy: a model for on-line application. Radiother Oncol 2005;75(3):271–8.

61. Kupelian P, Willoughby T, Mahadevan A, et al. Multi-institutional clinical experience with the Calypso System in localization and continuous, real-time monitoring of the prostate gland during external radiotherapy. Int J Radiat Oncol Biol Phys 2007;67(4):1088–98.

62. Peeters ST, Heemsbergen WD, Koper PC, et al. Dose-response in radiotherapy for localized prostate cancer: results of the Dutch multicenter randomized phase

III trial comparing 68 Gy of radiotherapy with 78 Gy. J Clin Oncol 2006;24(13): 1990–6.

63. Zietman AL, DeSilvio ML, Slater JD, et al. Comparison of conventional-dose vs high-dose conformal radiation therapy in clinically localized adenocarcinoma of the prostate: a randomized controlled trial. JAMA 2005;294(10):1233–9.

64. Dearnaley DP, Sydes MR, Graham JD, et al. Escalated-dose versus standard-dose conformal radiotherapy in prostate cancer: first results from the MRC RT01 randomised controlled trial. Lancet Oncol 2007;8(6):475–87.

65. Kuban DA, Tucker SL, Dong L, et al. Long-term results of the MD Anderson randomized dose-escalation trial for prostate cancer. Int J Radiat Oncol Biol Phys 2008;70(1):67–74.

66. Pollack A, Zagars GK, Starkschall G, et al. Prostate cancer radiation dose response: results of the MD Anderson phase III randomized trial. Int J Radiat Oncol Biol Phys 2002;53(5):1097–105.

67. Diez P, Vogelius IS, Bentzen SM. A new method for synthesizing radiation dose-response data from multiple trials applied to prostate cancer. Int J Radiat Oncol Biol Phys 2010;77(4):1066–71.

68. Viani GA, Stefano EJ, Afonso SL. Higher-than-conventional radiation doses in localized prostate cancer treatment: a meta-analysis of randomized, controlled trials. Int J Radiat Oncol Biol Phys 2009;74(5):1405–18.

69. Zietman AL, Bae K, Slater JD, et al. Randomized trial comparing conventional-dose with high-dose conformal radiation therapy in early-stage adenocarcinoma of the prostate: long-term results from Proton Radiation Oncology Group/American College of Radiology 95-09. J Clin Oncol 2010;28(7):1106–11.

70. Trofimov A, Nguyen PL, Coen JJ, et al. Radiotherapy treatment of early-stage prostate cancer with IMRT and protons: a treatment planning comparison. Int J Radiat Oncol Biol Phys 2007;69(2):444–53.

71. Sheets NC, Goldin GH, Meyer AM, et al. Intensity-modulated radiation therapy, proton therapy, or conformal radiation therapy and morbidity and disease control in localized prostate cancer. JAMA 2012;307(15):1611–20.

72. Nguyen PL, Gu X, Lipsitz SR, et al. Cost implications of the rapid adoption of newer technologies for treating prostate cancer. J Clin Oncol 2011;29(12):1517–24.

73. Turner SL, Adams K, Bull CA, et al. Sexual dysfunction after radical radiation therapy for prostate cancer: a prospective evaluation. Urology 1999;54(1): 124–9.

74. Zelefsky MJ, Cowen D, Fuks Z, et al. Long term tolerance of high dose three-dimensional conformal radiotherapy in patients with localized prostate carcinoma. Cancer 1999;85(11):2460–8.

75. Robinson JW, Moritz S, Fung T. Meta-analysis of rates of erectile function after treatment of localized prostate carcinoma. Int J Radiat Oncol Biol Phys 2002; 54(4):1063–8.

76. Sanda MG, Dunn RL, Michalski J, et al. Quality of life and satisfaction with outcome among prostate-cancer survivors. N Engl J Med 2008;358(12): 1250–61.

77. Incrocci L, Koper PC, Hop WC, et al. Sildenafil citrate (Viagra) and erectile dysfunction following external beam radiotherapy for prostate cancer: a randomized, double-blind, placebo-controlled, cross-over study. Int J Radiat Oncol Biol Phys 2001;51(5):1190–5.

78. Incrocci L, Slob AK, Hop WC. Tadalafil (Cialis) and erectile dysfunction after radiotherapy for prostate cancer: an open-label extension of a blinded trial. Urology 2007;70(6):1190–3.

79. Pezaro CJ, Mukherji D, De Bono JS. Abiraterone acetate: redefining hormone treatment for advanced prostate cancer. Drug Discov Today 2012;17(5–6): 221–6.

80. Denham JW, Steigler A, Lamb DS, et al. Short-term neoadjuvant androgen deprivation and radiotherapy for locally advanced prostate cancer: 10-year data from the TROG 96.01 randomised trial. Lancet Oncol 2011;12(5):451–9.

81. Pilepich MV, Winter K, John MJ, et al. Phase III radiation therapy oncology group (RTOG) trial 86-10 of androgen deprivation adjuvant to definitive radiotherapy in locally advanced carcinoma of the prostate. Int J Radiat Oncol Biol Phys 2001; 50(5):1243–52.

82. Bolla M, Van Tienhoven G, Warde P, et al. External irradiation with or without long-term androgen suppression for prostate cancer with high metastatic risk: 10-year results of an EORTC randomised study. Lancet Oncol 2010;11(11): 1066–73.

83. McGowan D, Hunt D, Jones C, et al. Short-term endocrine therapy prior to and during radiation therapy improves overall survival in patients with T1b-T2b adenocarcinoma of the prostate and PSA ≤20: initial results of RTOG 94-08. Int J Radiat Oncol Biol Phys 2010;77(1):1.

84. Pilepich MV, Winter K, Lawton CA, et al. Androgen suppression adjuvant to definitive radiotherapy in prostate carcinoma—long-term results of phase III RTOG 85-31. Int J Radiat Oncol Biol Phys 2005;61(5):1285–90.

85. Williams S, Buyyounouski M, Kestin L, et al. Predictors of androgen deprivation therapy efficacy combined with prostatic irradiation: the central role of tumor stage and radiation dose. Int J Radiat Oncol Biol Phys 2011;79(3):724–31.

86. Hanks GE, Pajak TF, Porter A, et al. Phase III trial of long-term adjuvant androgen deprivation after neoadjuvant hormonal cytoreduction and radiotherapy in locally advanced carcinoma of the prostate: the Radiation Therapy Oncology Group Protocol 92-02. J Clin Oncol 2003;21(21):3972–8.

87. Peters CA, Walsh PC. The effect of nafarelin acetate, a luteinizing-hormone–releasing hormone agonist, on benign prostatic hyperplasia. N Engl J Med 1987;317(10):599–604.

88. Zelefsky MJ, Leibel SA, Burman CM, et al. Neoadjuvant hormonal therapy improves the therapeutic ratio in patients with bulky prostatic cancer treated with three-dimensional conformal radiation therapy. Int J Radiat Oncol Biol Phys 1994;29(4):755–61.

89. National Guideline, C. ACR-ASTRO practice guideline for transperineal permanent brachytherapy of prostate cancer. Available at: http://www.guidelines.gov/content.aspx?id=32531&search=acr-astro+prostate+brachytherapy. Accessed on November 20, 2012.

90. Morris WJ, Keyes M, Spadinger I, et al. Population-based 10-year oncologic outcomes after low-dose-rate brachytherapy for low-risk and intermediate-risk prostate cancer. Cancer 2013;119(8):1537–46.

91. Potters L, Morgenstern C, Calugaru E, et al. 12-year outcomes following permanent prostate brachytherapy in patients with clinically localized prostate cancer. J Urol 2005;173(5):1562–6.

92. Grimm PD, Blasko JC, Sylvester JE, et al. 10-year biochemical (prostate-specific antigen) control of prostate cancer with 125I brachytherapy. Int J Radiat Oncol Biol Phys 2001;51(1):31–40.

93. Zelefsky MJ, Kuban DA, Levy LB, et al. Multi-institutional analysis of long-term outcome for stages T1-T2 prostate cancer treated with permanent seed implantation. Int J Radiat Oncol Biol Phys 2007;67(2):327–33.

94. Ash D, Al-Qaisieh B, Gould K, et al. Long term outcomes following iodine-125 monotherapy for localized prostate cancer: the Cookridge 10 year results. Clin Oncol (R Coll Radiol) 2007;19(Suppl 3):S18.

95. Stock RG, Cesaretti JA, Stone NN. Disease-specific survival following the brachytherapy management of prostate cancer. Int J Radiat Oncol Biol Phys 2006;64(3):810–6.

96. Critz FA, Benton JB, Shrake P, et al. 25 year disease free survival rate after irradiation of prostate cancer calculated with the prostate specific antigen definition of recurrence used for radical prostatectomy. J Urol 2013;189:878–83.

97. Stock RG, Cahlon O, Cesaretti JA, et al. Combined modality treatment in the management of high-risk prostate cancer. Int J Radiat Oncol Biol Phys 2004; 59(5):1352.

98. Bittner N, Merrick GS, Wallner KE, et al. Whole-pelvis radiotherapy in combination with interstitial brachytherapy: does coverage of the pelvic lymph nodes improve treatment outcome in high-risk prostate cancer? Int J Radiat Oncol Biol Phys 2010;76(4):1078–84.

99. Kubicek GJ, Naguib M, Redfield S, et al. Combined transperineal implant and external beam radiation for the treatment of prostate cancer: a large patient cohort in the community setting. Brachytherapy 2011;10(6):449–53.

100. Williams SG, Millar JL, Duchesne GM, et al. Factors predicting for urinary morbidity following 125iodine transperineal prostate brachytherapy. Radiother Oncol 2004;73(1):33–8.

101. Ash D, Bottomley D, Al-Qaisieh B, et al. A prospective analysis of long-term quality of life after permanent I-125 brachytherapy for localised prostate cancer. Radiother Oncol 2007;84(2):135–9.

102. Merrick GS, Butler WM, Wallner KE, et al. Dysuria after permanent prostate brachytherapy. Int J Radiat Oncol Biol Phys 2003;55(4):979–85.

103. Lee WR, Hall MC, McQuellon RP, et al. A prospective quality-of-life study in men with clinically localized prostate carcinoma treated with radical prostatectomy, external beam radiotherapy, or interstitial brachytherapy. Int J Radiat Oncol Biol Phys 2001;51(3):614–23.

104. Crook J, McLean M, Catton C, et al. Factors influencing risk of acute urinary retention after TRUS-guided permanent prostate seed implantation. Int J Radiat Oncol Biol Phys 2002;52(2):453–60.

105. Gutman S, Merrick GS, Butler WM, et al. Severity categories of the international prostate symptom score before, and urinary morbidity after, permanent prostate brachytherapy. BJU Int 2006;97(1):62–8.

106. Martens C, Pond G, Webster D, et al. Relationship of the international prostate symptom score with urinary flow studies, and catheterization rates following 125I prostate brachytherapy. Brachytherapy 2006;5(1):9–13.

107. Kollmeier MA, Stock RG, Cesaretti J, et al. Urinary morbidity and incontinence following transurethral resection of the prostate after brachytherapy. J Urol 2005;173(3):808–12.

108. Merrick GS, Butler WM, Galbreath RW, et al. Erectile function after permanent prostate brachytherapy. Int J Radiat Oncol Biol Phys 2002;52(4):893–902.

109. Khor R, Duchesne G, Tai KH, et al. Direct 2-arm comparison shows benefit of high-dose-rate brachytherapy boost vs external beam radiation therapy alone for prostate cancer. Int J Radiat Oncol Biol Phys 2013;85:679–85.

110. Demanes DJ, Martinez AA, Ghilezan M, et al. High-dose-rate monotherapy: safe and effective brachytherapy for patients with localized prostate cancer. Int J Radiat Oncol Biol Phys 2011;81:1286–92.

111. Barkati M, Williams SG, Foroudi F, et al. High-dose-rate brachytherapy as a monotherapy for favorable-risk prostate cancer: a phase II trial. Int J Radiat Oncol Biol Phys 2012;82:1889–96.
112. Ghadjar P, Keller T, Rentsch CA, et al. Toxicity and early treatment outcomes in low- and intermediate-risk prostate cancer managed by high-dose-rate brachytherapy as a monotherapy. Brachytherapy 2009;8(1):45–51.
113. Duchesne GM, Williams SG, Das R, et al. Patterns of toxicity following high-dose-rate brachytherapy boost for prostate cancer: mature prospective phase I/II study results. Radiother Oncol 2007;84(2):128–34.
114. Pellizzon AC, Salvajoli JV, Maia MA, et al. Late urinary morbidity with high dose prostate brachytherapy as a boost to conventional external beam radiation therapy for local and locally advanced prostate cancer. J Urol 2004;171(3):1105–8.
115. Martinez A, Gonzalez J, Spencer W, et al. Conformal high dose rate brachytherapy improves biochemical control and cause specific survival in patients with prostate cancer and poor prognostic factors. J Urol 2003;169(3):974–9 [discussion: 979–80].
116. Hindson BR, Millar JL, Matheson B. Urethral strictures following high-dose-rate brachytherapy for prostate cancer: analysis of risk factors. Brachytherapy 2013; 12:50–5.
117. Sullivan L, Williams SG, Tai KH, et al. Urethral stricture following high dose rate brachytherapy for prostate cancer. Radiother Oncol 2009;91(2):232–6.
118. Hoskin P, Rojas A, Ostler P, et al. OC-0051 quality of life after radical radiotherapy for prostate cancer: results from a randomised trial of EBRT±HDR-BT. Radiother Oncol 2012;103:S20.
119. Mitchell CR, Boorjian SA, Umbreit EC, et al. 20-year survival after radical prostatectomy as initial treatment for cT3 prostate cancer. BJU Int 2012;110:1709–13.
120. Freedland SJ, Partin AW, Humphreys EB, et al. Radical prostatectomy for clinical stage T3a disease. Cancer 2007;109(7):1273–8.
121. Carver BS, Bianco FJ Jr, Scardino PT, et al. Long-term outcome following radical prostatectomy in men with clinical stage T3 prostate cancer. J Urol 2006;176(2): 564–8.
122. Epstein J, Carmichael M, Partin A, et al. Is tumor volume an independent predictor of progression following radical prostatectomy? A multivariate analysis of 185 clinical stage B adenocarcinomas of the prostate with 5 years of followup. J Urol 1993;149(6):1478.
123. Myers RP, Fleming TR. Course of localized adenocarcinoma of the prostate treated by radical prostatectomy. Prostate 1983;4(5):461–72.
124. Pound CR, Partin AW, Eisenberger MA, et al. Natural history of progression after PSA elevation following radical prostatectomy. JAMA 1999;281(17):1591–7.
125. Freedland SJ, Humphreys EB, Mangold LA, et al. Risk of prostate cancer-specific mortality following biochemical recurrence after radical prostatectomy. JAMA 2005;294(4):433–9.
126. Connolly JA, Shinohara K, Presti JC Jr, et al. Local recurrence after radical prostatectomy: characteristics in size, location, and relationship to prostate-specific antigen and surgical margins. Urology 1996;47(2):225–31.
127. Kassabian V, Bottles K, Weaver R, et al. Possible mechanism for seeding of tumor during radical prostatectomy. J Urol 1993;150(4):1169.
128. Michalski JM, Lawton C, El Naqa I, et al. Development of RTOG consensus guidelines for the definition of the clinical target volume for postoperative conformal radiation therapy for prostate cancer. Int J Radiat Oncol Biol Phys 2010;76(2):361.

129. Sidhom MA, Kneebone AB, Lehman M, et al. Post-prostatectomy radiation therapy: consensus guidelines of the Australian and New Zealand Radiation Oncology Genito-urinary group. Radiother Oncol 2008;88(1):10–9.

130. Spiotto MT, Hancock SL, King CR. Radiotherapy after prostatectomy: improved biochemical relapse-free survival with whole pelvic compared with prostate bed only for high-risk patients. Int J Radiat Oncol Biol Phys 2007;69(1):54–61.

131. Feng M, Hanlon AL, Pisansky TM, et al. Predictive factors for late genitourinary and gastrointestinal toxicity in patients with prostate cancer treated with adjuvant or salvage radiotherapy. Int J Radiat Oncol Biol Phys 2007;68(5):1417–23.

132. Bolla M, van Poppel H, Tombal B, et al. Postoperative radiotherapy after radical prostatectomy for high-risk prostate cancer: long-term results of a randomised controlled trial (EORTC trial 22911). Lancet 2012;380:2018–27.

133. Wiegel T, Bottke D, Steiner U, et al. Phase III postoperative adjuvant radiotherapy after radical prostatectomy compared with radical prostatectomy alone in pt3 prostate cancer with postoperative undetectable prostate-specific antigen: ARO 96-02/AUO AP 09/95. J Clin Oncol 2009;27(18):2924–30.

134. Thompson IM, Tangen CM, Paradelo J, et al. Adjuvant radiotherapy for pathological T3N0M0 prostate cancer significantly reduces risk of metastases and improves survival: long-term followup of a randomized clinical trial. J Urol 2009; 181(3):956–62.

135. Daly T, Hickey BE, Lehman M, et al. Adjuvant radiotherapy following radical prostatectomy for prostate cancer. Cochrane Database Syst Rev 2011;(12):CD007234.

136. Stephenson AJ, Scardino PT, Kattan MW, et al. Predicting the outcome of salvage radiation therapy for recurrent prostate cancer after radical prostatectomy. J Clin Oncol 2007;25(15):2035–41.

137. Stephenson AJ, Shariat SF, Zelefsky MJ, et al. Salvage radiotherapy for recurrent prostate cancer after radical prostatectomy. JAMA 2004;291(11):1325–32.

138. King CR. The timing of salvage radiotherapy after radical prostatectomy: a systematic review. Int J Radiat Oncol Biol Phys 2012;84(1):104–11.

139. Messing EM, Manola J, Yao J, et al. Immediate versus deferred androgen deprivation treatment in patients with node-positive prostate cancer after radical prostatectomy and pelvic lymphadenectomy. Lancet Oncol 2006;7(6):472–9.

140. Bolla M, Van Tienhoven G, De Reijke T, et al. Concomitant and adjuvant androgen deprivation (ADT) with external beam irradiation (RT) for locally advanced prostate cancer: 6 months versus 3 years ADT—results of the randomized EORTC Phase III trial 22961. J Clin Oncol 2007;25(Suppl 18):5014.

141. Huang J, Kestin LL, Ye H, et al. Analysis of second malignancies after modern radiotherapy versus prostatectomy for localized prostate cancer. Radiother Oncol 2011;98(1):81–6.

142. Brenner DJ, Curtis RE, Hall EJ, et al. Second malignancies in prostate carcinoma patients after radiotherapy compared with surgery. Cancer 2000;88(2): 398–406.

143. Hall EJ, Wuu CS. Radiation-induced second cancers: the impact of 3D-CRT and IMRT. Int J Radiat Oncol Biol Phys 2003;56(1):83–8.

144. Vilanova JC, Barcelo J. Prostate cancer detection: magnetic resonance (MR) spectroscopic imaging. Abdom Imaging 2007;32(2):253–61.

145. Wefer AE, Hricak H, Vigneron DB, et al. Sextant localization of prostate cancer: comparison of sextant biopsy, magnetic resonance imaging and magnetic resonance spectroscopic imaging with step section histology. J Urol 2000;164(2): 400–4.

146. Arrayeh E, Westphalen AC, Kurhanewicz J, et al. Does local recurrence of prostate cancer after radiation therapy occur at the site of primary tumor? Results of a longitudinal MRI and MRSI study. Int J Radiat Oncol Biol Phys 2012;82(5): e787–93.

147. Pucar D, Hricak H, Shukla-Dave A, et al. Clinically significant prostate cancer local recurrence after radiation therapy occurs at the site of primary tumor: magnetic resonance imaging and step-section pathology evidence. Int J Radiat Oncol Biol Phys 2007;69(1):62–9.

148. van der Heide A, Korporaal J, Groenendaal G, et al. Functional MRI for tumor delineation in prostate radiation therapy. Imaging Med 2011;3(2):219–31.

149. Beauregard JM, Williams SG, Degrado TR, et al. Pilot comparison of F-fluorocholine and F-fluorodeoxyglucose PET/CT with conventional imaging in prostate cancer. J Med Imaging Radiat Oncol 2010;54(4):325–32.

150. Fricke E, Machtens S, Hofmann M, et al. Positron emission tomography with 11C-acetate and 18F-FDG in prostate cancer patients. Eur J Nucl Med Mol Imaging 2003;30(4):607–11.

151. Park H, Wood D, Hussain H, et al. Introducing parametric fusion PET/MRI of primary prostate cancer. J Nucl Med 2012;53(4):546–51.

152. Kupelian PA, Lee C, Langen KM, et al. Evaluation of image-guidance strategies in the treatment of localized prostate cancer. Int J Radiat Oncol Biol Phys 2008; 70(4):1151–7.

153. Arcangeli G, Saracino B, Gomellini S, et al. A prospective phase III randomized trial of hypofractionation versus conventional fractionation in patients with high-risk prostate cancer. Int J Radiat Oncol Biol Phys 2010;78(1):11–8.

154. Arcangeli G, Fowler J, Gomellini S, et al. Acute and late toxicity in a randomized trial of conventional versus hypofractionated three-dimensional conformal radiotherapy for prostate cancer. Int J Radiat Oncol Biol Phys 2011;79(4): 1013–21.

155. Dearnaley D, Syndikus I, Sumo G, et al. Conventional versus hypofractionated high-dose intensity-modulated radiotherapy for prostate cancer: preliminary safety results from the CHHiP randomised controlled trial. Lancet Oncol 2012; 13(1):43–54.

156. Pollack A, Hanlon AL, Horwitz EM, et al. Dosimetry and preliminary acute toxicity in the first 100 men treated for prostate cancer on a randomized hypofractionation dose escalation trial. Int J Radiat Oncol Biol Phys 2006;64(2): 518–26.

157. Lukka H, Hayter C, Julian JA, et al. Randomized trial comparing two fractionation schedules for patients with localized prostate cancer. J Clin Oncol 2005; 23(25):6132–8.

158. Yeoh EE, Holloway RH, Fraser RJ, et al. Hypofractionated versus conventionally fractionated radiation therapy for prostate carcinoma: updated results of a phase III randomized trial. Int J Radiat Oncol Biol Phys 2006;66(4): 1072–83.

159. Hadziahmetovic M, Loo BW, Timmerman RD, et al. Stereotactic body radiation therapy (stereotactic ablative radiotherapy) for stage I non-small cell lung cancer–updates of radiobiology, techniques, and clinical outcomes. Discov Med 2010;9(48):411–7.

160. Timmerman R, Paulus R, Galvin J, et al. Stereotactic body radiation therapy for inoperable early stage lung cancer. JAMA 2010;303(11):1070–6.

161. Freeman DE, King CR. Stereotactic body radiotherapy for low-risk prostate cancer: five-year outcomes. Radiat Oncol 2011;6:3.

162. de Bono JS, Logothetis CJ, Molina A, et al. Abiraterone and increased survival in metastatic prostate cancer. N Engl J Med 2011;364(21):1995–2005.

163. Scher HI, Beer TM, Higano CS, et al. Antitumour activity of MDV3100 in castration-resistant prostate cancer: a phase 1–2 study. Lancet 2010;375(9724):1437–46.

164. Scher HI, Fizazi K, Saad F, et al. Increased survival with enzalutamide in prostate cancer after chemotherapy. N Engl J Med 2012;367:1187–97.

Imaging in Prostate Carcinoma

Katherine Zukotynski, MD[a,b,]*, Masoom A. Haider, MD[a]

KEYWORDS

- Prostate cancer • Imaging • PET/CT • MRI

KEY POINTS

- Imaging is often used to guide biopsy at the time of clinical presentation and to stage men diagnosed with prostate cancer at risk of metastases so that appropriate therapy can be given.
- Nearly all men with a clinical suspicion of prostate cancer will have transrectal ultrasonography (TRUS) to guide biopsy.
- Magnetic resonance imaging (MRI) is becoming more ubiquitous to evaluate the primary malignancy and detect disease extension beyond the prostate capsule.
- Several imaging modalities including TRUS, MRI, and computed tomography (CT) can be helpful to detect spread of disease to lymph nodes, although detection of small nodal metastases remains problematic.
- MRI, CT, skeletal scintigraphy, and positron emission tomography (PET)/CT can detect distant metastatic disease.

INTRODUCTION

Prostate cancer is the most common cancer in men, excluding skin cancer. It is expected that 1 in 6 men will be diagnosed with prostate cancer during their lifetime and 1 in 36 will die of the disease. Although there has been a slight upward trend in the incidence of prostate cancer over the past 30 years, likely due to increasing early detection, the death rate has slightly decreased. It is estimated that 238,590 new cases of prostate cancer will be diagnosed in the United States in 2013 and that 29,720 men will die of the disease.[1] Nearly all metastatic disease becomes refractory to androgen deprivation therapy (ADT) and is referred to as castrate-resistant prostate cancer (CRPC). Most men who die of prostate cancer have castrate-resistant disease.

---

[a] Department of Medical Imaging, Sunnybrook Health Sciences Centre, University of Toronto, 2075 Bayview Avenue, Toronto, Ontario M4N 3M5, Canada; [b] Department of Radiology, Brigham and Women's Hospital, Harvard Medical School, 75 Francis Street, Boston, MA 02115, USA
* Corresponding author. Sunnybrook Health Sciences Centre, 2075 Bayview Avenue, Room AG-13, Toronto, Ontario M4N 3M5, Canada.
E-mail address: kzukotynski@partners.org

Hematol Oncol Clin N Am 27 (2013) 1163–1187
http://dx.doi.org/10.1016/j.hoc.2013.08.003
0889-8588/13/$ – see front matter © 2013 Elsevier Inc. All rights reserved.

Cancer within the prostate is often multifocal. The most common histology is adenocarcinoma, whereas less-common malignancies of the prostate gland include, for example, transitional cell carcinoma arising in the periurethral prostatic ducts and prostate sarcoma, either rhabdomyosarcoma or leiomyosarcoma. Investigation into the biologic behavior of prostate cancer has led to improved understanding of the spectrum of genetic alterations in the disease.[2] Furthermore, recent advances in our understanding of the molecular basis of disease have led to development of 6 agents that prolong longevity in men with CRPC: 2 cytotoxic agents (docetaxel[3] and cabazitaxel[4]), 2 hormonal therapies (abiraterone[5] and enzalutamide[6]), an alpha-emitting radiopharmaceutical (alpharadin[7]), and an immune therapy (sipuleucel-T[8]).

Imaging is often used to guide biopsy at the time of clinical presentation and to stage men diagnosed with prostate cancer so that appropriate therapy can be given, be it active surveillance, surgery, hormonal treatment, radiation therapy, or more recently radiofrequency ablation, cryoablation, or high intensity-focused ultrasound.

IMAGING MODALITIES COMMONLY USED TO EVALUATE PROSTATE CANCER

Multimodality imaging is often useful in the evaluation of men with prostate cancer. Nearly all men with a clinical suspicion of prostate cancer will have TRUS to guide biopsy; however, the sensitivity of routine gray-scale ultrasonography is limited to the detection of cancer and systematic biopsy is typically performed. Multiparametric MRI (mpMRI) is becoming more ubiquitous to evaluate the site of primary malignancy, guide needle biopsy, and detect disease extension beyond the prostate capsule. Anterior tumors, in particular, are often missed by routine TRUS biopsy, and MRI can help in detection and biopsy guidance for these tumors.[9,10] There is also growing evidence that MRI may improve risk stratification for enrollment onto active surveillance.[11] Several imaging modalities including TRUS, MRI, and CT can be helpful in detecting spread of disease to lymph nodes, although the detection of small nodal metastases remains problematic. ^{111}In-capromab pendetide single-photon emission computed tomography/CT (SPECT/CT) has been used for the detection of prostate cancer spread in the past but is rarely seen in routine clinical practice today. The predominant regional lymph nodes involved in the spread of prostate cancer are the obturator, sacral, external, internal, and common iliac lymph nodes. Detection of malignant disease spread to lymph nodes is important because this is a strong predictor of disease recurrence and progression. MRI, CT, skeletal scintigraphy, and PET/CT can detect distant metastatic disease. The skeleton is the most common site of prostate cancer metastases, via hematogenous spread, and although both lytic and sclerotic disease may be found, osteoblastic metastases are more common. MRI, CT, and PET/CT can also be used to identify metastatic disease to soft tissue throughout the body.

In recent years, for staging, there has been a shift away from imaging in the initial evaluation of prostate cancer, particularly if there is a low clinical risk of distant disease (prostate-specific antigen [PSA]<20 ng/mL, Gleason score>7, and/or clinical tumor stage below T3[12]). Indeed, the Cancer of the Prostate Strategic Urologic Research Endeavor reported a decrease in prostate cancer imaging from 1995 to 2002: by 63% in low-risk patients, 26% in intermediate-risk patients, and 11% in high-risk patients.[13] In general, imaging findings should be interpreted in the clinical context. Although guidelines regarding the appropriate use of imaging in prostate cancer have been proposed,[9] given recent developments of novel technologies, the optimal algorithm for prostate cancer imaging remains an area of active interest and research.

TRUS

TRUS is frequently the initial imaging modality used to assess pathologic condition of the prostate and is performed in all men with a clinical suspicion of prostate cancer as an adjunct to biopsy, because it does not have ionizing radiation, is inexpensive, and is easily accessible. The appearance of prostate cancer on TRUS is variable. Although a hypoechoic mass is often identified, the disease may be isoechoic to the adjacent gland. Increased contact between the mass and the prostatic capsule, particularly if associated with bulging and irregularity of the capsule, suggests extracapsular extension.[14] Seminal vesicle asymmetry or loss of fluid content may suggest invasion.[15] TRUS is not sufficient for local staging with a prediction of extracapsular extension accuracy ranging between 37% and 83%.[16–19] Furthermore, the sensitivity and specificity of TRUS for the detection of multifocal disease is approximately 40% to 50%.[19,20] The addition of color or power Doppler, contrast, or three-dimensional imaging may depict sites of increased vascularity and improve tumor detection, but have not yet been shown to have an impact on staging.[21–26] Overall, the known limitations of TRUS for the detection of prostate cancer has led to development of the traditional 8- to 12-core biopsy with samples taken from both sides (typically 4–6 per side) of the gland in a systematic manner.

MRI

MRI is an emerging modality for local prostate cancer staging in men with intermediate to high risk of local extension beyond the prostate capsule. Limited by issues related to expense and accessibility, MRI is not routinely used for staging in all centers. Although a magnetic field of 1.5 T is sufficient, 3 T provides improved spatial resolution.[9,27] To achieve the best image quality, it is generally accepted that an endorectal coil should be used.[28] However, the need for an endorectal coil at 3 T remains controversial.[29] The peripheral zone of the prostate gland contains most of the prostate glandular tissue, and 70% of cancers originate in this location. The peripheral zone has high signal intensity on T2-weighted images. The transitional zone is composed of the prostate tissue immediately adjacent to the proximal prostatic urethra, which is the site of benign prostatic hyperplasia and location of origin of 20% of prostate cancers. The central zone surrounds the transitional zone at the base of the prostate gland and accounts for 10% of prostate cancers. The central zone and transitional zone together form the central gland and have low or mixed signal intensity on T2-weighted images. The central gland is separated from the peripheral zone by a low-signal-intensity pseudocapsule (also called the surgical capsule). The prostate gland is separated from the periprostatic soft tissue by a 2 to 3 mm fibromuscular layer that has low signal intensity on T2-weighted images. The neurovascular bundles are located in the periprostatic soft tissue and have mixed signal intensity on T2-weighted images because of the relatively low signal intensity of the nerves when compared with the adjacent fat and the relatively high signal intensity of the vascular structures related to slow vascular flow. The seminal vesicles are composed of several lobules of high signal intensity surrounded by low-signal-intensity walls on T2-weighted images. T1-weighted images cannot distinguish the zonal anatomy of the prostate gland but are particularly helpful in identifying biopsy-related hemorrhage, which is hyperintense to normal parenchyma. T2-weighted imaging alone is insufficient to accurately localize cancer within the gland but is essential for delineating the overall anatomy and extraprostatic spread.

Staging includes characterization of the primary site of disease and detection of extracapsular extension and/or seminal vesicle invasion. On MRI, extracapsular extension is seen as direct tumor extension into the periprostatic fat; asymmetry or tumor envelopment of the neurovascular bundle; an angulated, speculated, or irregular prostate gland contour; and capsular retraction and/or obliteration of the rectoprostatic angle. Seminal vesicle extension involves direct tumor extension from the base of the prostate gland into and around the seminal vesicles, loss of normal seminal vesicle architecture, and/or the presence of low signal intensity within the seminal vesicles. Additional findings on MRI include the results of evaluation of the periprostatic lymph nodes and pelvic bone marrow.

The reported sensitivity and specificity of MRI for local staging varies considerably and has been reported to range from 15% to 100% and 67% to 100%, respectively,[27] with 13% to 91% and 49% to 99%, respectively, for the detection of extracapsular extension and 23% to 80% and 80% to 95%, respectively, for the detection of seminal vesicle invasion.[30–38] It has been shown that the accuracy of staging depends on the individual radiologist expertise.[39,40] A meta-analysis reported that the sensitivity and specificity of MRI for the detection of prostate cancer that had spread to the lymph nodes was approximately 40% and 80%, respectively.[41] This was increased to 90.5% with the use of lymphotropic ultrasmall superparamagnetic particles of iron oxide (USPIO, ferumoxtran-10), although the time to interpret studies was also significantly increased by this method.[42–44] USPIO particles are taken up by macrophages in normal lymph nodes, resulting in decreased signal intensity. Nodes that harbor malignancy do not accumulate USPIO, and, therefore, their signal intensity does not change. A comparison of pre-USPIO and post-USPIO images can show lymph node spread of malignant disease. Although the addition of diffusion-weighted imaging (DWI) to USPIO MRI did not result in further sensitivity improvement, it did reduce the time needed for image interpretation.[45] To date, however, there have been regulatory issues with the use of USPIO, and this is not available for routine clinical practice.

MRI is rarely performed in the setting of widespread disease or after therapy for prostate cancer, although it may be used to detect metastatic disease to bone or characterize recurrent disease. A recent prospective study reported that the sensitivity and specificity for the detection of bone metastases was 100% and 88%, respectively.[46]

The increasing evidence that using mpMRI can localize prostate cancer has resulted in a rapidly growing interest in the use of mpMRI to localize prostate cancer for biopsy and improve risk stratification. Further discussion of how mpMRI is used in clinical practice is detailed later in the article.

CT

Contrast-enhanced, multidetector CT has a limited role in the detection and staging of localized prostate cancer.[9,27] Although the specificity of CT for local staging is reported to be relatively high, the sensitivity is low and it is usually impossible to detect prostate cancer unless it has extended beyond the confines of the gland. The detection of lymph node metastases is also limited. CT can detect both osteolytic and osteoblastic skeletal metastases with sensitivity ranging from 71% to 100%.[47] In general, CT is performed in high-risk patients or patients with advanced disease for the assessment of the pelvic and retroperitoneal lymph nodes.[9,27]

Skeletal Scintigraphy (⁹⁹ᵐTc-MDP Bone Scan)

^{99m}Tc-Methylene Diphosphonate (MDP) bone scan is the current routine imaging modality used to assess the burden of skeletal disease in patients with prostate cancer. Although planar images are most commonly acquired, SPECT can significantly increase contrast as well as allow for more detailed anatomic localization. SPECT/CT may also be performed and can give additional information through the combination of both functional and anatomic imaging. However, due to increased radiation exposure and time for study acquisition and interpretation, this is rarely performed. Findings that suggest osseous metastatic disease result from osteoblastic activity, which typically occurs in reaction to tumor infiltration. The advantages of bone scans are the wide availability, low cost, and ability to image the entire skeleton. The principal drawback is that bone scans do not directly image metastatic disease, but rather the reaction of bone to metastases. Therefore, image interpretation can be confounded because osseous healing from trauma or cancer therapy can be difficult to distinguish from progressive osseous metastatic disease. Flare is defined as apparent "disease progression" on bone scan after 3 months of therapy based on increased lesion intensity or number in the setting of improved levels of PSA and subsequent stability or improvement of bone scan findings on repeat bone scan after 6 months of therapy. This occurs in men with prostate cancer and can lead to significant confusion when radiology reports suggest "progressive disease" rather than flare in the appropriate clinical setting.[48–50] Furthermore, it is difficult to accurately quantify the burden of osseous metastatic disease using ^{99m}Tc-MDP bone scans. The bone scan index was developed by Dennis and colleagues[51] to measure total skeletal disease by summing the product of the weight and fractional involvement of each of 158 individual bones, where each bone is expressed as a percentage of the entire skeleton. Unfortunately, this is time consuming and rarely used in clinical practice. To date, it remains difficult to reliably quantify response to therapy using ^{99m}Tc-MDP bone scans.

PET

PET/CT uses a radiotracer to detect a metabolic process with PET and fuses this with CT to determine the anatomic location of this process. PET/CT can detect metabolically active malignancy prior to anatomic change and can be helpful for the diagnosis and follow-up of patients with cancer. Two PET tracers readily available for clinical use are ^{18}F-labeled sodium fluoride (^{18}F-NaF) and ^{18}F-labeled 2-fluoro-2-deoxy-D-glucose (^{18}F-FDG).

^{18}F-NaF is a high-affinity bone-seeking agent with a higher affinity for osteoblastic activity and superior imaging characteristics than ^{99m}Tc-MDP. Furthermore, ^{18}F-NaF PET/CT has higher sensitivity and specificity for the detection of osseous malignancy than ^{99m}Tc-MDP bone scans. In a study comparing ^{99m}Tc-MDP bone scans and ^{18}F-NaF PET/CT in patients with localized high-risk or metastatic prostate cancer, Even-Sapir and colleagues[52] reported that the sensitivity and specificity of ^{99m}Tc-MDP planar bone scans was 70% and 57%, respectively, in patients being evaluated for metastases prior to local prostate cancer therapy, whereas for ^{18}F-NaF PET/CT it was 100% and 100%, respectively. However, both ^{18}F-NaF PET/CT and ^{99m}Tc-MDP bone scans rely on detecting bone turnover, not malignant cells themselves, and therefore generate an indirect marker of osseous malignancy.

^{18}F-FDG is taken up by tumor cells according to the glycolytic rate (Warburg effect) and directly assesses the extent of malignancy. Furthermore, ^{18}F-FDG PET/CT can be used to detect both soft tissue and osseous diseases. Although ^{18}F-FDG is the most common PET radiotracer in oncology today, early studies using ^{18}F-FDG conducted in patient populations with a heterogeneous spectrum of prostate cancer disease states (hormone-naïve prostate cancer and CRPC) revealed variable FDG uptake (from intense to negligible) across the spectrum of disease. Further radiotracer accumulation in the genitourinary tract may obscure the pathology in the prostate and/or adjacent lymph nodes, and therefore, a negative ^{18}F-FDG PET/CT does not exclude malignancy. Recent studies have focused on CRPC patient populations with more informative results regarding the utility of ^{18}F-FDG PET/CT. In particular, a study published by Morris and colleagues[53] in 2005 suggested that ^{18}F-FDG PET could serve as an outcome measure in patients being treated for CRPC. A total of 18 patients with evaluable ^{18}F-FDG PET at baseline and after 12 weeks of therapy revealed that ^{18}F-FDG PET was able to assess treatment effects usually described by a combination of PSA, ^{99m}Tc-MDP bone scan, and diagnostic anatomic imaging. In a recent study by Autio and colleagues,[54] the variability in ^{18}F-FDG uptake was able to provide prognostic information. Namely, patients with FDG-avid disease had hazard ratio 2.24 for shorter time to death than patients with non–FDG-avid tumors. Other investigators have independently reported an inverse relationship between intensity of ^{18}F-FDG uptake at sites of disease and overall survival and found that ^{18}F-FDG PET/CT was more sensitive than ^{99m}Tc-MDP bone scans in the detection of skeletal disease.[55]

Overall, reports on the utility of PET/CT in prostate cancer are mixed, and to date, PET/CT is not recommended for diagnosis or staging. However, PET/CT can complement anatomic imaging for the detection of malignancy and assessment of response to therapy. Research into PET/CT in prostate cancer and development of new PET radiotracers is ongoing and is discussed in the section on future directions.

IMAGING IN STAGING AND MANAGEMENT OF PROSTATE CANCER: LOCALIZED AND METASTATIC DISEASE

Once the diagnosis of prostate cancer has been established, typically following TRUS-guided biopsy, accurate patient staging is needed to determine appropriate management. In the past, imaging was limited and could not accurately identify men with extracapsular spread of disease or seminal vesicle invasion. For many years, nomograms based on the results of digital rectal examination (DRE), PSA, and Gleason score were used to estimate the probability of prostate cancer extending beyond the prostate gland.[56–59] At present, the relative risk of disease spread beyond the prostate gland is estimated and imaging is performed when considered beneficial. For example, imaging is often most valuable to provide accurate staging in men with intermediate to high risk of disease extension beyond the prostate gland. In particular, men with clinically localized disease and an intermediate to high probability of disease extension beyond the gland may benefit from referral to MRI for staging. In the right clinical setting, prostatectomy can significantly decrease the incidence of metastatic disease and prostate-related mortality, although the outcome is often complicated by morbidity such as sexual dysfunction or urinary incontinence.[60] When extracapsular tumor extension is present or there is invasion of the seminal vesicles, malignant adenopathy, or distant metastatic disease, hormonal therapy and radiation may be preferred. Therefore, intermediate- or high-risk men will likely benefit from MRI for local staging (**Fig. 1**) because detection of disease beyond the prostate gland capsule indicates stage III (T3a) disease or higher and results in management change.[61,62] More recently, MRI has been used to accurately define the site of extraprostatic extension and guide nerve-sparing surgery.[63] Men with nonpalpable disease, low PSA, low tumor volume, and low tumor grade based on TRUS-guided biopsy are more frequently being managed with active surveillance. It is thought that the incidence of extracapsular disease in these men is so low that imaging is of little benefit. Men placed on surveillance typically have serial DREs, PSA measurements, and annual biopsy. Results in the literature suggest, that in this way, up to 70% of men can avoid treatment altogether.[64]

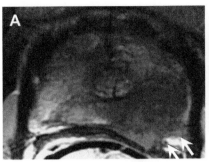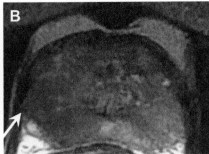

Fig. 1. The T2-weighted magnetic resonance images of 2 men both with pT3a disease. (*A*) Extraprostatic extension (*arrows*) in a man with positive digital rectal examination, PSA levels 4.5 ng/mL, and biopsy-proven Gleason 9 disease. (*B*) Extraprostatic extension (*arrow*) in a man with negative digital rectal examination, PSA levels of 3.7 ng/mL, and biopsy-proven Gleason 8 disease.

There is growing interest in the use of mpMRI for better risk stratification in patients eligible for active surveillance. Risk stratification is based on nonimaging parameters including PSA, number of positive cores, cancer length, and Gleason score. Reclassification of risk category can occur in 20% to 30% of patients, suggesting that significant cancer may have been missed by the TRUS biopsy approach initially.[7,8,65–68] Many of these tumors are anterior away from typical locations covered with the transrectal biopsy approach.[67] mpMRI has been shown to perform well in detecting these cancers.[10] Patients on active surveillance with a demonstrated lesion had a hazard ratio of 4.0 for Gleason score upgrading compared to those without such lesions.[69] Thus mpMRI offers the potential for better patient selection for active surveillance and the potential for better monitoring while on active surveillance; however, further prospective trials are needed to establish the optimal role for imaging in this setting.

Skeletal scintigraphy is commonly performed in men with prostate cancer when there is a clinical suspicion of osseous disease or when bone pain is present (**Fig. 2**). Although the point at which skeletal scintigraphy should be performed to assess for osseous disease remains debatable, the most recent EU guidelines state that skeletal scintigraphy may not be indicated in asymptomatic patients if the serum PSA level is less than 20 ng/mL, in the presence of well or moderately differentiated disease.[70] Indeed, in one study, only 1% of men in a series with PSA less than 50 ng/mL, clinical stage T2b disease or less, and Gleason score less than 8 had osseous disease detected on skeletal scintigraphy.[71] Contrast-enhanced CT of the abdomen and pelvis has limited value in initial staging and determining local disease extent in low-risk to intermediate-risk patients. It is typically reserved for use in men with a high probability of metastatic disease (**Fig. 3**).[9]

Recurrent prostate cancer after therapy is relatively common. It has been suggested that up to 33% of men postradical prostatectomy develop local recurrence or metastatic disease.[72] Imaging can be helpful for the detection of local recurrence, the detection of distant metastatic disease, and planning optimal therapy. However, imaging postsurgery is typically performed to detect distant metastatic disease rather than local recurrence alone. With PSA levels less than 10 ng/mL, it is rare to see radiographic evidence of disease. The challenge is that men with localized recurrence in the prostate bed may benefit from targeted radiotherapy to this area, but we are limited to postprostatectomy PSA level, prostatectomy pathologic condition, and PSA doubling time to predict which men have only localized disease and will benefit

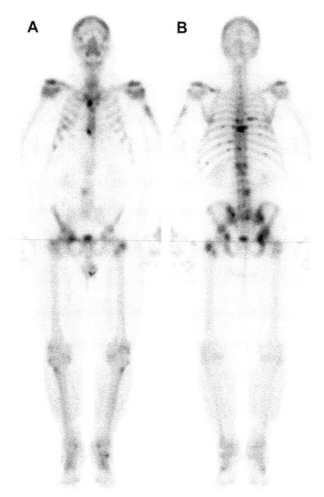

Fig. 2. A 57-year-old man with prostate cancer and bone pain. (*A*) Anterior and (*B*) posterior planar images from a ^{99m}Tc-MDP bone scan show widespread osseous disease involving the axial and appendicular skeleton.

from radiation therapy.[73] MRI may be helpful after brachytherapy to evaluate seed placement and identify sites of developing disease.[74]

FUTURE DIRECTIONS

In recent years, several technical developments have been suggested to improve image-guided prostate gland biopsy at the time of diagnosis. There has also been a paradigm shift in oncologic imaging from traditional anatomic assessment (ie, measurements of tumor size and extent of disease) toward a combined anatomic and functional evaluation, including the use of perfusion, diffusion, and metabolic characterization with MRI and PET/CT. With the growing number of available therapies for castrate-resistant disease, an unmet clinical need is to develop imaging strategies to identify patients with CRPC who are destined to benefit from a given therapy while

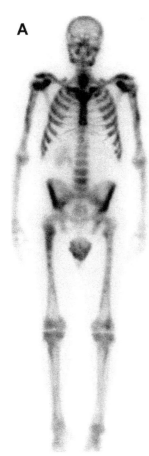

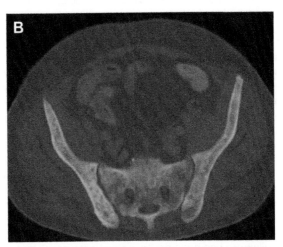

Fig. 3. A 70-year-old man has prostate cancer, rising PSA levels, and suspicion of bone metastases. Anterior planar image from a ^{99m}Tc-MDP bone scan (*A*) shows widespread osseous disease involving the axial and appendicular skeletons. A single axial image from a CT scan of the same patient at the level of the sacroiliac joints (*B*) shows diffuse sclerotic osseous disease in the sacrum and both iliac bones.

avoiding expensive, futile, and in some cases, toxic therapy. At present, patients are treated and analyzed as a group where a new therapy is ultimately approved if it provides a clinical benefit (most often measured in terms of overall survival) to the entire group. This results in some patients achieving significant improvement with acceptable toxicity, some with significant improvement but substantial toxicity, and some with no benefit and sometimes with significant toxicity. It would be ideal if a noninvasive biomarker could be used to individualize therapy and avoid prolonged exposure to toxic, futile, and expensive treatment. The use of circulating tumor cells has led to advances in this area and can provide prognostic information. However, this technology has not been universally adopted because it does not direct therapy. To date, there is no reliable early imaging method to assess efficacy and avoid futile therapy.

At the Society of Urologic Oncology 2012 annual meeting,[75] enhanced ultrasonographic techniques that could improve TRUS were reviewed; however, to date these are not readily available or approved by the US Food and Drug Administration. mpMRI and MRI-guided biopsy or MRI/ultrasonography coregistration were also discussed as methods to provide better anatomic detail and identify lesions that may be missed with the traditional 12-core biopsy. Several new imaging techniques are providing noninvasive characterization of prostate cancer biology, aggressiveness, and therapy response such as dynamic contrast-enhanced (DCE) MRI, magnetic resonance spectroscopic imaging (MRSI), DWI and novel PET tracers. The state-of-the-art interpretation of prostate MRI now includes mpMRI, which is a combination of T2-weighted imaging with two or more of DWI, DCE-MRI, or MRSI. This has been shown to provide information related to local staging and improved determination of tumor location in the prostate to guide biopsy and therapy. The advantages and limitations of each of these techniques are discussed.

DCE-MRI

DCE protocols have been used in combination with MRI to detect metastatic bone disease and evaluate tumor vascularity and response to antiangiogenic therapy in a variety of primary tumor types, including prostate cancer. In this technique, diffusion of contrast from the intravascular to the extracellular space permits quantitative assessment of tumor microvasculature. A series of T1-weighted magnetic resonance images are acquired before, during, and over several minutes after the administration of a bolus of gadolinium-based contrast media. Several values are then determined based on these data points including intratumoral vascular fraction, tumor blood flow, vascular permeability-surface area product, and accessible extravascular-extracellular space. These calculations depend both on the MRI acquisition protocol and the compartment model used to analyze the data, which are not standardized, limiting broad application and reproducibility. Furthermore, the relative contribution of vessel permeability and tumor blood flow to the overall signal intensity changes observed on DCE-MRI studies is frequently unknown, making the calculation of tumor perfusion challenging and possibly erroneous. In DCE-MRI, K^{trans} is a commonly cited measure of interest, a parameter describing the transfer constant between the intravascular and extravascular spaces. A change greater than 40% in K^{trans} from baseline to follow-up has been proposed as being consistent with a drug effect in pharmacodynamic studies.[76]

Prostate cancer shows early, rapid enhancement and washout on DCE-MRI. Although small, low-grade tumors may be missed because of an essentially normal enhancement pattern and false-positive results may occur related to benign conditions such as prostatitis, the addition of DCE-MRI to conventional MRI improves staging accuracy compared with the use of each technique alone.[77]

MRSI

MRSI uses the fact that different metabolites have different resonant frequencies to detect cancer. In prostate cancer, evaluation of the ratio of several metabolites including choline, citrate and creatine levels are calculated within a chosen tissue voxel. MRSI may result in improved tumor detection sensitivity and estimation of tumor volume. At 1.5 T, the resonance frequency of choline can not be distinguished from that of creatine but can be discriminated from that of citrate. The normal prostate gland contains low levels of choline and creatine but high levels of citrate, a situation that is revered in prostate cancer, likely because of increased cell membrane turnover associated with elevated cell proliferation, cellularity, and growth. Thus, a ratio of (choline + creatinine)/citrate greater than 0.75 suggests the presence of prostate cancer.[78] Indeed, this ratio is also thought to be related to the Gleason score and therefore may serve as a marker of tumor aggressiveness.

DWI

DWI is an MRI technique garnering interest for the assessment and characterization of primary tumors and in the detection of osseous metastatic disease. DWI is a technique based on the premise that the diffusion of water molecules is restricted in highly cellular areas (tumor) in contrast to less-cellular (nontumor) tissues. DWI-MRI can be used to detect prostate cancer, where signal intensity is increased on diffusion-weighted images and reduced on the apparent diffusion coefficient (ADC) map at the site of malignancy, reflecting increased restriction. Recent results in the literature suggest improvement in the detection of seminal vesicle invasion when DWI-MRI is combined with conventional MRI of the prostate.[79,80] In a recent meta-analysis comparing T2-weighted imaging, DWI, and DCE-MRI, DWI was shown to be the most accurate for cancer localization within the gland.[81] The ADC measurement that is derived for the DWI images has also been shown to be negatively correlated with the Gleason score[82] and predict progression while on active surveillance.[83]

mpMRI

There is growing interest in determining the location of the dominant and most aggressive site of cancer within the prostate gland to direct biopsy and plan focal therapy. With current random biopsies using TRUS, undergrading of cancer remains an issue.[84] mpMRI (**Fig. 4**) is showing the most promise in the accurate detection of the dominant site of cancer. The European Society of Uroradiology has recently proposed guidelines for the performance of mpMRI and a scoring scheme for cancer localization (Pi-Rads).[85,86] This is gaining wider acceptance with validation studies recently published.[87] Multiple studies are showing the improved detection of prostate cancer with mpMRI-directed biopsies in patients with repeated negative results of biopsy and elevated levels of PSA with a median of only 4-core biopsy.[88] Studies also suggest better detection of occult higher Gleason grade tumors with MRI-directed biopsy in low-risk patients on active surveillance.[11] The American College of Radiology now classifies mpMRI as a usually appropriate test in the setting of multiple negative biopsies where there is concern for cancer based on rising or persistently elevated serum markers, suggesting malignancy.[9]

PET

Although the role of PET/CT in the setting of prostate cancer is under investigation, there is growing interest in determining the value of established tracers such as ^{18}F-FDG, ^{18}F-NaF, and ^{18}F- or ^{11}C-labeled choline as well as in the development, supply, and assessment of novel tracers such as 16β-^{18}F-fluoro-5α-dihydrotestosterone (^{18}F-FDHT), I-amino-3-^{18}F-fluorocyclobutane-1-carboxylic acid (^{18}F-FACBC), and prostate specific membrane antigen (PSMA) probes among others.

^{18}F-FDG is the most common PET radiotracer used in clinical oncology today. An indicator of glycolysis, ^{18}F-FDG uptake is variable in prostate cancer and is confounded by uptake in benign prostate pathology and physiologic activity in the genitourinary tract. In general, ^{18}F-FDG PET/CT is thought to have limited value in men with suspected prostate cancer at presentation. Minamimoto and colleagues[89] found that ^{18}F-FDG PET/CT had a sensitivity of only 37% for the detection of prostate cancer in asymptomatic men without a known history of malignancy. Watanabe and colleagues[90] reported that ^{18}F-FDG PET/CT had a significantly lower sensitivity (31%) compared with MRI (88%) for the detection of prostate cancer in men suspected to have the disease. Results in the literature have also suggested limited value

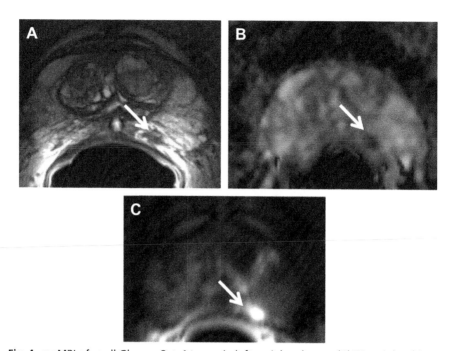

Fig. 4. mpMRI of small Gleason 3 + 4 tumor in left peripheral zone: (*A*) T2-weighted image shows a subtle tumor (focal T2 dark nodule, *arrow*) in the left peripheral zone of the prostate gland. (*B*) The ADC map shows a correlating focal area of restricted diffusion (*arrow*). (*C*) Dynamic contrast-enhanced image shows a focal area of early enhancement corresponding to the area of restricted diffusion confirming with certainty the tumor location (*arrow*). Biopsy showed a Gleason 3 + 4 tumor occupying 18% of one core in the left medial peripheral zone. No extraprostatic extension was seen at pathologic examination or on imaging at prostatectomy.

of ^{18}F-FDG PET/CT in men with suspected biochemical prostate cancer recurrence.[91,92] Of note, Minamimoto and colleagues[93] published an article studying 50 men with elevated serum PSA levels and ^{18}F-FDG PET/CT before biopsy that reported a low sensitivity and specificity when the entire cohort was considered, but a positive predictive value of 87% in the subset of men older than 70 years with serum PSA levels greater than 12 ng/mL. Thus, although the sensitivity of ^{18}F-FDG for the initial detection of prostate cancer is low, the study may have value in a subset of men with aggressive disease (**Fig. 5**). An area where ^{18}F-FDG PET/CT has significant potential is identifying response to therapy and predicting outcome in men with aggressive prostate cancer. ^{18}F-FDG uptake depends, at least in part, on the expression of GLUT1. In vitro studies suggest that GLUT1 expression is higher in poorly differentiated prostate cancer cell lines (ie, DU145 and PC-3) compared with well-differentiated lines (ie, LNCaP).[94] ^{18}F-FDG uptake can also be seen in hormone-dependent cell lines such as CWR22 and may decrease after ADT.[95] It is thought that GLUT1 expression is seen more frequently at the center of a neoplastic growth, possibly related to hypoxia at the center of a highly proliferative mass.[96] Further GLUT1 gene expression may correlate with Gleason score.[97] In 2002, Oyama and colleagues[98] reported that primary prostate cancer with high ^{18}F-FDG uptake had a worse prognosis than cancer with low uptake. In 2005, Morris and colleagues[53]

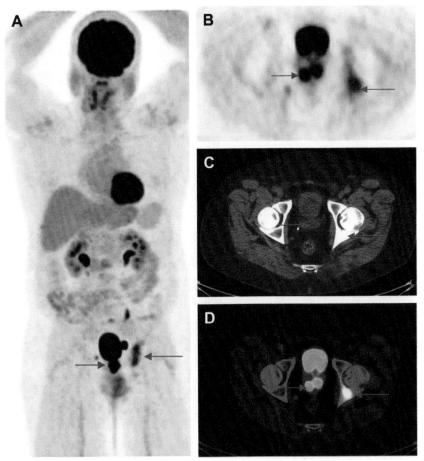

Fig. 5. A 61-year-old man with aggressive prostate cancer. ^{18}F-FDG PET/CT shows both osseous and soft tissue metastatic prostate cancer on the maximum intensity projection image (A), axial ^{18}F-FDG PET (B), CT (C), and fused ^{18}F-FDG PET/CT images (D). The red arrows point to malignant soft tissue disease in the prostate bed and to osseous metastatic disease in the left acetabulum.

showed that the appearance of new lesions or an increase of more than 33% in the average maximum standardized uptake value measurement from up to 5 lesions could be used to categorize men with castrate-resistant metastatic disease on antimicrotubule chemotherapy into progressors versus nonprogressors. In 2010, Meirelles and colleagues[55] suggested that FDG avidity was an independent prognostic factor in a multivariate analysis of men with metastatic prostate cancer. In 2012, Jadvar and colleagues[99] reported preliminary results from a prospective analysis in men with metastatic CRPC and showed that more intensely FDG-avid disease was an independent prognostic factor in a multivariate Cox regression analysis.

^{18}F-NaF is taken up by bone via chemisorption with exchange of ^{18}F$^-$ for OH$^-$ on the surface of the hydroxyapatite matrix of bone to form fluoroapatite. Recently, the use of ^{18}F-NaF PET/CT in prostate cancer (**Fig. 6**) has been gaining attention because of accessibility, high sensitivity, and high specificity for the detection of osseous disease,

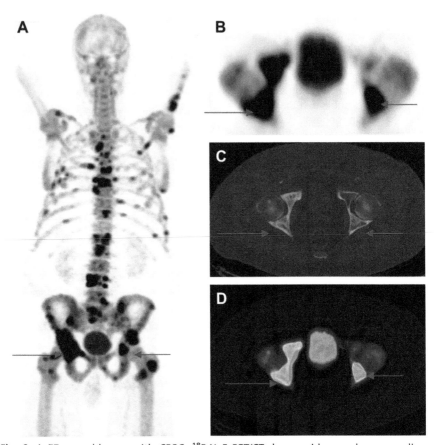

Fig. 6. A 57-year-old man with CRPC: ^{18}F-NaF PET/CT shows widespread osseous disease involving the axial and appendicular skeleton on the maximum intensity projection image (*A*), axial ^{18}F-NaF PET (*B*), CT (*C*), and fused ^{18}F-NaF PET/CT images (*D*). The red arrows point to areas of disease seen on all images.

particularly when combined with the anatomic information generated by the CT portion of the study. Furthermore, a semiquantitative analysis can be done with ^{18}F-NaF PET/CT to assess treatment response. For example, a pilot study of 5 men with CRPC imaged before and after [223]radium chloride therapy suggested that ^{18}F-NaF PET/CT was more accurate than a qualitative comparison of ^{99m}Tc-MDP bone scans in assessing osseous response.[100] Radiotracer kinetic studies can also show the combined effects of skeletal blood flow and osteoblastic turnover, thereby allowing characterization of skeletal disease according to regional metabolic parameters.[101–103] Of note, a drawback of the wide adoption of ^{18}F-NaF PET/CT in routine clinical practice is the increased cost and time needed for interpretation compared with ^{99m}Tc-MDP bone scans. Also, ^{18}F-NaF assesses osseous response to disease rather than the disease itself and is subject to the flare phenomenon.[104]

Over the years, several additional PET radiotracers have been developed. For example, [11]C- or ^{18}F-labeled choline have been used for imaging men with prostate cancer. Choline is associated with cell membrane synthesis and is increased in cancer cells in which choline kinase activity has been upregulated. According to the literature, the sensitivity and specificity of ^{11}C-choline PET for the detection of primary disease ranges from 55% to 100% and 62% to 86%, respectively.[105–108] It has been reported that ^{11}C-choline PET/CT understages prostate cancer[109] and that the ability of ^{11}C-choline PET/CT to assess extraprostatic extension is limited.[110] Furthermore, there has been no significant correlation found between intensity of ^{11}C-choline uptake, Gleason score, and/or PSA.[111] Also, results are mixed regarding the utility of ^{11}C-choline in the evaluation of pelvic adenopathy in men with prostate cancer.[112–114] In general, ^{11}C-choline PET/CT and MRI are complementary for detecting and staging primary prostate cancer. ^{11}C-choline PET/CT has shown promise for the detection of recurrent disease after primary therapy[115,116] and is likely more useful in this context than ^{18}F-FDG.[117] Moreover, ^{11}C-choline PET/CT can be used to evaluate therapy response.[118,119] ^{18}F-labeled choline has the advantage of a longer half life than ^{11}C-choline and therefore the potential for greater accessibility. A few studies evaluating the utility of ^{18}F-choline in prostate cancer staging have shown relatively limited sensitivity[120–122] and have concluded that ^{18}F-choline PET/CT had little value in the initial evaluation of men with prostate cancer. Although ^{18}F-choline has utility in the assessment of men with biochemical recurrent disease, several studies have reported low sensitivity when the PSA is low,[123–126] and it has been suggested that ^{18}F-choline PET/CT be considered if the PSA level is greater than 2 ng/mL, PSA doubling time is 6 months or less, and PSA velocity is greater than 2 ng/mL/y.[127] ^{11}C-choline PET/CT is likely slightly more specific than skeletal scintigraphy and slightly less sensitive for the detection of osseous disease.[128] ^{18}F-choline PET/CT may be slightly more specific than ^{18}F-NaF PET/CT for the detection of osseous disease with similar sensitivity.[129] It has been suggested that [11]C- or [18]F- labeled choline PET/CT are complementary to skeletal scintigraphy or ^{18}F-NaF PET/CT for the detection of bone disease.

Similar to [11]C- or ^{18}F-labeled choline, [11]C- or ^{18}F-labeled acetate uptake reflects cell membrane phospholipid metabolism and is elevated in malignant cells with increased cellular growth. In general, [11]C- or ^{18}F-labeled acetate may be helpful to detect primary, recurrent, and metastatic prostate cancer. However, experience is limited and results in the literature suggest relatively low sensitivity with improved detection when the PSA level is greater than 3 ng/mL.[130] Overall, this radiotracer seems to be comparable/complementary to other radiotracers.[131–135]

[18]F-3'-deoxy-3'-fluorothymidine (^{18}F-FLT) is a thymidine analog that is phosphorylated by thymidine kinase 1 and provides a noninvasive measure of cellular proliferation by following the thymidine salvage DNA pathway. Although preclinical studies have suggested that ^{18}F-FLT may be useful in the evaluation of prostate cancer, to date, there is little supportive clinical information. [18]F-2'-fluoro-5-methyl-L-β-D-arabinofuranosyluracil (^{18}F-FMAU) is also a thymidine analog, which is preferentially phosphorylated by thymidine kinase 2 rather than thymidine kinase 1 as in the case of ^{18}F-FLT. A potential strength of ^{18}F-FMAU is that, unlike ^{18}F-FLT, ^{18}F-FMAU does not physiologically accumulate in bone marrow. A pilot study using ^{18}F-FMAU in men with locally recurrent prostate cancer suggested this tracer could detect sites of recurrent disease and sites of osseous metastases.[136]

Recently, there has been growing excitement around the use of androgen receptor targeting PET probes. Androgen receptors are thought to be present in all histologic types of prostate cancer, recurrent disease, and metastases, and androgen deprivation resistance is thought to result from mutations in the androgen receptor. ^{18}F-FDHT has been studied in a few small pilot series of men with metastatic prostate cancer and has shown changes after antiandrogen therapy,[137] suggesting that this tracer could be used as a pharmacodynamic biomarker rather than a marker of therapy response.[138,139]

Another radiotracer that has been used in the realm of prostate cancer imaging research is ^{11}C-methionine. ^{11}C-methionine uptake reflects amino acid transport and protein synthesis, which is typically elevated in malignancy. In a few small pilot studies, ^{11}C-methionine showed promising results compared with ^{18}F-FDG in men with progressing/recurrent prostate cancer for detecting disease at a lower grade.[140–142] Anti-^{18}F-FACBC is a synthetic L-leucine analog that reflects amino acid transport, which is typically elevated in prostate cancer. Schuster and colleagues[143,144] have found promising results suggesting that ^{18}F-FACBC is able to detect primary prostate cancer, metastatic lymph node disease, and recurrent disease.

Several novel probes are also under investigation. For example, there are both PET and SPECT probes targeting PSMA, a cell surface transmembrane glycoprotein that is overexpressed in prostate cancer cells. This has potential not only for the detection of disease but also for the assessment of therapy response.[145–147] Bombasin is a 14-amino acid analog of the human gastrin-releasing peptide that binds Gastrin–releasing peptide receptor, which is overexpressed in prostate cancer. To date, there is little clinical data available to predict the value of PSMA and bombasin in prostate cancer evaluation and management.

There are numerous radiotracers available for imaging prostate cancer, the majority of which are under investigation and currently lack definitive clinical data. The value of these radiotracers in the assessment and treatment of men with prostate cancer is a topic of research. Of note, the availability of multiple radiotracers has underlined the heterogeneity of the underlying biology. For example, certain sites of prostate cancer may accumulate only one radiotracer, whereas others accumulate multiple radiotracers concurrently. There has been growing interest in identifying the optimal imaging strategy for men with prostate cancer. Continued study is needed before the techniques discussed in this section are available for routine clinical practice and this is an active area of research.

SUMMARY

Imaging is a powerful tool in the detection, diagnosis, characterization, management, and follow-up of prostate carcinoma. Anatomic imaging alone is limited in detecting disease extent and response to therapy. Multimodality imaging including both anatomic and functional components typically provides complementary information in the assessment of primary and recurrent disease and is important for the development of noninvasive biomarkers. In particular, mpMRI and PET/CT present promising tools for prostate cancer staging and follow-up, especially with the use of diffusion-weighted sequences, contrast enhancement, 3T magnets, and novel PET radiotracers. mpMRI is showing promise in localizing the dominant site of disease within the prostate gland and has the potential to improve accurate risk stratification for patients with prostate cancer. Further work on standardization of techniques, increasing the availability of imaging modalities, and decreasing the cost for assessment is needed and is a dynamic area of research that is expanding to meet growing clinical and therapeutic needs.

REFERENCES

1. American Cancer Society Website. Cancer facts and figures. Available at: http://www.cancer.org/Research/CancerFactsFigures/index. Accessed March 21, 2013.
2. Bryś M, Migdalska-Sęk M, Pastuszak-Lewandoska D, et al. Diagnostic value of DNA alteration: loss of heterozygosity or allelic imbalance-promising for molecular staging of prostate cancers. Med Oncol 2013;30(1):391.

3. Tannock IF, de Wit R, Berry WR, et al. Docetaxel plus prednisone or mitoxantrone plus prednisone for advanced prostate cancer. N Engl J Med 2004;351: 1502–12.
4. de Bono JS, Oudard S, Ozguroglu M, et al. Prednisone plus cabazitaxel or mitoxantrone for metastatic castration-resistant prostate cancer progressing after docetaxel treatment: a randomised open-label trial. Lancet 2010;376:1147–54.
5. de Bono JS, Logothetis CJ, Molina A, et al. Abiraterone and increased survival in metastatic prostate cancer. N Engl J Med 2011;364:1995–2005.
6. Scher H, Fizazi K, Saad S, et al. MDV3100, an androgen receptor signaling inhibitor (ARSI), improves overall survival in patients with prostate cancer post docetaxel; results from the Phase 3 AFFIRM Study. GU ASCO 2012. J Clin Oncol 2012;30(suppl 5) [abstract LBA1].
7. Parker C, Heinrich D, O'Sullivan JM, et al. Overall survival benefit of radium-223 chloride (alpharadin) in the treatment of patients with symptomatic bone metastases in castration-resistant prostate cancer (CRPC): a phase III randomised trial (ALSYMPCA). Proceedings of ECCO/ESMO Annual Meeting. Stockholm, Sweden. September 23 to 27, 2011.
8. Kantoff PW, Higano CS, Shore ND, et al. Sipuleucel-T immunotherapy for castration-resistant prostate cancer. N Engl J Med 2010;363:411–22.
9. Eberhardt SC, Carter S, Casalino DD, et al. ACR appropriateness criteria prostate cancer-pretreatment detection, staging, and surveillance. J Am Coll Radiol 2013;10:83–92.
10. Lawrentschuk N, Haider MA, Daljeet N, et al. 'Prostatic evasive anterior tumours': the role of magnetic resonance imaging. BJU Int 2010;105(9):1231–6.
11. Margel D, Yap SA, Lawrentschuk N, et al. Impact of multiparametric endorectal coil prostate magnetic resonance imaging on disease reclassification among active surveillance candidates: a prospective cohort study. J Urol 2012;187(4):1247–52.
12. O'Dowd GJ, Veltri RW, Orozco R, et al. Update on the appropriate staging evaluation for newly diagnosed prostate cancer. J Urol 1997;158:687–98.
13. Cooperberg MR, Lubeck DP, Grossfeld GD, et al. Contemporary trends in imaging test utilization for prostate cancer staging: data from the cancer of the prostate strategic urologic research endeavor. J Urol 2002;168:491–5.
14. Ukimura O, Troncoso P, Ramirez EI, et al. Prostate cancer staging: correlation between ultrasound determined tumor contact length and pathologically confirmed extraprostatic extension. J Urol 1998;159:1251–9.
15. Ohori M, Egawa S, Shinohara K, et al. Detection of microscopic extracapsular extension prior to radical prostatectomy for clinically localized prostate cancer. Br J Urol 1994;74:72–9.
16. Hamper UM, Sheth S, Walsh PC, et al. Carcinoma of the prostate: value of transrectal sonography in detecting extension into the neurovascular bundle. AJR Am J Roentgenol 1990;155:1015–9.
17. Hamper UM, Sheth S, Walsh PC, et al. Capsular transgression of prostatic carcinoma: evaluation with transrectal US with pathologic correlation. Radiology 1991;178:791–5.
18. McSherry SA, Levy F, Schiebler ML, et al. Preoperative prediction of pathological tumor volume and stage in clinically localized prostate cancer: comparison of digital rectal examination, transrectal ultrasonography and magnetic resonance imaging. J Urol 1991;146:85–9.
19. Rifkin MD, Zerhouni EA, Gatsonis CA, et al. Comparison of magnetic resonance imaging and ultrasonography in staging early prostate cancer. Results of a multi-institutional cooperative trial. N Engl J Med 1990;323:621–6.

20. Beerlage HP, Aarnink RG, Ruijter ET, et al. Correlation of transrectal ultrasound, computer analysis of transrectal ultrasound and histopathology of radical prostatectomy specimen. Prostate Cancer Prostatic Dis 2001;4:56–62.

21. Sauvain JL, Palascak P, Bourscheid D, et al. Value of power Doppler and 3D vascular sonography as a method for diagnosis and staging prostate cancer. Eur Urol 2003;44:21–30.

22. Cornud F, Hamida K, Flam T, et al. Endorectal color Doppler sonography and endorectal MR imaging features of nonpalpable prostate cancer: correlation with radical prostatectomy findings. AJR Am J Roentgenol 2000;175:1161–8.

23. Sedelaar JP, van Leenders GJ, Goossen TE, et al. Value of contrast ultrasonography in the detection of significant prostate cancer: correlation with radical prostatectomy specimens. Prostate 2002;53:246–53.

24. Mitterberger M, Pinggera GM, Horninger W, et al. Comparison of contrast enhanced color Doppler targeted biopsy to conventional systematic biopsy: impact on Gleason score. J Urol 2007;178:464–8.

25. Mitterberger M, Pinggera GM, Pallwein L, et al. The value of three-dimensional transrectal ultrasonography in staging prostate cancer. BJU Int 2007;100:47–50.

26. Aigner F, Mitterberger M, Rehder P, et al. Status of transrectal ultrasound imaging of the prostate. J Endourol 2010;24:685–91.

27. Turkbey B, Albert PS, Kurdzie K, et al. Imaging localized prostate cancer: current approaches and new developments. AJR Am J Roentgenol 2009;192:1471–80.

28. Beyersdorff D, Taymoorian K, Knosel T, et al. MRI of prostate cancer at 1.5 and 3.0 T: comparison of image quality in tumor detection and staging. AJR Am J Roentgenol 2005;185(5):1214–20.

29. Sosna J, Pedrosa I, Dewolf WC, et al. MR imaging of the prostate at 3 Tesla: comparison of an external phased-array coil to imaging with an endorectal coil at 1.5 Tesla. Acad Radiol 2004;11(8):857–62.

30. Sala E, Akin O, Moskowitz CS, et al. Endorectal MR imaging in the evaluation of seminal vesicle invasion: diagnostic accuracy and multivariate feature analysis. Radiology 2006;238:929–37.

31. Bartolozzi C, Menchi I, Lencioni R, et al. Local staging of prostate carcinoma with endorectal coil MRI: correlation with whole mount radical prostatectomy specimens. Eur Radiol 1996;6:339–45.

32. Cornud F, Flam T, Chauveinc L, et al. Extraprostatic spread of clinically localized prostate cancer: factors predictive of pT3 tumor and of positive endorectal MR imaging examination results. Radiology 2002;224:203–10.

33. Ikonen S, Karkkainen P, Kivisaari L, et al. Magnetic resonance imaging of clinically localized prostatic cancer. J Urol 1998;159:915–9.

34. Ikonen S, Karkkainen P, Kivisaari L, et al. Endorectal magnetic resonance imaging of prostatic cancer: comparison between fat suppressed T2 -weighted fast spin echo and three-dimensional dual-echo, steady-state sequences. Eur Radiol 2001;11:236–41.

35. May F, Treumann T, Dettmar P, et al. Limited value of endorectal magnetic resonance imaging and transrectal ultrasonography in the staging of clinically localized prostate cancer. BJU Int 2001;87:66–9.

36. Perrotti M, Kaufman RP Jr, Jennings TA, et al. Endo-rectal coil magnetic resonance imaging in clinically localized prostate cancer: is it accurate? J Urol 1996;156:106–9.

37. Presti JC, Hricak H, Narayan PA, et al. Local staging of prostatic carcinoma: comparison of transrectal sonography and endorectal MR imaging. AJR Am J Roentgenol 1996;166:103–8.

38. Rorvik J, Halvorsen OJ, Albrektsen G, et al. MRI with an endorectal coil for staging of clinically localized prostate cancer prior to radical prostatectomy. Eur Radiol 1999;9:29–34.
39. Schiebler ML, Yankaskas BC, Tempany C, et al. MR imaging in adenocarcinoma of the prostate: interobserver variation and efficacy for determining stage C disease. AJR Am J Roentgenol 1992;158:559–62.
40. Mullerad M, Hricak H, Wang L, et al. Prostate cancer: detection of extracapsular extension by genitourinary and general body radiologists at MR imaging. Radiology 2004;232:140–6.
41. Hövels AM, Heesakkers RA, Adang EM, et al. The diagnostic accuracy of CT and MRI in the staging of pelvic lymph nodes in patients with prostate cancer: a meta-analysis. Clin Radiol 2008;63:387–95.
42. Pouliot F, Johnson M, Wu L. Non-invasive molecular imaging of prostate cancer lymph nodes metastases. Trends Mol Med 2009;15:254–60.
43. Harisinghani MG, Barentsz J, Hahn PF, et al. Noninvasive detection of clinically occult lymph-node metastases in prostate cancer. N Engl J Med 2003;348: 2491–9.
44. Zahee A, Cho SY, Pomper MG. New agents and techniques for imaging prostate cancer. J Nucl Med 2009;50:1387–90.
45. Thoeny HC, Triantafyllou M, Birkhaeuser FD, et al. Combined ultra small super-paramagnetic particles of iron oxide-enhanced and diffusion-weighted magnetic resonance imaging reliably detect pelvic lymph node metastases in normal sized nodes of bladder and prostate cancer patients. Eur Urol 2009; 55:761–9.
46. Leucovet FE, Geukens D, Stainer A, et al. Magnetic resonance imaging of the axial skeleton for detecting bone metastases in patients with high-risk prostate cancer: diagnostic and cost-effectiveness and comparison with current detection strategies. J Clin Oncol 2007;25:3281–7.
47. Messiou C, Cook G, de Souza NM. Imaging metastatic bone disease from carcinoma of the prostate. Br J Cancer 2009;101:1225–32.
48. Cook GJ, Venkitaraman R, Sohaib AS. The diagnostic utility of the flare phenomenon on bone scintigraphy in staging prostate cancer. Eur J Nucl Med Mol Imaging 2011;38:7–13.
49. Pollen JJ, Witztum KF, Ashburn WL. The flare phenomenon on radionuclide bone scan in metastatic prostate cancer. AJR Am J Roentgenol 1984;142:773–6.
50. Coleman RE, Mashiter G, Whitaker KB, et al. Bone scan flare predicts successful systemic therapy for bone metastases. J Nucl Med 1988;29:1354–9.
51. Dennis ER, Jia X, Mezheritskiy IS, et al. Bone scan index: a quantitative treatment response biomarker for castration-resistant metastatic prostate cancer. J Clin Oncol 2012;30:519–24.
52. Even-Sapir E, Metser U, Mishani E, et al. The detection of bone metastases in patients with high-risk prostate cancer: 99mTc-MDP Planar bone scintigraphy, single- and multi-field-of-view SPECT, 18F-fluoride PET, and 18F-fluoride PET/CT. J Nucl Med 2006;47:287–97.
53. Morris MJ, Akhurst T, Larson SM, et al. Fluorodeoxyglucose positron emission tomography as an outcome measure for castrate metastatic prostate cancer treated with antimicrotubule chemotherapy. Clin Cancer Res 2005;11:3210–6.
54. Autio K, Jia X, Heller G, et al. 18F-16β-fluoro-5α-dihydrotestosterone (FDHT) PET as a prognostic biomarker for survival in patients with metastatic castrate-resistant prostate cancer (mCRPC). J Clin Oncol 2012;30(Suppl) [abstract 4517].

55. Meirelles GS, Schoder H, Ravizzini GC, et al. Prognostic value of baseline [18F] fluorodeoxyglucose positron emission tomography and 99mTc-MDP bone scan in progressing metastatic prostate cancer. Clin Cancer Res 2010;16:6093–9.

56. Partin AW, Kattan MW, Subong EN, et al. Combination of prostate-specific antigen, clinical stage, and Gleason score to predict pathological stage of localized prostate cancer. A multi-institutional update. JAMA 1997;277:1445–51.

57. Presti JC Jr. Prostate cancer: assessment of risk using digital rectal examination, tumor grade, prostate-specific antigen, and systemic biopsy. Radiol Clin North Am 2000;38:49–58.

58. Partin AW, Mangold LA, Lamm DM, et al. Contemporary update of prostate cancer staging nonograms (Partin tables) for the new millennium. Urology 2001;58: 843–8.

59. D'Amico AV, Schnall M, Whittington R, et al. Endorectal coil MRI identifies locally advanced prostate cancer in select patients with clinically localized disease. Urology 1998;51:449–54.

60. Holmberg L, Bill-Axelson A, Helgesen F, et al. A randomized trial comparing radical prostatectomy with watchful waiting in early prostate cancer. N Engl J Med 2002;347:781–9.

61. Jager GJ, Severens JL, Thornbury JR, et al. Prostate cancer staging: should MR imaging be used? A decision analytic approach. Radiology 2000;215:445–51.

62. Langlotz CP. Benefits and costs of MR imaging of prostate cancer. Magn Reson Imaging Clin N Am 1996;4:533–44.

63. McClure TD, Margolis DJ, Reiter RE, et al. Use of MR imaging to determine preservation of the neurovascular bundles at robotic-assisted laparoscopic prostatectomy. Radiology 2012;262:874–83.

64. Carter HB, Walsh PC, Landis P, et al. Expectant management of non-palpable prostate cancer with curative intent: preliminary results. J Urol 2002;167:1231–4.

65. Berglund RK, Masterson TA, Vora KC, et al. Pathological upgrading and up staging with immediate repeat biopsy in patients eligible for active surveillance. J Urol 2008;180(5):1964–7.

66. Klotz L, Zhang L, Lam A, et al. Clinical results of long-term follow-up of a large, active surveillance cohort with localized prostate cancer. J Clin Oncol 2010; 28(1):126–31.

67. Duffield AS, Lee TK, Miyamoto H, et al. Radical prostatectomy findings in patients in whom active surveillance of prostate cancer fails. J Urol 2009;182(5): 2274–8.

68. Porten SP, Whitson JM, Cowan JE, et al. Changes in prostate cancer grade on serial biopsy in men undergoing active surveillance. J Clin Oncol 2011;29(20): 2795–800.

69. Fradet V, Kurhanewicz J, Cowan JE, et al. Prostate cancer managed with active surveillance: role of anatomic MR imaging and MR spectroscopic imaging. Radiology 2010;256(1):176–83.

70. European Association of Urology Guidelines 2012. Available at: http://www.uroweb.org/guidelines/. Accessed March 21, 2013.

71. Lee N, Fawaaz R, Olsson CA, et al. Which patients with newly diagnosed prostate cancer need a bone scan? An analysis based on 631 patients. Int J Radiat Oncol Biol Phys 2000;48:1443–6.

72. Leventis AK, Shariat SF, Slawin KM. Local recurrence after radical prostatectomy: correlation of US features with prostatic fossa biopsy findings. Radiology 2001;219:432–9.

73. Ornstein DK, Oh J, Herschman JD, et al. Evaluation and management of the man who has failed primary curative therapy for prostate cancer. Urol Clin North Am 1998;25:591–601.
74. Coakley FV, Hricak H, Wefer AE, et al. Brachytherapy for prostate cancer: endorectal MR imaging of local treatment-related changes. Radiology 2001;219:817–21.
75. Gulley JL, Emberton M, Kurhanewicz J, et al. Progress in prostate cancer imaging. Urol Oncol 2012;30:938–9.
76. Jackson A, O'Connor JP, Parker GJ, et al. Imaging tumor vascular heterogeneity and angiogenesis using dynamic contrast-enhanced magnetic resonance imaging. Clin Cancer Res 2007;13:3449–59.
77. Bloch BN, Furman-Haran E, Helbich TH, et al. Prostate cancer: accurate determination of extracapsular extension with high-spatial resolution dynamic contrast-enhanced and T2-weighted MR imaging – initial results. Radiology 2007;245:176–85.
78. Yu KK, Scheidler J, Hricak H, et al. Prostate cancer: prediction of extracapsular extension with endorectal MR imaging and three-dimensional proton MR spectroscopic imaging. Radiology 1999;213:481–8.
79. Kim CK, Park BK, Kim B. Diffusion-weighted MRI at 3T for the evaluation of prostate cancer. AJR Am J Roentgenol 2010;194:1461–9.
80. Kim CK, Choi D, Park BK, et al. Diffusion-weighted MR imaging for the evaluation of seminal vesicle invasion in prostate cancer: initial results. J Magn Reson Imaging 2008;28:963–9.
81. Tan CH, Wei W, Johnson V, et al. Diffusion-weighted MRI in the detection of prostate cancer: meta-analysis. AJR Am J Roentgenol 2012;199:822–9.
82. Hambrock T, Somford DM, Huisman HJ, et al. Relationship between apparent diffusion coefficients at 3.0-T MR imaging and Gleason grade in peripheral zone prostate cancer. Radiology 2011;259:453–61.
83. Giles SL, Morgan VA, Riches SF, et al. Apparent diffusion coefficient as a predictive biomarker of prostate cancer progression: value of fast and slow diffusion components. AJR Am J Roentgenol 2011;196(3):586–91.
84. Rajinikanth A, Manoharan M, Soloway CT, et al. Trends in Gleason score: concordance between biopsy and prostatectomy over 15 years. Urology 2008;72:177–82.
85. Barentsz JO, Richenberg J, Clements R, et al. ESUR prostate MR guidelines 2012. Eur Radiol 2012;22:746–57.
86. Dickinson L, Ahmed HU, Allen C, et al. Magnetic resonance imaging for the detection, localisation, and characterisation of prostate cancer: recommendations from a European consensus meeting. Eur Urol 2011;59:477–94.
87. Portalez D, Mozer P, Cornud F, et al. Validation of the European Society of Urogenital Radiology scoring system for prostate cancer diagnosis on multiparametric magnetic resonance imaging in a cohort of repeat biopsy patients. Eur Urol 2012;62:986–96.
88. Hambrock T, Somford DM, Hoeks C, et al. Magnetic resonance imaging guided prostate biopsy in men with repeat negative biopsies and increased prostate specific antigen. J Urol 2010;183:520–7.
89. Minamimoto R, Senda M, Jinnouchi S, et al. The current status of an FDG-PET cancer screening program in Japan based on a 4-year (2006–2009) nationwide survey. Ann Nucl Med 2013;27:46–57.
90. Watanabe H, Kanematsu M, Kondo H, et al. Preoperative detection of prostate cancer: a comparison with 11C-choline PET, 18F-fluorodeoxyglucose PET, and MR imaging. J Magn Reson Imaging 2010;31:1151–6.

91. Schöder H, Herrmann K, Gönen M, et al. 2-[18F]fluoro-2-deoxyglucose positron emission tomography for detection of disease in patients with prostatespecific antigen relapse after radical prostatectomy. Clin Cancer Res 2005;11: 4761–9.

92. Jadvar H, Desai B, Ji L, et al. Prospective evaluation of 18FNaF and 18F-FDG PET/CT in detection of occult metastatic disease in biochemical recurrence of prostate cancer. Clin Nucl Med 2012;37:637–43.

93. Minamimoto R, Uemura H, Sano F, et al. The potential of FDG PET/CT for detecting prostate cancer in patients with an elevated serum PSA level. Ann Nucl Med 2011;25:21–7.

94. Effert P, Beniers AJ, Tamimi Y, et al. Expression of glucose transporter 1 (GLUT-1) in cell lines and clinical specimen from human prostate adenocarcinoma. Anticancer Res 2004;24:3057–63.

95. Kukuk D, Reischl G, Raguin O, et al. Assessment of PET tracer uptake in hormone-independent and hormone-dependent xenograft prostate cancer mouse models. J Nucl Med 2011;52:1654–63.

96. Reinicke K, Sotomayor P, Cisterna P, et al. Cellular distribution of Glut-1 and Glut-5 in benign and malignant human prostate tissue. J Cell Biochem 2012; 113:553–62.

97. Stewardt GD, Gray K, Pennington CJ, et al. Analysis of hypoxia-associated gene expression in prostate cancer: lysyl oxidase and glucose transporter 1 expression correlate with Gleason score. Oncol Rep 2008;20:1561–7.

98. Oyama N, Akino H, Suzuki Y, et al. Prognostic value of 2-deoxy-2-[F-18]fluoro-D-glucose positron emission tomography imaging for patients with prostate cancer. Mol Imaging Biol 2002;4:99–104.

99. Jadvar H, Desai B, Ji L, et al. Prognostic utility of FDG PET/CT in men with castrate-resistant metastatic prostate cancer. J Nucl Med 2012;53(Suppl 1): 116.

100. Cook GJ, Parker C, Chua S, et al. 18F-fluoriode: changes in uptake as a method to assess response in bone metastases from castrate-resistant prostate cancer patients treated with 223Ra-chloride (Alpharadin). EJNMMI Res 2011;1:4.

101. Blake GM, Park-Holohan SJ, Cook GJ, et al. Quantitative studies of bone with the use of 18F-fluoride and 99mTc-methylene diphosphonate. Semin Nucl Med 2001;31:28–49.

102. Cook GJ, Blake GM, Marsden PK, et al. Quantification of skeletal kinetic indices in Paget's disease using dynamic 18F-fluoride positron emission tomography. J Bone Miner Res 2002;17:854–9.

103. Siddique M, Blake GM, Frost ML, et al. Estimation of regional bone metabolism from whole-body 18F-fluoride PET static images. Eur J Nucl Med Mol Imaging 2012;39(2):337–43.

104. Wade AA, Scott JA, Kuter I, et al. Flare response in 18F-fluoride ion PET bone scanning. AJR Am J Roentgenol 2006;186:1783–6.

105. Scher B, Seitz M, Albinger W, et al. Value of 11C-choline PET and PET-CT in patients with suspected prostate cancer. Eur J Nucl Med Mol Imaging 2007; 34:45–53.

106. Farsad M, Schiavina R, Castellucci P, et al. Detection and localization of prostate cancer: correlation of (11C)C-choline PET/CT with histopathologic step-section analysis. J Nucl Med 2005;46:1642–9.

107. Testa C, Schiavina R, Lodi R, et al. Prostate cancer: sextant localization with MR imaging, MR spectroscopy, and 11C-choline PET-CT. Radiology 2007;244: 797–806.

108. Yamaguchi T, Lee J, Uemura H, et al. Prostate cancer: a comparative study of 11C-choline PET and MR imaging combined with proton MR spectroscopy. Eur J Nucl Med Mol Imaging 2005;32:742–8.

109. Rinnab L, Blumstein NM, Mottaghy FM, et al. 11C-choline positron emission tomography/computed tomography and transrectal ultrasonography for staging localized prostate cancer. BJU Int 2007;99:1421–6.

110. Martorana G, Schaivina R, Cort B, et al. 11C-choline positron emission tomography/computed tomography for tumor localization of primary prostate cancer in comparison with 12-core biopsy. J Urol 2006;176:954–60.

111. Giovacchini G, Picchio M, Coradesschi E, et al. 11C-choline uptake with PET/CT for the initial diagnosis of prostate cancer: relation to PSA levels, tumor stage and anti-androgenic therapy. Eur J Nucl Med Mol Imaging 2008;35:1065–73.

112. de Jong IJ, Pruim J, Elsinga PH, et al. Preoperative staging of pelvic lymph nodes in prostate cancer by ^{11}C-choline PET. J Nucl Med 2003;44:331–5.

113. Schiavina R, Scattoni V, Castellucci P, et al. (11)C-choline positron emission tomography/computerized tomography for preoperative lymph node staging in intermediate- risk and high-risk prostate cancer: comparison with clinical staging nomograms. Eur Urol 2008;54:392–401.

114. Budiharto T, Joniau S, Lerut E, et al. Prospective evaluation of (11)C-choline positron emission tomography and diffusion weighted magnetic resonance imaging for the nodal staging of prostate cancer with a high risk of lymph node metastases. Eur Urol 2011;60:125–30.

115. Krause BJ, Souvatzpglou M, Tuncel M, et al. The detection rate of [(11)C] choline-PET/CT depends on the serum PSA-value in patients with biochemical recurrence of prostate cancer. Eur J Nucl Med Mol Imaging 2008;35:18–23.

116. Castellucci P, Fuccio C, Nanni C, et al. Influence of trigger PSA and PSA kinetics on 11C-choline PET/CT detection rate in patients with biochemical relapse after radical prostatectomy. J Nucl Med 2009;50:1394–400.

117. Richter JA, Rodríguez M, Rioja J, et al. Dual tracer 11C-choline and FDG-PET in the diagnosis of biochemical prostate cancer relapse after radical treatment. Mol Imaging Biol 2010;12:210–7.

118. Fuccio C, Schiavina R, Castellucci P, et al. Androgen deprivation therapy influences the uptake of 11C-choline in patients with recurrent prostate cancer: the preliminary results of a sequential PET/CT study. Eur J Nucl Med Mol Imaging 2011;38:1985–9.

119. Emonds KM, Swinnen JV, van Weerden WM, et al. Do androgens control the uptake of 18F-FDG, 11C-choline and 11C-aceatte in human prostate cancer cell lines? Eur J Nucl Med Mol Imaging 2011;38:1842–53.

120. Beheshti M, Imamovic L, Broinger G, et al. 18 F-choline PET/CT in the preoperative staging of prostate cancer in patients with intermediate or high risk of extracapsular disease: a prospective study of 130 patients. Radiology 2010;254:925–33.

121. Steuber T, Scholomm T, Heinzer H, et al. [F(18)]-fluoroethylcholine combined inline PET-CT scan for detection of lymph node metastasis in high risk prostate cancer patients prior to radical prostatectomy: preliminary results from a prospective histology-based study. Eur J Cancer 2010;2:449–55.

122. Poulsen MH, Bouchelouche K, Gerke O, et al. [F(18)]-fluorocholine positron-emission/computed tomography for lymph node staging of patients with prostate cancer: preliminary results of a prospective study. BJU Int 2010;106:639–43.

123. Picchio M, Briganti A, Fanti S, et al. The role of choline positron emission tomography/computed tomography in the management of patients with

prostate-specific antigen progression after radical treatment of prostate cancer. Eur Urol 2011;59:51–60.

124. Pelosi E, Arena V, Skanjeti A, et al. Role of whole-body (18F)-choline PET/CT in disease detection in patients with biochemical relapse after radical treatment for prostate cancer. Radiol Med 2008;113:895–904.

125. Heinisch M, Dirisamer A, Loidl W, et al. Positron emission tomography/computed tomography with F-18 fluorocholine for restaging of prostate cancer patients: meaningful at PSA < 5 ng/mL? Mol Imaging Biol 2006;8:43–8.

126. Graute V, Jansen N, Ubeleis C, et al. Relationship between PSA kinetics and 18F-fluorolcholine PET/CT detection rates of recurrence in patients with prostate cancer after total prostatectomy. Eur J Nucl Med Mol Imaging 2012;39:271–82.

127. Schillaci O, Calabria F, Tavolozza M, et al. Influence of PSA, PSA velocity, and PSA doubling time on contrast-enhanced (18)F-choline PET/CT detection rate in patients with rising PSA after radical prostatectomy. Eur J Nucl Med Mol Imaging 2012;39:589–96.

128. Picchio M, Spinapolice EG, Fallanca F, et al. [11C]choline PET/CT detection of bone metastases in patients with PSA progression after primary treatment for prostate cancer: comparison with bone scintigraphy. Eur J Nucl Med Mol Imaging 2012;39:13–26.

129. Langsteger W, Balogova S, Huchet V, et al. Fluorocholine (18F) and sodium fluoride (18F) PET/CT in the detection of prostate cancer: prospective comparison of diagnostic performance determined by masked reading. Q J Nucl Med Mol Imaging 2011;55:448–57.

130. Oyama N, Miller TR, Dehdashti F, et al. 11C-acetate PET imaging of prostate cancer: detection of recurrent disease at PSA relapse. J Nucl Med 2003;44:549–55.

131. Oyama N, Akino H, Kanamaru H, et al. 11C-acetate PET imaging of prostate cancer. J Nucl Med 2002;43:181–6.

132. Yu EY, Muzi M, Hackenvracht JA. C11-aceatte and F-18 FDG PET for men with prostate cancer bone metastases: relative findings and response to therapy. Clin Nucl Med 2011;36:192–8.

133. Kotzerke J, Volkmer BG, Neumaier B, et al. Carbon-11 acetate positron emission tomography can detect local recurrence of prostate cancer. Eur J Nucl Med Mol Imaging 2002;29:1380–4.

134. Sandblom G, Sorensen J, Lundin N, et al. Positron emission tomography with 11C-acetate for tumor detection and localization in patients with prostate specific antigen relapse after radical prostatectomy. Urology 2006;67:996–1000.

135. Kotzerke J, Volkmer BG, Glatting G, et al. Intraindividual comparison of [11C]acetate and [11C] choline PET for detection of metastases of prostate cancer. Nuklearmedizin 2003;42:25–30.

136. Sun H, Sloan A, Mangner TJ, et al. Imaging DNA synthesis with [18F]FMAU and positron emission tomography in patients with cancer. Eur J Nucl Med Mol Imaging 2005;32:15–22.

137. Dehdashti F, Picus J, Michalski J, et al. Positron tomographic assessment of androgen receptors in prostatic carcinoma. Eur J Nucl Med Mol Imaging 2005;32:344–50.

138. Fox J, Morris MJ, Larson SM, et al. Developing imaging strategies for castration resistant prostate cancer. Acta Oncol 2011;50(Suppl 1):39–48.

139. Scher HI, Beer TM, Higano CS, et al. Antitumor activity of MDV3100 in castration-resistant prostate cancer: a phase 1-2 study. Lancet 2010;375:1437–46.

140. Macapinlac HA, Humm JL, Akhurst T, et al. Differential metabolism and pharmacokinetics of L-[1-(11C)]-methionine and 2-[(18F)F]fluoro-2-deoxy-D-glucose

(FDG) in androgen independent prostate cancer. Clin Positron Imaging 1999;2: 173–81.

141. Nunez R, Macapinlac HA, Yeung HW, et al. Combined 18F-FDG and 11C-methionine PET scans in patients with newly progressive metastatic prostate cancer. J Nucl Med 2002;43:46–55.

142. Shiiba M, Ishihara K, Kimura G, et al. Evaluation of primary cancer using (11C)-methionine-PET/CT and (18)F-FDG-PET/CT. Ann Nucl Med 2011;26: 138–45.

143. Schuster DM, Votaw JR, Nieh PT, et al. Initial experience with the radiotracer anti-1-amino-3-18F-fluorocyclobutane-1-carboxylic acid with PET/CT in prostate carcinoma. J Nucl Med 2007;48:56–63.

144. Schuster DM, Savir-Baruch B, Nieh PT, et al. Detection of recurrent prostate carcinoma with anti-1-amino-3-18F fluorocyclobutane-1-carboxylic acid PET/CT and 111In-capromab pendetide SPECT/CT. Radiology 2011;259:852–61.

145. Bouchelouche K, Choyke PL, Capala J. Prostatespecific membrane antigen: a target for imaging and therapy with radionuclides. Discov Med 2010;9:55–61.

146. Evans MJ, Smith-Jones PM, Wongvipat J, et al. Noninvasive measurement of androgen receptor signaling with positron emitting radiopharmaceutical that targets prostate-specific membrane antigen. Proc Natl Acad Sci U S A 2011;108: 9578–82.

147. Barrett JA, Coleman RE, Goldsmith SJ, et al. First-in-man evaluation of 2 high-affinity PSMA-avid small molecules for imaging prostate cancer. J Nucl Med 2013;54:380–7.

Neoadjuvant and Adjuvant Hormonal and Chemotherapy for Prostate Cancer

Elaine T. Lam, MD*, L. Michael Glodé, MD

KEYWORDS

- Prostate cancer • Neoadjuvant therapy • Adjuvant therapy • Chemotherapy

KEY POINTS

- Adjuvant androgen deprivation therapy is well-established in conjunction with RT for intermediate- and high-risk disease.
- The role of hormone therapy is less clear in patients who undergo a prostatectomy.
- Further exploration and patient selection is needed to better define the roles of ADT alone, androgen-AR axis modifications, and chemotherapy in the adjuvant setting.

INTRODUCTION

Among the 241,000 men who are diagnosed with prostate cancer each year, 82% will have localized disease and 11% will have regional or locally advanced disease.[1] Most men treated with radical prostatectomy or radiation therapy (RT) will be cured of prostate cancer. However, some men will experience treatment failure. The factors that increase the risk of cancer recurrence after primary therapies include extraprostatic (T3 or T4) disease, pretreatment prostate-specific antigen (PSA) greater than 20 ng/mL, Gleason score of 8 or more, perineural invasion on biopsy, and seminal vesicle involvement or positive margins in the prostatectomy specimen.[2–7] Androgen deprivation therapy (ADT) is well established in the treatment of metastatic prostate cancer. Adjuvant hormone therapy, following prostatectomy and/or radiotherapy, has been studied in the high-risk prostate cancer setting to try to reduce the risk of recurrence and improve patient outcomes. Its role in localized cancer is well established in conjunction with RT for intermediate- and high-risk disease but is far less clear in patients who undergo a prostatectomy.

Division of Medical Oncology, University of Colorado Anschutz Medical Campus, Mailstop 8117, 12801 East 17th Avenue, Aurora, CO 80045, USA
* Corresponding author.
E-mail address: elaine.lam@ucdenver.edu

Hematol Oncol Clin N Am 27 (2013) 1189–1204
http://dx.doi.org/10.1016/j.hoc.2013.08.004
0889-8588/13/$ – see front matter Published by Elsevier Inc.
hemonc.theclinics.com

ADJUVANT HORMONE THERAPY FOLLOWING PROSTATECTOMY

There have been limited studies evaluating the role of adjuvant hormone therapy following prostatectomy (**Table 1**). The Eastern Cooperative Oncology Group study (ECOG 3886) evaluated immediate versus deferred ADT in men with node-positive prostate cancer. Between 1988 and 1993, 98 men who underwent a radical prostatectomy and pelvic lymphadenectomy and found to have microscopic lymph node metastases were randomized to receive immediate lifelong ADT or to be observed and receive ADT on symptomatic recurrence or detection of distant metastatic disease. At a median follow-up of 11.9 years, the men assigned to the immediate ADT arm had a significant improvement in overall survival (hazard ratio [HR] 1.84, 95% confidence interval [CI] 1.01–3.35, $P = .04$), prostate cancer–specific survival (HR 4.09, CI 1.76–9.49, $P = .0004$), and progression-free survival (PFS) (HR 3.42, CI 1.96–5.98, $P<.0001$).[8] In this study, patients in the observation arm were initiated on ADT only after the development of symptomatic recurrence or detectable metastatic disease and not at the time of biochemical recurrence, which can occur at a median of 8 years before the onset of radiologic evidence of metastatic disease.[9]

A separate retrospective observational study using Surveillance, Epidemiology, and End Results (SEER)–Medicare data was done to evaluate the impact of adjuvant ADT for patients who have node-positive prostate cancer in the contemporary era of postoperative PSA surveillance to detect biochemical recurrence. Wong and colleagues[10] used the SEER-Medicare database to construct a cohort of men with lymph node–positive disease who had undergone radical prostatectomy between 1991 and 1999 and classified them as receiving adjuvant ADT (within 120 days of radical prostatectomy) or not receiving adjuvant ADT (subsequent ADT initiated >120 days from surgery or no ADT). Among the 731 men identified, 209 had received ADT within 120 days of radical prostatectomy. After adjusting for potential confounders of receiving adjuvant ADT (ie, tumor characteristics, extent of nodal disease, demographics, receipt of RT), there was no statistically significant difference in the overall survival between the adjuvant ADT and non-ADT group (HR 0.97, 95% CI 0.71–1.27). Additionally, there was no statistically significant survival difference when various definitions of adjuvant ADT (90, 150, 180, and 365 days) were tested. One important limitation of this study is that the indication for ADT (adjuvant vs salvage) was not available through the database.

In the SWOG (Southwest Oncology Group) S9921 trial, 983 men with high-risk prostate cancer (extraprostatic extension, positive nodes, positive margin Gleason 7 or Gleason grade >7) received adjuvant therapy with ADT (goserelin and bicalutamide for 2 years) alone or in combination with 6 cycles of mitoxantrone chemotherapy after a prostatectomy. For the 481 men who received ADT only, the estimated 5-year biochemical failure-free survival was 92.5% (95% CI 90–95) and the 5-year overall survival was 95.9% (95% CI 93.9–97.9). This trial was closed to accrual in January 2007 after 3 cases of acute myelogenous leukemia were reported in the mitoxantrone treatment arm. The final analysis of the primary end point of overall survival comparing the 2 arms for this trial has not been reported; however, the results seen in the ADT-only arm make a compelling argument to counsel patients with high-risk prostate cancer about adjuvant ADT after a prostatectomy.[11] This study represents the largest prospective cohort of patients with high-risk prostate cancer receiving adjuvant ADT and showed favorable results.

The use of antiandrogen therapy alone in the adjuvant setting has also been investigated. Wirth and colleagues[12] studied the role of adjuvant flutamide therapy in 309 patients with locally advanced, lymph node–negative prostate cancer who were randomized to receive either flutamide or observation after a prostatectomy. At a median

Table 1
Adjuvant hormonal therapy after prostatectomy

Study	ECOG 3886 (Messing)		SEER Retrospective (Wong)		Adjuvant Flutamide (Wirth)		Adjuvant Bicalutamide (Iverson)	
Design	Immediate vs deferred ADT		Adjuvant ADT vs no ADT		Flutamide vs observation		Bicalutamide vs observation	
	Immediate	Deferred	Adjuvant	No adjuvant	Flutamide	Observation	Bicalutamide	Placebo
Median Biochemical PFS (y)	13.9	2.4 (P<.0001)	Not reported	Not reported	10.8	9.9 (P = .0041)	6.6	3.7 (P = .001)
	HR 3.42 (95% CI 1.96–5.98)		—		HR 0.51 (95% CI 0.32–0.81)		HR 0.85 (95% CI 0.79–0.91)	
Median Disease-Specific Survival (y)	Not reached	12.3 (P = .0004)	Not reached (NS)		Not reported	Not reported	Not reported	Not reported
	HR 4.09 (95% CI 1.76–9.49)		HR 0.97 (95% CI 0.56–1.68)		—		—	
Median Overall Survival (y)	13.9	11.3 (P = .04)	Not reached (NS)		11[a]	Not reached (NS)	Not reached	Not reached (NS)
	HR 1.84 (95% CI 1.01–3.35)		HR 0.95 (95% CI 0.71–1.27)		HR 1.04 (95% CI 0.53–2.02)		HR 1.01 (95% CI 0.94–1.09)	

Abbreviations: ADT, androgen deprivation therapy; CI, confidence interval; HR, hazard ration; NS, not statistically significant; PFS, progression-free survival; SEER, Surveillance, Epidemiology, and End Results.

[a] Data not reported in primary article and estimated from available survival curves.

follow-up of 6.1 years, flutamide treatment was associated with considerable toxicity; although it showed improved recurrence-free survival (P = .0041), it did not improve the overall survival (P = .92). The Early Prostate Cancer Program was an international program consisting of 3 randomized, double-blind, placebo-controlled clinical trials. Men with localized or locally advanced prostate cancer were randomized to receive either oral bicalutamide 150 mg once daily or oral placebo in addition to standard care with radical prostatectomy, radiotherapy, or watchful waiting.[13] In all, 8113 patients with localized (T1–2, N0/Nx) or locally advanced (T3–4, any N; or any T, N+) prostate cancer (all M0) were enrolled in 3 complementary double-blind, placebo-controlled trials. At a median follow-up of 9.7 years, bicalutamide significantly improved PFS (HR 0.85, 95% CI 0.79–0.91, P = .001) compared with placebo; however, there was no difference in overall survival (HR 1.01, P = .77). Moreover, the improvement in PFS was observed in patients with locally advanced prostate cancer but not in patients with localized disease. In a subset analysis, the overall survival benefit was demonstrated in patients with locally advanced disease undergoing radiotherapy (P = .031).[14]

Based on data from the ECOG 3886 and the SWOG S9921 studies, it may be reasonable to consider adjuvant ADT in some patients with lymph node–positive or high-risk prostate cancer after a prostatectomy, especially in patients who may not be candidates for adjuvant radiation (discussed later). Given the lack of an overall survival benefit from the flutamide and bicalutamide studies, the use of antiandrogen therapy alone in the adjuvant setting is generally not recommended.

ADJUVANT RT FOLLOWING PROSTATECTOMY

The use of adjuvant RT alone for high-risk disease following prostatectomy has been studied by the European Organization for Research and Treatment of Cancer (EORTC) 22911 and SWOG 8794 trials and the Arbeitsgemeinschaft Radiologische Onkologie und Urologische Onkologie of the German Cancer Society (ARO 96-02/AUO AP 09/95). **Table 2** summarizes these trials.

EORTC 22911 was a phase III trial comparing immediate postoperative RT (60 Gy conventional) versus the wait-and-see approach in which patients underwent RT at the time of biochemical recurrence (PSA >0.2, confirmed >2 weeks apart). There were 1005 patients enrolled in this study. At 10.6 years of follow-up, 39.4% in the immediate RT group experienced biochemical progression, clinical progression, or death compared with 61.8% in the wait-and-see group. There was no difference in overall survival between the treatment groups (HR 1.18, 95% CI 0.91–1.53, P = .2024), with a 10-year survival of 76.9% (95% CI 72.4–80.8) in the postoperative irradiation group compared with 80.7% (76.4–84.3) in the wait-and-see group. There was an increase in late effects seen in patients treated with immediate postoperative RT.[15]

SWOG S8794 evaluated 425 men with pathologically advanced prostate cancer who had undergone radical prostatectomy, randomized to receive 60 to 64 Gy of external beam radiotherapy delivered to the prostatic fossa (n = 214) or usual care plus observation (n = 211). The primary outcome was metastasis-free survival; the secondary outcomes included PSA relapse, recurrence-free survival, overall survival, freedom from hormonal therapy, and postoperative complications. At a median follow-up of 10.6 years (interquartile range 9.2–12.7 years), 76 (35.5%) of 214 men in the adjuvant radiotherapy group were diagnosed with metastatic disease or died (median metastasis-free estimate 14.7 years) compared with 91 (43.1%) of 211 (median metastasis-free estimate 13.2 years) of those in the observation group (HR 0.75, 95% CI 0.55–1.02, P = .06). Radiotherapy also significantly reduced the rates

Table 2
Adjuvant RT after prostatectomy

Study	EORTC 22911 (Bolla)		SWOG S8794 (Thompson)		ARO 96-02/AUO AP 09/95 (Wiegel)	
Design	Immediate postoperative irradiation vs wait-and-see approach		Immediate postoperative irradiation vs observation		Immediate postoperative irradiation vs wait-and-see approach	
	Postoperative irradiation (60 Gy)	Wait-and-see	Postoperative irradiation (60–64 Gy)	Observation	Postoperative irradiation (60 Gy)	Wait-and-see
Median Biochemical PFS (y)	6.12 HR 0.49 (95% CI 0.41–1.59)		10.3 HR 0.43 (95% CI 0.31–0.58, $P<.001$)	3.1	Not reported Biochemical NED at 10 y 56% vs 35% (HR 0.51, $P = .00002$)	Not reported
Median DSS (y)	Not reported DSS at 10 y 96.1% vs 94.6%, HR 0.78 (95% CI 0.46–1.33, $P = .3407$)		13.8 HR 0.62 (95% CI 0.46–0.82, $P = .001$)	9.9	Not reported —	Not reported
Median OS (y)	Not reached OS at 10 y 76.9% vs 80.7% ($P = .2024$)	15.6[a]	15.2 (HR, 0.72, 95% CI 0.55–0.96, $P = .023$)	13.3	Not reached $P = .59$	Not reached

Abbreviations: ARO, Arbeitsgemeinschaft Radiologische Onkologie; AUO, Arbeitsgemeinschaft Urologische Onkologie; DSS, disease-specific survival; EORTC, European Organization for Research and Treatment of Cancer; NED, No evidence of disease; OS, overall survival; SWOG, Southwest Oncology Group.

[a] Data not reported in primary article and estimated from available survival curves.

of PSA relapse (median PSA relapse-free survival 10.3 years for radiotherapy vs 3.1 years for observation, HR 0.43, 95% CI 0.31–0.58, P<.001) and disease recurrence (median recurrence-free survival 13.8 years for radiotherapy vs 9.9 years for observation, HR 0.62, 95% CI 0.46–0.82, P = .001).[16] With a longer follow-up of 12.7 years for the radiotherapy arm and 12.5 years for the observation arm, a survival advantage was seen. The median overall survival was 13.3 years in the observation arm and 15.2 years in the radiotherapy arm (HR 0.72, 95% CI 0.55–0.96, P = .023).[3]

The ARO German study (96-02/AUO AP 09/95) randomly assigned 192 men with PT3N0 prostate cancers who achieved undetectable PSA to receive immediate postoperative RT (60 Gy) or the wait-and-see approach. At 5 years, the biochemical PFS was significantly improved in the RT group compared with observation (72% vs 54%, P = .0015).[17] At 10 years, RT improved biochemical control by 49% (freedom from biochemical failure [bNED] 56% vs 35%, HR 0.51, P = .00002). There was no difference in metastases-free survival (P = .56) or overall survival (P = .59), although the study was not powered to detect differences in overall survival.[18]

The timing of radiotherapy after radical prostatectomy is still controversial. Studies are ongoing to determine the best setting (adjuvant vs salvage) for radiotherapy, including the Trans-Tasman Radiation Oncology Group Radiotherapy, Adjuvant versus Early Salvage (RAVES) study (ClinicalTrials.gov, identifier NCT00860652) and the Medical Research Council Radiation Therapy and Androgen Deprivation Therapy in Treating Patients Who Have Undergone Surgery for Prostate Cancer (RADICALS) study (ClinicalTrials.gov, identifier NCT00541047).

ADJUVANT ANDROGEN DEPRIVATION THERAPY IN COMBINATION WITH RT

The benefit of combining ADT to external beam RT (EBRT), compared with EBRT alone in patients with clinically localized prostate cancer with prostate gland intact, has been demonstrated repeatedly in multiple trials.[19–25] However, the optimum duration of ADT in this setting is still controversial and varies based on the risk category. **Table 3** summarizes the clinical trials evaluating adjuvant ADT in combination with RT.

The Radiation Therapy Oncology Group (RTOG) 85-31 study evaluated the effectiveness of adjuvant ADT versus salvage ADT in patients with extraprostatic or lymph node–positive prostate cancer treated with definitive EBRT. The minimal target dose to the prostatic target volume was 65 Gy in definitively treated patients and 60 Gy in postoperatively treated patients. The daily dose was 1.8 to 2.0 Gy given 4 to 5 times weekly. Patients who had undergone definitive prostatectomy were also eligible if they had extracapsular extension involving the resection margin or seminal vesicle involvement. Between 1987 and 1992, 977 patients were randomized to receive adjuvant goserelin (initiated during the last week of EBRT and continued indefinitely or until signs of progression) or observation and initiation of goserelin at the time of locoregional or metastatic relapse. The 10-year overall survival rate was significantly greater for the adjuvant arm than for the control arm (49% vs 39%, P = .002). The 10-year local failure rate was 23% for the adjuvant arm versus 38% for the control arm (P<.0001). At 10 years, the incidence of distant metastases and disease-specific mortality was 24% versus 39% (P<.001) and 16% versus 22% (P = .0052), respectively, both in favor of the adjuvant arm.[25]

The RTOG 86-10 study randomized 456 patients with T2 to T4 and N0 to N1 prostate cancer to receive EBRT alone or EBRT plus short-term (4 month) neoadjuvant and concurrent ADT. The minimum target doses to the regional lymphatics and the prostatic target volume were 44 Gy and 65 Gy, respectively. The maximum target dose (defined as the greatest dose in target volume delivered to an area greater than

2 cm^2) was 50 Gy for the regional lymphatics target volume and 72 Gy for the prostatic boost target volume. The daily doses were 1.8 to 2.0 Gy given 4 to 5 times a week. The 10-year overall survival (43% vs 34%, $P = .12$) and median overall survival (8.7 vs 7.3 years) did not reach statistical significance. However, the 10-year disease-specific mortality (23% vs 36%, $P = .01$), rate of distant metastasis (35% vs 47%, $P = .006$), disease-free survival (DFS) (11% vs 3%, $P<.0001$), and rate of biochemical failure (65% vs 80%, $P<.0001$) favored the EBRT-plus-ADT arm compared with the EBRT-alone arm.[19,20]

The RTOG 92-02 study randomized 1554 patients with T2c-T4, N0 prostate cancer to receive EBRT plus 4 months of neoadjuvant/concurrent ADT (short-term androgen deprivation) versus EBRT plus 2 years of neoadjuvant/concurrent/adjuvant ADT (long-term androgen deprivation [LTAD]). The prostate was to receive 65 to 70 Gy for T2c tumors and 67.5 to 70.0 Gy for T3 to T4 tumors, at 1.8 to 2.0 Gy per day. The regional lymphatics were to receive 44 to 46 Gy in 1.8- to 2.0-Gy fractions. Higher doses, up to 50.0 Gy, were permitted. The 10-year overall survival was not statistically different for the intent-to-treat population (52% vs 54%, $P = .36$) but was improved in a post hoc subset analysis of patients with Gleason 8 to 10 cancer (32% vs 45%, $P = .0061$). There were statistically significant improvements in 10-year DFS (13% vs 23%, $P<.0001$), disease-specific survival (84% vs 89%, $P = .0042$), local progression (22% vs 12%, $P<.0001$), distant metastasis (23% vs 15%, $P<.0001$), and biochemical failure (68% vs 52%, $P<.0001$) favoring the EBRT-plus-LTAD arm.[21,22]

The EORTC 22,863 study comparing EBRT versus EBRT plus 3 years of ADT in 415 patients with T1–2 high-grade or T3–4 prostate cancer showed statistically significant improvements in 5-year overall survival (62% vs 78%, $P = .0002$), DFS (40% vs 74%, $P = .0001$), disease-specific survival (79% vs 94%, $P = .0001$), locoregional failures (16% vs 2%, $P<.0001$), and distant metastasis (29% vs 10%, $P<.0001$), all favoring the EBRT-plus-ADT arm.[23] Patients were treated once a day, 5 days a week, for 7 weeks; the first planning target volume was irradiated up to 50 Gy and the second received an additional 20 Gy. At the 10-year follow-up, the differences remained statistically significant. Comparing the EBRT alone and EBRT-plus-LTADT arms, the 10-year clinical DFS was 22.7% versus 47.7% (HR 0.42, 95% CI 0.33–0.55, $P<.0001$), 10-year overall survival was 39.8% versus 58.1% (HR 0.60, 95% CI 0.45–0.80, $P = .0004$), and 10-year prostate-cancer mortality was 30.4% versus 10.3% (HR 0.38, 95% CI 0.24–0.60, $P<.0001$). Moreover, there was no significant increase in late cardiovascular toxicity in the EBRT plus long-term ADT arm compared with the EBRT-alone arm.[26]

The follow-up on the EORTC study, EORTC 22961, compared radiotherapy and short-term (6 months) versus long-term (3 years) androgen suppression in patients with locally advanced prostate cancer (T1c-T2b, N1 or N2; or T2c-T4, N0-N2). A total of 970 patients who had received EBRT plus 6 months of ADT were randomized to receive no further treatment (short-term suppression) or 2.5 years of further treatment with a luteinizing hormone-releasing hormone agonist (long-term suppression). Treatment was provided once a day, 5 days a week, for 7 weeks at a dose of 50 Gy for the first planned target volume and an additional dose of 20 Gy for the second planned target volume. The 5-year overall mortality for short-term and long-term suppression was 19.0% and 15.2%, respectively (HR 1.42, upper 95.71% confidence limit 1.79, $P = .65$ for noninferiority).[27] Also, the group reported the 2-sided 95.71% CI of 1.09 to 1.85 is a post hoc indication that short-term suppression was inferior, for overall survival, to long-term suppression in this high-risk group. Longer-term follow-up is awaited.

The results of a randomized, multicenter, phase III study assessing the duration of androgen blockade combined with pelvic irradiation in high-risk (T3 or T4, Gleason

Table 3
Adjuvant ADT in combination with RT

Study	RTOG 85-31 (Pilepich)	RTOG 86-10 (Pilepich, Roach)	RTOG 92-02 (Horwitz)	EORTC 22863 (Bolla)
Design	EBRT + adjuvant ADT vs EBRT + salvage ADT (65–70 Gy if no prior RP, 60–65 Gy if prior RP)	EBRT alone vs EBRT + ST ADT (65–72 Gy)	EBRT plus ST (4 mo) vs LT ADT (2 y) (65–70 Gy)	EBRT alone vs EBRT + LT ADT (3 y) (70 Gy)
	Adjuvant — Salvage	EBRT alone — EBRT + ST ADT	ST ADT — LT ADT	EBRT alone — EBRT + LT ADT
Median Biochemical PFS (y)	Not reached — Not reported; PFS at 10 y, 37% vs 23% (P<.0001)	Not reported — Not reported; PFS at 10 y, 11.2% vs 3.4% (P<.0001) HR 1.97 (95% CI 1.61–2.42)	2.5[a] — 7.5[a]; PFS at 10 y, 13% vs 23% (P<.0001)	Not reported — Not reported; Median clinical PFS 4[a] y vs 9[a] y, clinical PFS at 10 y, 23% vs 48% (P<.0001), HR 0.42 (95% CI 0.33–0.55)
Median DSS (y)	Not reached — Not reached; DSS at 10 y, 84% vs 78% (P = .0052)	Not reached — Not reached; DSS at 10 y, 77% vs 64% (P = .01), HR 1.52 (95% CI 1.09–2.13)	Not reached — Not reached; DSS at 10 y, 84% vs 89% (P = .0042), HR 0.657 (95% CI 0.504–0.857)	Not reached — Not reached; DSS at 10 y, 70% vs 90% (P<.0001), HR 0.38 (95% CI 0.24–0.60)
Median OS (y)	10[a] — 8[a]; OS at 10 y, 49% vs 39% (P = .002)	7.3 — 8.7 (NS); OS at 10 y, 43% vs 34% (P = .12), HR 1.05 (95% CI 0.84–1.31)	Not reached — Not reached; OS at 10 y, 52% vs 54% (P = .36), HR 0.922 (95% CI 0.904–1.057)	7[a] — 11[a]; OS at 10 y, 40% vs 58% (P = .0004), HR 0.60 (95% CI 0.45–0.80)

Study	EORTC 22961 (Bolla)	D'Amico 2008	TROG 96.01 (Denham)
Design	EBRT plus ST (6 mo) vs LT ADT (3 y) ADT (70 Gy)	EBRT alone vs EBRT + ST (6 mo) ADT	EBRT alone vs EBRT + 3 mo ADT vs EBRT + 6 mo
	ST ADT — LT ADT	EBRT alone — EBRT + ST ADT	EBRT alone — EBRT + 3 mo ADT — EBRT + 6 mo ADT

	Study (5 y)	Study (8 y)	Study (10 y, ADT)
Median Biochemical PFS (y)	Not reported. Median *clinical* PFS 7.5 y vs not reached, clinical PFS at 5 y, 69% vs 80%, HR 1.77 (95% CI 1.4–2.24)	Not reported	Not reported. Cumulative PSA progression at 10 y, 73.8% RT alone vs 60.4% 3-mo ADT (HR 0.72, 95% CI 0.57–0.90, P = .003) vs 52.3% 6-mo ADT (HR 0.57, 95% CI 0.46–1.72, P<.0001)
Median DSS (y)	Not reached. DSS at 5 y, 95% vs 98% (P = .002), HR 1.71 (95% CI 1.14–2.57)	Not reached. DSS at 8 y, 87% vs 96% (P = .01), HR 4.1 (95% CI 1.4–12.1)	Not reached. DSS at 10 y, 11.4% RT alone vs 18.9% 3-mo ADT (HR 0.86, 95% CI 0.60–1.23, P = .398) vs 22% 6-mo ADT (HR 0.49, 95% CI 0.32–0.74, P = .008)
Median OS (y)	Not reached. OS at 5 y, 81% vs 85% (NS), HR 1.42 (95% CI 1.09–1.85)	9[a]. OS at 8 y, 61% vs 74% (P = .01), HR 1.8 (95% CI 1.1–2.9)	12[a]. OS at 10 y, 29.2% RT alone vs 36.7% 3-mo ADT (HR 0.84, 95% CI 0.65–1.08, P = .18) vs 42.5% 6-mo ADT (HR 0.63, 95% CI 0.48–0.83, P = .008).

Study		RTOG 94-08 (Jones)
Design	EBRT alone vs EBRT plus ST (4 mo); EBRT alone	EBRT + ST ADT
Median Biochemical PFS (y)	Not reported	Biochemical failure at 10 y, 41% RT alone vs 26% RT + ST ADT (HR 1.74, 95% CI 1.48–2.04, P<.001)
Median DSS (y)	Not reached	DSS at 10 y, 92% RT alone vs 96% RT + ST ADT (HR 1.87, 95% CI 1.27–2.74, P = .001)
Median OS (y)		11.8[a]. OS at 10 y, 38% RT alone vs 43% RT + ST ADT (HR 1.17, 95% CI 1.01–1.35, P = .03)

Abbreviations: DSS, disease-specific survival; LT, long-term; NS, not statistically significant; RP, radical prostatectomy; RTOG, The Radiation Therapy Oncology Group; ST, short-term.

[a] Data not reported in primary article and estimated from available survival curves.

8–10, or PSA >20 ng/mL) prostate cancers (ClinicalTrials.gov, identifier NCT00223171) was recently presented at the 2013 American Society of Clinical Oncology (ASCO) Genitourinary Cancers Symposium. In this study, 630 patients were randomized to either 18 months or 36 months of androgen deprivation therapy and all had 70 Gy of radiation. At a median follow-up of 77 months, 71 of 310 patients (22.9%) in the 36-month arm and 76 of 320 (23.8%) in the 18-month arm had died ($P = .802$). There were no significant differences in the rates of biochemical, regional, or distant failure between arms.[28]

D'Amico and colleagues[24] completed a study of EBRT versus EBRT plus 6 months of ADT in 206 patients with T1–4, N0 prostate cancer with at least one unfavorable prognostic feature (PSA >10 ng/mL, Gleason ≥7, T3a or T3b disease by magnetic resonance imaging) and found an increased overall survival in the EBRT-plus-ADT arm among patients with no or minimal comorbidities (HR 4.2, $P<.001$) but not among patients with moderate or severe comorbidities (HR 0.54, $P = .08$).

The TROG (Trans-Tasman Radiation Oncology Group) 96.01 trial evaluated 3-month and 6-month short-term neoadjuvant ADT in patients with locally advanced prostate cancer (T2b, T2c, T3, and T4 N0 M0). Between 1996 and 2000, 818 men were randomized to receive radiotherapy alone, radiotherapy with 3 months of ADT, or radiotherapy with 6 months of ADT. The radiotherapy dose for all groups was 66 Gy, delivered to the prostate and seminal vesicles (excluding pelvic nodes) in 33 fractions of 2 Gy per day. Neoadjuvant ADT consisted of goserelin given monthly and 250 mg flutamide given orally 3 times a day, beginning 2 months before radiotherapy for the 3-month group and 5 months before radiotherapy for the 6-month group. Primary end points were prostate cancer–specific mortality and all-cause mortality. Compared with radiotherapy alone, 3-month ADT had no effect on distant progression (HR 0.89, CI 0.60–1.31, $P = .550$), prostate cancer–specific mortality (HR 0.86, CI 0.60–1.23, $P = .398$), or all-cause mortality (HR 0.84, CI 0.65–1.08, $P = .180$). However, 6-month ADT demonstrated decreased distant progression (HR 0.49, CI 0.31–0.6, $P = .001$), prostate cancer–specific mortality (HR 0.49, CI 0.32–0.74, $P = .0008$), and all-cause mortality (HR 0.63, CI 0.48–0.83, $P = .0008$) compared with radiotherapy alone.[29]

The RTOG 94-08 study evaluated radiotherapy alone versus radiotherapy plus 4 months of neoadjuvant ADT, starting 2 months before radiotherapy, in patients with low- and intermediate-risk (T1b–T2b prostate cancer and PSA <20 mg/mL) prostate cancer. Radiotherapy, administered in daily 1.8-Gy fractions, consisted of 46.8 Gy delivered to the pelvis (prostate and regional lymph nodes), followed by 19.8 Gy to the prostate, for a total dose of 66.6 Gy. Between 1994 and 2001, 1979 patients were randomized with overall survival as the end point. The 10-year rate of overall survival was 62% in the RT-plus-short-term-ADT arm and 57% in the RT-alone arm (HR 1.17, $P = .03$).[30]

From these studies, it seems that for cancer-specific survival, at least 6 months of ADT is needed for a survival benefit in patients with intermediate-risk disease and treatment to 66.6 Gy. For higher-risk disease with 65 to 70 Gy used, 24 and 36 months have been shown to possibly be better than 4 and 6 months. More recently, the study of 18 months versus 36 months of ADT using 70 Gy has suggested 18 months may be clinically similar to 36 months. Prolonged duration of ADT needs to be balanced with the adverse effects of ADT.

The benefit of short-term ADT versus long-term ADT in the contemporary era of being able to deliver high-dose RT (HDRT) is still being investigated. RTOG 94-06 was a phase I/II trial evaluating dose-escalated 3-dimensional conformal RT to treat men with clinically localized (T1–T3) prostate cancer, with a primary objective to establish the maximum tolerated dose of RT that can be delivered safely to the prostate gland and surrounding tissue. In this study, some patients also received neo-adjuvant and/or adjuvant ADT at the treating investigators' discretion.[31–33] Data from this radiation dose-escalation study were used in a post hoc subset analysis to evaluate the bNED and DFS in men receiving HDRT of greater than 73.8 Gy. This analysis was carried out by stratifying the outcome into risk groups and hormone therapy use. When the patients were stratified by risk groups (and after adjusting for pretreatment PSA, biopsy Gleason score, and T stage), there was not a significant effect on bNED or DFS from the addition of hormone therapy to HDRT. bNED and DFS did approach significance in the high-risk patient subgroup.[34] Prospective studies are needed to fully evaluate the duration of adjuvant ADT in the era of HDRT.

ADJUVANT CHEMOTHERAPY

Chemotherapy alone, and in combination with RT and/or ADT, has been evaluated in numerous (mostly phase II, single arm) clinical trials in the neoadjuvant and adjuvant settings for high-risk prostate cancer.

In the neoadjuvant setting, many trials evaluated docetaxel or paclitaxel either as monotherapy or in combination with hormone therapy. Although there were definite decreases in PSA noted, the incidence of pathologic complete responses was generally very low. Depending on the combinations studied, some trials revealed a markedly increased incidence of severe toxicities, whereas others showed reasonable tolerability.[35–41]

In the adjuvant setting, the largest prospective adjuvant chemotherapy trial was the SWOG S9921 trial, which evaluated mitoxantrone plus ADT versus ADT alone. However, as noted previously, accrual to this study was halted after determination of 3 cases of acute myelogenous leukemia in the mitoxantrone arm.[11] The survival results are not expected to be reported until 2015 based on the current event rate. In a French study of 47 patients with high-risk prostate cancer who were randomized to receive 3 years of adjuvant ADT alone versus ADT plus adjuvant paclitaxel (100 mg/m^2 weekly for 8 weeks), the preliminary results showed that the combination was feasible, reasonably tolerated, and did not adversely affect quality of life. Survival data for this study are not yet mature.[42]

To date, there have been no trials demonstrating a survival benefit of neoadjuvant or adjuvant chemotherapy; therefore, its use in this setting is still investigational. However, there are numerous trials evaluating the role of neoadjuvant/adjuvant chemotherapy. One such trial is a phase III clinical trial investigating the role of neoadjuvant ADT in combination with docetaxel before radical prostatectomy versus surgery alone in patients with clinically localized high-risk prostate cancer (also known as Cancer and Leukemia Group B 90203, PUNCH [Preoperative Use of Neoadjuvant ChemoHormonal Therapy], ClinicalTrials.gov, identifier NCT00430183). Other trials include a phase I study of cabazitaxel and adjuvant radiation in stage 3 prostate cancer after prostatectomy (ClinicalTrials.gov, identifier NCT01650285); a phase II study of neoadjuvant cabazitaxel and ADT followed by salvage surgery for high-risk PSA failure with biopsy-proven recurrence after initial definitive radiotherapy (ClinicalTrials.gov, identifier NCT01531205); a phase II study of EBRT and 6-month androgen suppression with or without docetaxel in patients with high-risk localized or locally advanced prostate cancer (ClinicalTrials.gov, identifier NCT00116142); the phase III GETUG (Groupe D'Etude des Tumeurs Uro-Genitales) 12 trial of adjuvant hormonal therapy with and without docetaxel and estramustine in patients with advanced prostate cancer or with a high risk of relapse (ClinicalTrials.gov, identifier NCT00055731); and the Veterans

Affairs Cooperative Study 553 designed to evaluate early adjuvant docetaxel versus standard of care for postprostatectomy patients who are at a high risk of relapse (pT3b or T4, pT3a and Gleason ≥7, pT2 with positive surgical margins and Gleason 8–10, or PSA >20 ng/mL [ClinicalTrials.gov, identifier NCT00132301]).

NEOADJUVANT AND ADJUVANT APPROACHES WITH NEW HORMONAL AGENTS

Abiraterone acetate, an androgen biosynthesis inhibitor, is currently approved for metastatic castrate resistant prostate cancer (mCRPC), both in the predocetaxel and postdocetaxel setting. In the phase III, randomized, double blind, placebo-controlled COU-AA-302 study of 1088 patients with mCRPC without previous chemotherapy, abiraterone acetate was associated with improved radiographic PFS (16.5 months vs 8.3 months, HR 0.53, 95% CI 0.45–0.62, P<.001) and a trend toward improved overall survival (median not reached vs 27.2 months, HR 0.75, 95% CI 0.61–0.93, P = .01).[43] In the phase III COU-AA-301 study of 1195 patients with mCRPC with progression after docetaxel therapy, abiraterone acetate significantly prolonged the overall survival compared with placebo (15.8 months vs 11.2 months, HR 0.74, 95% CI 0.64–0.86, P<.0001).[44] There is an ongoing phase II trial evaluating the role of neoadjuvant abiraterone acetate plus ADT versus ADT alone in men with localized high-risk prostate cancer on the effects of serum and prostate tissue androgen levels (ClinicalTrials.gov, identifier NCT00924469). Results of the secondary end points of PSA and pathologic complete response (pCR) rates were presented at the 2012 ASCO Annual Meeting. Neoadjuvant ADT plus abiraterone acetate was associated with higher and earlier PSA (<0.2) declines compared with ADT alone. A pCR or near pCR was seen in 10 of 29 (34%) patients after 24 weeks of neoadjuvant ADT plus abiraterone acetate was (34%). After 12 weeks of combined treatment, pCR/near pCR was seen in 4 of 27 (15%) patients.[45] A similar study of neoadjuvant abiraterone acetate plus ADT versus ADT alone, with a primary end point of change in pathologic stage is also underway (ClinicalTrials.gov, identifier NCT01088529).

Enzalutamide is an antiandrogen that targets multiple steps in the androgen receptor signaling pathway. Enzalutamide is currently approved for the treatment of mCRPC in the postdocetaxel setting. In the AFFIRM (A Safety and Efficacy Study of MDV3100 in Patients With Castration-Resistant Prostate Cancer Who Have Been Previously Treated With Docetaxel-based Chemotherapy) trial, 1199 men with castrate-resistant disease that was progressive after chemotherapy were randomized to receive enzalutamide in a 2:1 fashion. Enzalutamide exhibited superior overall survival compared with placebo (18.4 months vs 13.6 months, HR 0.63, 95% CI 0.53–0.75, P<.001) as well as the proportion of patients with PSA reduction by 50% or more (54% vs 2%, P<.001), soft tissue response rate (29% vs 4%, P<.001), time to PSA progression (8.3 months vs 3 months, HR 0.25, P<.001), radiographic PFS (8.3 months vs 2.9 months, HR 0.40, P<.001), and time to the first skeletal-related event (16.7 months vs 13.3 months, HR 0.69, P<.001).[46] The PREVAIL (A Safety and Efficacy Study of Oral MDV3100 in Chemotherapy-Naive Patients With Progressive Metastatic Prostate Cancer) trial evaluates enzalutamide in patients with mCRPC in the prechemotherapy setting (ClinicalTrials.gov, identifier NCT01212991). Accrual to this trial has completed, but mature data are not yet available. Evaluation of enzalutamide in the neoadjuvant setting is under way. There is an ongoing phase II trial comparing 6 months of neoadjuvant use of enzalutamide alone or in combination with leuprolide and dutasteride in patients with localized prostate cancer looking at a primary end point of the pathologic response rate (ClinicalTrials.gov, identifier NCT01547299).

An ongoing phase III trial is investigating the role of enhanced androgen suppression with the addition of orteronel (TAK-700), a CYP17A1 inhibitor that blocks androgen synthesis, in patients undergoing definitive RT and neoadjuvant/concurrent/adjuvant ADT for high-risk localized prostate cancer. This study will enroll 900 patients who will be randomized to receive dose-escalated RT and 2 years of ADT (GNRH agonist plus antiandrogen) with or without 2 years of orteronel (ClinicalTrials.gov, identifier NCT01546987). The Medical Reserve Council's (MRC) Systemic Therapy in Advancing or Metastatic Prostate Cancer: Evaluation of Drug Efficacy (STAMPEDE) study has a cohort of ADT plus radiation with or without abiraterone.

The success of the newer hormonal agents in metastatic castrate-resistant disease has spurred much interest in evaluating the role of these agents much earlier in the treatment of prostate cancer. Any potential benefit of neoadjuvant and adjuvant therapies for prostate cancer will have to be balanced with the expected and significant side effects of ADT and the potential impacts on quality of life.

FUTURE DIRECTIONS

The development and validation of predictive biomarkers of response to ADT may be one strategy to optimize the benefit and minimize the harm to patients with localized high-risk prostate cancer. The mechanisms that promote androgen receptor reactivation are being identified and may help in the selection of appropriate therapeutic research and intervention.[47] Potential novel predictors of ADT response may be found in somatic alterations in androgen receptor (AR) pathway genes, which influence AR activity or in germline variants in androgen-AR axis genes.[48] There has also been some preliminary work done to evaluate predictive markers of response to adjuvant chemotherapy. Antonarakis and colleagues[49] performed a post hoc analysis examining PTEN and other protein markers in primary tumors of patients with high-risk prostate cancer who participated in the TAX2501 adjuvant docetaxel trial. PTEN loss was observed in 61% of patients and was associated with lower preoperative PSA levels, higher clinical stage, low Ki67 expression, and presence of p53 and ERG. In a multivariate analysis, PTEN loss (P = .035), MYC expression (P = .001), and Ki67 expression ($P<.001$) emerged as independent prognostic factors for PFS in these patients with high-risk prostate cancer who received docetaxel after prostatectomy.[49]

The role of adjuvant ADT in the setting of postoperative RT is best established. Further exploration and patient selection is needed to better define the roles of ADT alone, androgen-AR axis modifications, and chemotherapy in the adjuvant setting and, it is hoped, to decrease the number of men who relapse and get salvage therapy and, more importantly, decrease the number of men who die of prostate cancer after localized therapy.

REFERENCES

1. Siegel R, Naishadham D, Jemal A. Cancer statistics, 2012. CA Cancer J Clin 2012;62:10–29.
2. Carver BS, Bianco FJ Jr, Scardino PT, et al. Long-term outcome following radical prostatectomy in men with clinical stage T3 prostate cancer. J Urol 2006;176: 564–8.
3. Thompson IM, Tangen CM, Paradelo J, et al. Adjuvant radiotherapy for pathological T3N0M0 prostate cancer significantly reduces risk of metastases and improves survival: long-term followup of a randomized clinical trial. J Urol 2009; 181:956–62.

4. Swanson GP, Goldman B, Tangen CM, et al. The prognostic impact of seminal vesicle involvement found at prostatectomy and the effects of adjuvant radiation: data from Southwest Oncology Group 8794. J Urol 2008;180:2453–7 [discussion: 2458].

5. Van der Kwast TH, Bolla M, Van Poppel H, et al. Identification of patients with prostate cancer who benefit from immediate postoperative radiotherapy: EORTC 22911. J Clin Oncol 2007;25:4178–86.

6. Roehl KA, Han M, Ramos CG, et al. Cancer progression and survival rates following anatomical radical retropubic prostatectomy in 3,478 consecutive patients: long-term results. J Urol 2004;172:910–4.

7. Shelley MD, Kumar S, Coles B, et al. Adjuvant hormone therapy for localised and locally advanced prostate carcinoma: a systematic review and meta-analysis of randomised trials. Cancer Treat Rev 2009;35:540–6.

8. Messing EM, Manola J, Yao J, et al. Immediate versus deferred androgen deprivation treatment in patients with node-positive prostate cancer after radical prostatectomy and pelvic lymphadenectomy. Lancet Oncol 2006;7:472–9.

9. Pound CR, Partin AW, Eisenberger MA, et al. Natural history of progression after PSA elevation following radical prostatectomy. JAMA 1999;281:1591–7.

10. Wong YN, Freedland S, Egleston B, et al. Role of androgen deprivation therapy for node-positive prostate cancer. J Clin Oncol 2009;27:100–5.

11. Dorff TB, Flaig TW, Tangen CM, et al. Adjuvant androgen deprivation for high-risk prostate cancer after radical prostatectomy: SWOG S9921 study. J Clin Oncol 2011;29:2040–5.

12. Wirth MP, Weissbach L, Marx FJ, et al. Prospective randomized trial comparing flutamide as adjuvant treatment versus observation after radical prostatectomy for locally advanced, lymph node-negative prostate cancer. Eur Urol 2004;45: 267–70 [discussion: 270].

13. See WA, Wirth MP, McLeod DG, et al. Bicalutamide as immediate therapy either alone or as adjuvant to standard care of patients with localized or locally advanced prostate cancer: first analysis of the early prostate cancer program. J Urol 2002;168:429–35.

14. Iversen P, McLeod DG, See WA, et al. Antiandrogen monotherapy in patients with localized or locally advanced prostate cancer: final results from the bicalutamide Early Prostate Cancer programme at a median follow-up of 9.7 years. BJU Int 2010;105:1074–81.

15. Bolla M, van Poppel H, Tombal B, et al. Postoperative radiotherapy after radical prostatectomy for high-risk prostate cancer: long-term results of a randomised controlled trial (EORTC trial 22911). Lancet 2012;380:2018–27.

16. Thompson IM Jr, Tangen CM, Paradelo J, et al. Adjuvant radiotherapy for pathologically advanced prostate cancer: a randomized clinical trial. JAMA 2006;296: 2329–35.

17. Wiegel T, Bottke D, Steiner U, et al. Phase III postoperative adjuvant radiotherapy after radical prostatectomy compared with radical prostatectomy alone in pT3 prostate cancer with postoperative undetectable prostate-specific antigen: ARO 96-02/AUO AP 09/95. J Clin Oncol 2009;27:2924–30.

18. Wiegel T, Bottke D, Bartkowiak D, et al. Phase III results of adjuvant radiotherapy (RT) versus wait-and-see (WS) in patients with pT3 prostate cancer following radical prostatectomy (RP) (ARO 96–02/AUO AP 09/95): ten years follow-up. J Clin Oncol 2013;31(Suppl 6) [abstract: 4].

19. Pilepich MV, Winter K, John MJ, et al. Phase III radiation therapy oncology group (RTOG) trial 86-10 of androgen deprivation adjuvant to definitive radiotherapy in

locally advanced carcinoma of the prostate. Int J Radiat Oncol Biol Phys 2001;50: 1243–52.

20. Roach M 3rd, Bae K, Speight J, et al. Short-term neoadjuvant androgen deprivation therapy and external-beam radiotherapy for locally advanced prostate cancer: long-term results of RTOG 8610. J Clin Oncol 2008;26:585–91.

21. Hanks GE, Pajak TF, Porter A, et al. Phase III trial of long-term adjuvant androgen deprivation after neoadjuvant hormonal cytoreduction and radiotherapy in locally advanced carcinoma of the prostate: the Radiation Therapy Oncology Group Protocol 92-02. J Clin Oncol 2003;21:3972–8.

22. Horwitz EM, Bae K, Hanks GE, et al. Ten-year follow-up of radiation therapy oncology group protocol 92-02: a phase III trial of the duration of elective androgen deprivation in locally advanced prostate cancer. J Clin Oncol 2008; 26:2497–504.

23. Bolla M, Collette L, Blank L, et al. Long-term results with immediate androgen suppression and external irradiation in patients with locally advanced prostate cancer (an EORTC study): a phase III randomised trial. Lancet 2002;360:103–6.

24. D'Amico AV, Chen MH, Renshaw AA, et al. Androgen suppression and radiation vs radiation alone for prostate cancer: a randomized trial. JAMA 2008;299: 289–95.

25. Pilepich MV, Winter K, Lawton CA, et al. Androgen suppression adjuvant to definitive radiotherapy in prostate carcinoma–long-term results of phase III RTOG 85-31. Int J Radiat Oncol Biol Phys 2005;61:1285–90.

26. Bolla M, Van Tienhoven G, Warde P, et al. External irradiation with or without long-term androgen suppression for prostate cancer with high metastatic risk: 10-year results of an EORTC randomised study. Lancet Oncol 2010;11:1066–73.

27. Bolla M, de Reijke TM, Van Tienhoven G, et al. Duration of androgen suppression in the treatment of prostate cancer. N Engl J Med 2009;360:2516–27.

28. Nabid A, Carrier N, Martin A, et al. High-risk prostate cancer treated with pelvic radiotherapy and 36 versus 18 months of androgen blockade: results of a phase III randomized study. J Clin Oncol 2013;31(Suppl 18):LBA4510.

29. Denham JW, Steigler A, Lamb DS, et al. Short-term neoadjuvant androgen deprivation and radiotherapy for locally advanced prostate cancer: 10-year data from the TROG 96.01 randomised trial. Lancet Oncol 2011;12:451–9.

30. Jones CU, Hunt D, McGowan DG, et al. Radiotherapy and short-term androgen deprivation for localized prostate cancer. N Engl J Med 2011;365:107–18.

31. Michalski JM, Winter K, Purdy JA, et al. Toxicity after three-dimensional radiotherapy for prostate cancer with RTOG 9406 dose level IV. Int J Radiat Oncol Biol Phys 2004;58:735–42.

32. Ryu JK, Winter K, Michalski JM, et al. Interim report of toxicity from 3D conformal radiation therapy (3D-CRT) for prostate cancer on 3DOG/RTOG 9406, level III (79.2 Gy). Int J Radiat Oncol Biol Phys 2002;54:1036–46.

33. Michalski JM, Bae K, Roach M, et al. Long-term toxicity following 3D conformal radiation therapy for prostate cancer from the RTOG 9406 phase I/II dose escalation study. Int J Radiat Oncol Biol Phys 2010;76:14–22.

34. Valicenti RK, Bae K, Michalski J, et al. Does hormone therapy reduce disease recurrence in prostate cancer patients receiving dose-escalated radiation therapy? An analysis of Radiation Therapy Oncology Group 94-06. Int J Radiat Oncol Biol Phys 2011;79:1323–9.

35. Rosenthal SA, Bae K, Pienta KJ, et al. Phase III multi-institutional trial of adjuvant chemotherapy with paclitaxel, estramustine, and oral etoposide combined with long-term androgen suppression therapy and radiotherapy versus long-term

androgen suppression plus radiotherapy alone for high-risk prostate cancer: preliminary toxicity analysis of RTOG 99-02. Int J Radiat Oncol Biol Phys 2009;73:672–8.

36. Patel AR, Sandler HM, Pienta KJ. Radiation Therapy Oncology Group 0521: a phase III randomized trial of androgen suppression and radiation therapy versus androgen suppression and radiation therapy followed by chemotherapy with docetaxel/prednisone for localized, high-risk prostate cancer. Clin Genitourin Cancer 2005;4:212–4.

37. Kumar P, Perrotti M, Weiss R, et al. Phase I trial of weekly docetaxel with concurrent three-dimensional conformal radiation therapy in the treatment of unfavorable localized adenocarcinoma of the prostate. J Clin Oncol 2004;22:1909–15.

38. Perrotti M, Doyle T, Kumar P, et al. Phase I/II trial of docetaxel and concurrent radiation therapy in localized high risk prostate cancer (AGUSG 03-10). Urol Oncol 2008;26:276–80.

39. Sanfilippo NJ, Taneja SS, Chachoua A, et al. Phase I/II study of biweekly paclitaxel and radiation in androgen-ablated locally advanced prostate cancer. J Clin Oncol 2008;26:2973–8.

40. Hussain M, Smith DC, El-Rayes BF, et al. Neoadjuvant docetaxel and estramustine chemotherapy in high-risk/locally advanced prostate cancer. Urology 2003; 61:774–80.

41. Hirano D, Nagane Y, Satoh K, et al. Neoadjuvant LHRH analog plus estramustine phosphate combined with three-dimensional conformal radiotherapy for intermediate- to high-risk prostate cancer: a randomized study. Int Urol Nephrol 2010;42: 81–8.

42. Ploussard G, Paule B, Salomon L, et al. Pilot trial of adjuvant paclitaxel plus androgen deprivation for patients with high-risk prostate cancer after radical prostatectomy: results on toxicity, side effects and quality-of-life. Prostate Cancer Prostatic Dis 2010;13:97–101.

43. Ryan CJ, Smith MR, de Bono JS, et al. Abiraterone in metastatic prostate cancer without previous chemotherapy. N Engl J Med 2013;368:138–48.

44. Fizazi K, Scher HI, Molina A, et al. Abiraterone acetate for treatment of metastatic castration-resistant prostate cancer: final overall survival analysis of the COU-AA-301 randomised, double-blind, placebo-controlled phase 3 study. Lancet Oncol 2012;13:983–92.

45. Taplin ME, Montgomery RB, Logothetis C, et al. Effect of neoadjuvant abiraterone acetate (AA) plus leuprolide acetate (LHRHa) on PSA, pathological complete response (pCR), and near pCR in localized high-risk prostate cancer (LHRPC): results of a randomized phase II study. J Clin Oncol 2012;30(Suppl) [abstract 4521].

46. Scher HI, Fizazi K, Saad F, et al. Increased survival with enzalutamide in prostate cancer after chemotherapy. N Engl J Med 2012;367:1187–97.

47. Knudsen KE, Kelly WK. Outsmarting androgen receptor: creative approaches for targeting aberrant androgen signaling in advanced prostate cancer. Expert Rev Endocrinol Metab 2011;6:483–93.

48. Kohli M, Qin R, Jimenez R, et al. Biomarker-based targeting of the androgen-androgen receptor axis in advanced prostate cancer. Adv Urol 2012;2012: 781459.

49. Antonarakis ES, Keizman D, Zhang Z, et al. An immunohistochemical signature comprising PTEN, MYC, and Ki67 predicts progression in prostate cancer patients receiving adjuvant docetaxel after prostatectomy. Cancer 2012;118: 6063–71.

Management of Patients with Biochemical Recurrence After Local Therapy for Prostate Cancer

Channing J. Paller, MD, Emmanuel S. Antonarakis, MD,
Mario A. Eisenberger, MD, Michael A. Carducci, MD*

KEYWORDS

- Rising prostate-specific antigen • Prostate cancer • Hormonal therapy
- Androgen-deprivation therapy • Biochemical recurrence

KEY POINTS

- Nearly three-quarters of a million American men who have been treated with prostatectomy and/or radiation therapy experience an increasing prostate-specific antigen (PSA) level, a condition known as biochemical recurrence (BCR).
- Post localized therapy, some of these men develop distant metastases with time, but many years may pass before signs of clinical progression appear.
- Although androgen-deprivation therapy remains a reasonable option for some men with BCR, deferring androgen ablation or offering nonhormonal therapies may be appropriate in patients where the risk of clinical/metastatic progression and prostate cancer–specific death is low.
- Drug development in this space is a challenge because of the heterogeneous and prolonged natural history of biochemically recurrent prostate cancer, and the lack of short-term, validated surrogate end points for overall survival.

INTRODUCTION

Approximately 239,000 men will be diagnosed with prostate cancer in 2013, but 88% of these men will ultimately die from ischemic heart disease or other nonprostate cancer causes.[1,2] An estimated 60,000 to 70,000 men are diagnosed in the United States each year with biochemical recurrence (BCR), a state defined as rising prostate-specific antigen (PSA) after radical prostatectomy (RP) or radiation treatment,[3] and overall, three-quarters of a million men are estimated to be living with rising PSA after local therapy without evidence of overt metastatic disease.[4]

Prostate Cancer Research Program, Sidney Kimmel Comprehensive Cancer Center at Johns Hopkins, 1650 Orleans Street, CRB1-1M59, Baltimore, MD 21287, USA
* Corresponding author.
E-mail address: carducci@jhmi.edu

Hematol Oncol Clin N Am 27 (2013) 1205–1219
http://dx.doi.org/10.1016/j.hoc.2013.08.005
0889-8588/13/$ – see front matter © 2013 Elsevier Inc. All rights reserved.
hemonc.theclinics.com

The optimal management of patients with nonmetastatic, hormone-naive, biochemically relapsed prostate cancer remains largely unestablished at this time because of the lack of prospective randomized trials designed to address standards of care.[5] Treatment decisions remain largely intuitive at the present time. Recognizing the deficiency, this article describes a logical risk-based approach for therapeutic considerations and clinical research in this relatively common subset of patients. The approach is based on extensive data on the natural history of these patients at the Johns Hopkins Hospital (JHH). This article discusses this and other existing datasets and defines potential risk-benefit ratios of existing modalities of treatment.

DEFINITION OF BCR

The definition of BCR after local therapy varies based on the primary modality of treatment. After surgery, PSA levels greater than 0.2 ng/mL or greater than 0.4 ng/mL and rising are often considered evidence of BCR.[3] However, in 2007, the American Urological Association (AUA) reported on a review of more than 13,000 citations referencing BCR in patients with prostate cancer and found 54 different definitions of BCR after surgery and 99 different definitions of BCR after radiation therapy (RT).[6] The lack of consistently applied definitions of BCR limits the interpretation of data on natural history and some of the therapeutic considerations in these patients. Such inconsistencies are especially challenging for the interpretation and design of clinical trials.

BCR After RP

Among the 54 definitions of BCR after prostatectomy discovered by the AUA researchers, the most common was a PSA of greater than 0.2 ng/mL or a close variation. The authors, who were also members of the AUA Prostate Guideline Update Panel,[6] recommended that practitioners use a single definition of BCR after RP as follows:

> It is recommended that biochemical (PSA) recurrence following radical prostatectomy be defined as a serum PSA of 0.2 ng/mL or greater, with a second confirmatory level of PSA of >0.2 ng/mL. The first postoperative PSA should be obtained between 6 weeks and 3 months following therapy. The date of failure should be defined as the date of the first detectable PSA level once this value has been confirmed.

In establishing this recommended definition, however, the panel added two caveats. First, the higher levels of PSA (>0.4 ng/mL) would have much greater specificity for clinical and/or radiographic recurrence and progression, but the authors justified the use of 0.2 ng/mL by arguing it had "provided high sensitivity for recurrence as well as the greatest generalizability." Second, this definition is not an effective predictor of death from prostate cancer, suggesting that prognosis should be based on nomograms that consider Gleason score and PSA kinetics, although available nomograms have not been prospectively validated.

The panel acknowledged the appropriateness of reporting biochemical outcomes using additional PSA thresholds. Although some researchers who have designed clinical trials enrolling patients with BCR have adopted this AUA definition,[7] other researchers use 0.4 ng/mL and rising as the eligibility criterion, arguing that the higher value is more specific for future risk of clinical and radiologic progression.[8] For trial purposes, the authors consider PSA levels greater than 0.4 ng/mL and rising as evidence of BCR after surgery.

BCR After RT

The AUA researchers found 99 definitions of BCR after RT, among which the most common was the American Society of Therapeutic Radiology and Oncology (ASTRO) definition: "the mid-point between PSA nadir and the first of three consecutive rises in PSA."[6] Despite a recommendation by the AUA for its adoption, the ASTRO definition is problematic because it requires backdating the time of BCR and because of its failure to use the PSA level at nadir as a risk factor. The Phoenix definition ("nadir + 2 ng/mL, with the failure date defined as the date the rise in PSA is noted") offers greater accuracy in predicting future clinical failures compared with the ASTRO definition.[9–11] However, the Phoenix definition provides substantially lower estimates of BCR at 5 years and substantially higher estimates of BCR at 10 years than the ASTRO definition.[12] The choice of definition can impact the findings of adjuvant treatment trials; the ASTRO definition would be likely to show a greater number of people experiencing BCR after treatment. The AUA retains its recommendation to use the ASTRO definition of BCR after RT alone (no hormonal therapy), whereas the Phoenix definition can be applied after RT with or without hormonal therapy, and avoids the need for backdating. As a result the Phoenix definition has gained wider acceptance in determining BCR for clinical decisions. Patients whose PSA dynamics meet the Phoenix definition and who have evidence of rapid PSA doubling time (PSADT; less than 10 months) may initiate treatment, whereas patients with evidence of slow PSADT may defer further therapy. To ensure comparability with future trial results, it is important to continue to use the Phoenix definition to set criteria for trial entry for patients with BCR after RT.

NATURAL HISTORY OF PATIENTS WITH PROSTATE CANCER EXPERIENCING BCR AFTER SURGERY OR RT

The natural history of patients with prostate cancer at JHH with evidence of BCR after RP has been extensively reported over the past 15 years. In 1999, Pound and colleagues[13] first described the natural history of 304 men who had undergone RP at Johns Hopkins between April 1982 and April 1997, who demonstrated subsequent evidence of BCR (PSA$\geq$0.2 ng/mL), and who did not receive androgen deprivation therapy (ADT) until there was evidence of metastatic disease. The researchers found that the median time from BCR to metastasis in all patients was 8 years and the median time from metastasis to death was 5 years. In this report, time to biochemical progression, pathologic Gleason score, and PSADT were significant predictors of metastasis-free survival (MFS) over 3-, 5-, and 7-year periods. Freedland and colleagues[14] published a study in 2005 describing cancer-specific mortality of the same Johns Hopkins prostate cancer cohort, with 5 additional years of follow-up. Of 379 patients who had experienced BCR, 66 died from prostate cancer, and the overall median survival had not been reached after 16 years. This analysis found that the same three factors—PSADT (<3, 3–8.9, and 9–14.9, and $\geq$15 months), Gleason score ($\leq$7 vs 8–10), and time from surgery to BCR (<3 vs >3 years)—were significant predictors of prostate cancer–specific mortality. In the most recent analysis of this same cohort, Antonarakis and colleagues[15] provided updated information on the natural history and markers predictive of MFS in an expanded cohort of patients from the JHH database including 450 men with BCR after RP, and reported that median overall MFS was 10 years after BCR (**Table 1**). However Antonarakis and colleagues[15] also found that only two of the predictors reported previously were significantly predictive of MFS: PSADT (<3, 3–8.9, and 9–14.9, and $\geq$15 months) and Gleason score (<6 vs 7 vs 8–10) (**Table 2**). In this updated analysis, time to BCR was not a significant predictor of metastasis. Several

Table 1
MFS after PSA recurrence following radical prostatectomy

	Median MFS, y (95% CI)	Metastasis-free Rate at 5 y, % (95% CI)	Metastasis-free Rate at 10 y, % (95% CI)
Pathologic Gleason Score			
8–10	4 (2, 6)	43 (32, 54)	19 (9, 33)
7	11 (9, >17)	71 (63, 78)	52 (41, 62)
4–6	>15 (14, >15)	94 (86, 98)	94 (86, 98)
PSADT			
<3 mo	1 (0, 1)	5 (1, 21)	n/a
3–9 mo	4 (2, 4)	27 (16, 39)	7 (1, 22)
9–15 mo	13 (6, >15)	77 (63, 86)	51 (34, 66)
>15 mo	15 (15, >17)	91 (85, 95)	72 (59, 83)

Abbreviations: CI, confidence interval; MFS, metastasis-free survival.

Data from Antonarakis ES, et al. The natural history of metastatic progression in men with prostate-specific antigen recurrence after radical prostatectomy: long-term follow-up. BJU Int 2012;109:32–9.

other analyses identified PSADT as a primary predictor of MFS and prostate cancer–specific mortality (see **Table 2**).

A study published by Zhou and colleagues[16] in 2005 described the natural history of 498 patients treated with RP at other institutions, including the University of California at San Francisco (the CaPSURE database), military hospitals, and the Virginia Mason Medical Center (the Department of Defense Center for Prostate Disease Research Multicenter National Prostate Cancer Database). Zhou and colleagues[16] reported that only PSADT and not time to BCR or Gleason score were significant predictors of time to prostate cancer–specific mortality. Both continuous and categorical (PSADT <3 vs >3 months) models confirmed these results. Zhou and colleagues also studied 661 patients who had undergone primary RT, and reported that PSADT is a significant predictor of time to prostate cancer–specific mortality for RT patients in the continuous and categorical models. Gleason score was also a significant predictor in the continuous model and in the categorical model for Gleason scores of 8 to 10, but not for lower Gleason scores.

DIAGNOSTIC EVALUATION AFTER PSA RECURRENCE

At this time there are no clear-cut guidelines regarding the frequency of follow-up, PSA determinations, and frequency of imaging procedures. These are dependent on various factors including physicians' routines, patients' requests, and other clinical and comorbid states. The JHH series described previously relied on PSA measurement every 6 months in the first year followed by yearly PSAs and bone scans and physical examinations that included a digital rectal examination. Patients with rapid PSADTs (≤3 months) are seen more frequently than patients with longer PSADTs. At JHH, technetium-99m bone scans and computed tomography scans of the abdomen and pelvis are scheduled annually in patients with PSADT greater than 3 months unless there are symptoms to suggest the need for additional work-up, except for those in clinical trials where the frequency and type of follow-up are determined by the study protocol. Based on clinical history of the patient, evaluation (endorectal magnetic resonance imaging or ultrasound) and possible biopsy of the prostate bed may also be considered if local relapse is suspected on digital rectal examination. Potential treatment objectives and therapeutic options, risk stratified by PSADT, are listed in **Table 3**.

SALVAGE RADIATION FOR BCR

Although adjuvant radiotherapy immediately after RP in patients with high-risk disease has been shown to reduce the risk of BCR in three trials and to lengthen MFS and overall survival in one of the three trials,[17–19] there have been no prospective studies of radiation deferred until BCR, known as salvage radiotherapy.

A retrospective analysis of 1540 patients with prostate cancer in 17 tertiary care hospitals showed that salvage radiation prolonged the time to PSA recurrence in men with lower Gleason (4–7) scores and increased PSADT (>6 months). These men, with more indolent disease, may have local-only recurrence and are those expected to benefit most from salvage radiation. Men with higher Gleason scores and shorter PSADT also benefited from salvage radiation, but to a lesser degree.[20] Paradoxically, a second retrospective study of 635 patients who underwent prostatectomy at JHH suggests that salvage radiotherapy improves prostate cancer–specific survival only in men with PSADT less than 6 months and only if salvage radiotherapy was administered within 2 years from BCR.[21] Although morbidities including gastrointestinal and genitourinary dysfunction are not uncommon with salvage radiotherapy, the incidence of severe toxicities reported was low.[17,22,23] Long-term toxicities include urethral strictures and radiation cystitis in approximately 4% to 8% of patients.[24,25] Based on these studies, salvage radiation is offered to patients who have PSA recurrence after RP, who have the greatest likelihood of benefit.

SALVAGE PROSTATECTOMY POSTRADIATION

Local persistence of prostate cancer is found in 40% to 70% of prostatic biopsies in men who have undergone RT,[26,27] and 30% to 50% of men experience BCR after RT.[28,29] Local disease growth after radiation has been associated with decreased time to metastatic progression and increased prostate cancer–specific mortality[30,31] and may also be associated with urologic morbidity including hematuria, bladder outlet obstruction, and chronic pain.[32] Salvage prostatectomy is the only salvage therapy for radiation failure shown to provide long-term cancer control with a 10-year cancer-specific survival of 70% to 77%.[33,34] The likelihood of benefit from salvage prostatectomy correlates with the original likelihood of cure had surgery been the preferred option. Patients with PSA less than 10 ng/mL show significantly better disease-free progression than patients with higher PSA values.[33] Salvage radiation is indicated only if there is biopsy-proved local recurrence without evidence of nodal or distant metastases. Furthermore, the Gleason score for the repeat biopsy should be the same or lower than the original Gleason score. A negative postradiation biopsy, however, creates clinical uncertainty. Options include clinical trials, ADT, or observation, or more aggressive work-up including endorectal magnetic resonance imaging and/or magnetic resonance spectroscopy, or a repeat biopsy.

Because of fibrosis arising from radiation, a high perioperative morbidity is associated with salvage RP with urinary incontinence rate of 32% and major complications including rectal injury or anastomotic injury in 17% to 32% of cases.[29] High levels of morbidity combined with the challenging nature of the procedure mean that highly experienced surgeons are crucial to success and low morbidity, and the procedure should be considered only for patients without radiographic evidence of metastases, PSA lower than 10 ng/mL, and favorable preradiation characteristics.

Table 2
Selected studies summarizing predictors of the natural history of prostate cancer after biochemical recurrence

Study	N (BCR/Total Number RP and/or RT)	End Point (Number with M1/Number PCSD)	MFS by PSADT Subgroup HR or MFS (95% CI)	PCSM by PSADT Subgroup HR or Mortality (95% CI)	OS by PSADT Subgroup HR (95% CI)	Significant Predictors
Primary treatment: radical prostatectomy						
Pound et al,[13] 1999	304/1997	MFS (103 M1 pts of 304)	PSADT <10 mo predictive of MFS (P<.001)	na	na	PSADT, Gleason score, time to BCR
D'Amico et al,[58] 2003	611/5918	PCSM, OS (154 ACD and 111 PCSD for RT + PR)	na	<3 mo HR 62.9 18.8–210.1) >3 mo HR 0.61 (0.51–0.73)	<3 mo HR 18.2 (8.9–37.2) >3 mo HR 0.84 (0.78–0.90)	PSADT
Freedland et al,[14] 2005	379/na	PCSM (66 PCSD of 379)	na	<3 mo: HR 27.5 (CI, 10.7–70.9) 3–8.9 mo: HR 8.8 (CI, 3.7–20.5) 9–14.9 mo: HR 2.44 (CI, 0.9–6.8) ≥15 mo: HR 1	na	PSADT, Gleason score, time to BCR
Zhou et al,[16] 2005	498/8669 (RT + RP)	PCSM (25 PCSD of 498)	na	<3 mo PCSM 31% (17%–45%) ≥3 mo PCSM 1% (0%–2%)	na	PSADT
Antonarakis et al,[15] 2012	450/na	MFS (134 M1 pts of 450)	Median MFS: <3 mo: 1 mo (CI, 0–1) 3–8.9 mo: 4 mo (CI, 2–4) 9–14.9 mo: 13 mo (CI, 6 to >15) ≥15 mo: 15 mo (CI, 15 to >17)	na	na	PSADT, Gleason score

Antonarakis et al,[59] 2011	346/na	MFS, OS (39 M1 pts of 190 with MFS data) (63 PCSD of 346)	<3 mo: HR 7.77 (CI, 2.65–22.76) 3–8.8 mo: HR 1.95 (CI, 1.04–3.66) ≥9 mo: HR 1	na	<3 mo: HR 27.4 (8.70–86.38) 3–8.8 mo: HR 6.16 (3.00–12.64) ≥9 mo: HR 1	PSADT
Primary treatment: radiotherapy						
D'Amico et al,[60] 2002	94/381	PCSM (20 PCSD of 94)	na	≤12 mo predictive of time to PCSD (P = .003)	PSADT ≤12 mo predictive of time to ACD (P = .02)	PSADT, delayed use of ADT
D'Amico et al,[58] 2003	840/2751	PCSM, OS (154 ACD and 111 PCSD for RT + PR)	na	<3 mo HR 12.2 (7.5–20.1) >3 mo HR 0.83 (0.78–0.87)	<3 mo HR 4.8 (3.4–7) >3 mo HR 0.95 (0.93–0.98)	PSADT
Zhou et al,[16] 2005	661/8669 (RT + RP)	PCSM (77 PCSD of 661)	na	<3 mo PCSM 75% (59%–92%) ≥3 mo PCSM 35% (24–47)	na	PSADT, Gleason score
Buyyounouski et al,[61] 2008	211/1578	MFS, PCSM (53 M1 pts of 211) (29 PCSD on 211)	<3 mo MFS HR 2.87 (P = .001) ≥3 mo MFS HR 1	na	na	IBF alone for PCSM; IBF, Gleason score, PSA nadir, PSADT for MFS

Abbreviations: ACD, any cause death; BCR, biochemical recurrence; DM, distant metastasis; IBF, interval to biochemical failure; M1, metastatic disease; MFS, metastasis-free survival; na, not available; OS, overall survival; PCSD, prostate cancer-specific deaths; PCSM, prostate cancer-specific mortality; PSADT, PSA doubling time; RP, radical prostatectomy; RT, radiation therapy.

Table 3
Potential treatment objectives and therapeutic options for patients risk stratified according to PSADT[14]

	PSADT <9 mo	PSADT ≥ 9 mo
Primary treatment objectives	Prevent progression and increase overall survival	Delay progression while limiting cumulative toxicity
Treatment options	More proactive and early implementation of androgen deprivation; intermittent or continuous based on close monitoring of PSA/PSADT Clinical trials (with more aggressive approaches)	Androgen deprivation, preferably intermittent, used at relatively high thresholds Clinical trials (natural compounds, immunotherapy, antimetastatic, targeted compounds, immunotherapy, and so forth)

HORMONAL THERAPY FOR BIOCHEMICALLY RECURRENT PROSTATE CANCER

The use of hormonal therapy in treating patients with prostate cancer has increased substantially over the past two decades. Between 1990 and 2007, for example, the use of adjuvant ADT has increased threefold to fivefold with brachytherapy and external-beam radiation, and high-risk patients are increasingly receiving multimodal therapy, often including ADT.[35] For patients with evidence of BCR, however, the impact of ADT on overall survival and quality of life remains unestablished primarily because of the lack of data derived from well-designed controlled trials.[25] The evidence available is primarily based on retrospective analyses or extrapolation of studies in distinct patient populations. The CaPSURE database indicates that of 620 men who underwent primary therapy with RP, and of the 430 men who underwent primary therapy with external-beam radiation (during the period 1989–2004), ADT was used as the next salvage therapy for 59% and 93% of the men, respectively.[36]

Early initiation of ADT is associated with a decline of PSA, frequently below detectable levels, and delayed time to metastases.[37,38] The impact of early initiation of ADT in patients without evidence of metastasis on overall survival, prostate cancer–specific survival, and quality of life has not been subjected to randomized controlled trials. In a retrospective review of 248 men who had undergone RT and who experienced BCR and had PSADT less than or equal to 12 months, the use of hormones at time of BCR prolonged MFS. No similar benefit was seen in men with PSADT greater than 12 months.[39] These results were confirmed according to the CaPSURE database from 1988 to 2002.[40] A third large retrospective analysis included men treated with ADT treatment at different PSA levels after RP (adjuvant, PSA of 0.4 ng/mL, PSA of 1 ng/mL, and PSA of 2 ng/mL, and at radiographic progression). Adjuvant ADT treatment was associated with a benefit in cancer-specific survival (98% vs 95%; $P = .009$) but not in overall survival. That benefit of ADT is lost, however, when ADT initiation was triggered by BCR at PSA values of 0.4 or 1 or 2 ng/mL, with nonsignificant trends showing longer time to metastatic disease and better cancer-specific survival for the untreated groups, although that effect may be an artifact of the patient population in the retrospective analysis.[41] No definitive statements can be made based on the retrospective nature of the analyses.

Three ongoing clinical trials are exploring the timing of adjuvant ADT initiation after radiation: Radiation Therapy and Androgen Deprivation Therapy in Treating Patients Who Have Undergone Surgery for Prostate Cancer (NCT00541047); the Australian and New Zealand Timing of Androgen Deprivation trial (NCT00110162); and the

Canadian Early versus Late Androgen Ablation Therapy trial (NCT0043975). These should provide important information regarding the benefits of ADT in patients with BCR.

Continuous Versus Intermittent Administration of ADT

A second decision arises for patients and their physicians who decide to use ADT: whether to administer ADT continuously or to use a cyclical process called intermittent androgen deprivation (IAD). IAD uses ADT treatment until a maximum PSA response is achieved, and then suspends treatment. ADT is reinitiated when the PSA reaches a predetermined level, usually between 4 and 10 ng/mL. Intermittent administration of ADT is used in the hope of prolonging time to castration resistance, decreasing acute and chronic side effects for patients who could be on hormonal therapy for extended periods, and minimizing costs.

Two phase III clinical trials, with a total enrollment of more than 2000 men with biochemically recurrent prostate cancer, have found IAD to be noninferior to continuous androgen deprivation (CAD) with respect to overall survival. A multicenter, international trial randomized 1386 men experiencing BCR after RT (with or without prior RP) into IAD and CAD arms. The IAD arm received 8 months of ADT followed by withdrawal, and then repeated the 8-month cycle when PSA reached greater than or equal to 10 ng/mL. Overall survival for the IAD arm was noninferior to the CAD arm after a median follow-up of 6.9 years. The IAD arm had more prostate cancer–related deaths (122 vs 97 deaths) but fewer noncancer-related deaths (134 vs 146 deaths). Median overall survival was 8.8 years on the IAD arm and 9.1 years on the CAD arm for a hazard ratio (HR) of 1.02 (95% confidence interval [CI], 0.86–1.21). Testosterone levels recovered during each off-treatment period and bone mass loss, hot flashes, fatigue, and erectile dysfunction were reduced, and libido was increased in the IAD arm.[42] Based on the lack of difference in overall survival, lower cost, and improvement in quality of life in the IAD arm, the authors recommend that physicians who choose to administer ADT to patients with BCR use IAD.

A second phase III trial enrolling 425 southern European men with BCR and 191 men with metastatic disease found no difference in overall survival between IAD and CAD. The overall survival HR for the BCR subgroup was 0.86 (95% CI, 0.65–1.14) in favor of CAD but the difference was not significant. For the metastatic subgroup the overall survival HR was 1.26 (95% CI, 0.90–1.78), but was also not significant. Better sexual function was reported by men in the IAD arm; however, this was not reported separately for the BCR subgroup.[43,44] The role of IAD for metastatic disease was also studied using a noninferiority design with 1500 patients (Southwest Oncology Group Study [S9346]). In contrast to the European study, S9346 reported an overall survival advantage of 9.2 years for CAD versus 7.1 years for IAD. However, IAD was not definitively shown to be noninferior to CAD in that study.[34] In sum, the use of IAD is not as well supported in metastatic disease as it is in biochemically recurrent disease and the timing and methodology and patient selection for IAD remain controversial.[45] Further research is exploring the association between ADT outcomes and predictive markers, such as PSADT, which may help guide treatment.[46]

Concerns About Adverse Effects of ADT

Given the long periods of MFS experienced by patients with BCR, they may undergo prolonged treatment with ADT and experience potential long-term side effects. These potential side effects, including sexual dysfunction and loss of libido, memory loss, poor metabolic health,[47,48] cardiovascular disease,[49] fracture risk, and bone loss,[50] are important considerations in the decision-making process on when to initiate

ADT, and whether to use intermittent or continuous ADT. Increased rates of diabetes and cardiovascular disease associated with ADT may be explained, in part, by significantly higher rates of poor metabolic health including insulin resistance experienced by men with BCR and/or metastatic prostate cancer who have been treated with ADT for at least 12 months, compared with age-matched men with BCR not being treated with ADT.[47] This is not surprising because cross-sectional studies have shown that men with low testosterone have higher prevalence of insulin resistance and in some cases metabolic syndrome after controlling for other risk factors.[51]

In 2010, the US Food and Drug Administration asked manufacturers of gonadotropin-releasing hormone (GnRH) agonists to add new warnings to labeling that would alert patients and their health care professionals to the potential risk of heart disease and diabetes in men treated with these medications. A 2006 study by Keating and coworkers[52] confirmed that patients prescribed GnRH agonists experienced increased risk of incident diabetes (adjusted HR, 1.44; $P<.001$); coronary heart disease (adjusted HR, 1.16; $P<.001$); myocardial infarction (adjusted HR, 1.11; $P<.03$); and sudden cardiac death (adjusted HR, 1.16; $P<.004$).

DRUG DEVELOPMENT END POINTS FOR PATIENTS WITH BIOCHEMICALLY RECURRENT PROSTATE CANCER

The heterogeneous and prolonged natural history of BCR and the lack of validated end points make drug development challenging for this patient population. Lengthy and highly variable periods of time before metastasis and death mean that the trials often must last for a decade or more before clinically relevant end points are reached. Although MFS is most likely a clinically relevant end point it has not been shown to be a surrogate for overall survival.[53] Clinical trials comparing no treatment or a placebo with a therapeutic intervention are challenging; most patients and physicians are reluctant to continue protocol-assigned treatment (treatment vs placebo) until metastases develop. Furthermore, researchers are limited by the lack of early biomarkers that are predictive of clinically relevant outcomes. The use of PSA dynamics (eg, PSADT, PSA slope, PSA velocity) is of unestablished clinical significance, and is often highly variable as observed even on placebo arms of trials.[54] In addition, the impact of modulating PSA kinetics on clinically defined end points (eg, MFS) remains uncertain.[55]

Treatment-induced changes in PSADT or other measures of PSA kinetics are even more problematic as end points because of the high variability of these measures. In three separate randomized controlled trials, patients on the placebo arms experienced a significant increase in PSADT: 73% of placebo patients experienced greater than 100% increase in PSADT and 31% experienced greater than 200% in a study of rosiglitazone,[56] 78% of placebo patients experienced a lengthening of PSADT in a study of atrasentan,[57] and 20% of placebo patients experienced greater than 200% increase of PSADT in a study of celecoxib.[7] For trials involving patients with BCR to provide clinically meaningful results, far more information is needed on the natural history and variation of PSADT in that patient population.[54] Despite these challenges, trials in this patient population can provide important information on drug activity, pharmacokinetics, and pharmacodynamics.

The ultimate treatment of patients with BCR is one that delays metastasis and death from prostate cancer without significant morbidities, such as those associated with long-term pharmacologic castration. The long-term impact of shorter courses (6–18 months) of ADT combined with other approaches, such as immunotherapy, antiangiogenesis, or novel hormonal agents, which aim to eradicate micrometastatic disease, are being evaluated. A currently emphasized potential end point is the observation of an undetectable PSA over time after an initial treatment course post-prostatectomy. Although an undetectable PSA has never been shown to be associated with longer MFS or overall survival, this potential end point is being actively evaluated in clinical trials designed to screen potential candidate treatments for subsequent randomized studies in the phase III setting. This novel end point is now being used in the design of upcoming trials with androgen receptor targeted approaches that combine GnRH agonists/antagonists with other hormonal agents (eg, abiraterone, enzalutamide) to completely inhibit androgen signaling.

SUMMARY

Risk stratification based on PSADT and Gleason score is the primary determinant of metastatic progression and prostate cancer–specific mortality and should help determine the frequency of diagnostic evaluation and timing of treatment initiation. From a clinical and trial design perspective, determination of BCR should be made using the AUA definition after prostatectomy and the Phoenix definition after radiation. It is important to emphasize that clinical trials remain the gold standard especially at this time when newer effective compounds and modalities have been approved in patients with more advanced disease.

REFERENCES

1. American Cancer Society. Cancer facts & figures. 2013. Atlanta.
2. Epstein MM, Edgren G, Rider JR, et al. Temporal trends in cause of death among Swedish and US men with prostate cancer. J Natl Cancer Inst 2012; 104:1335–42.
3. Moul JW, Banez LL, Freedland SJ. Rising PSA in nonmetastatic prostate cancer. Oncology (Williston Park) 2007;21:1436–45 [discussion: 1449, 1452, 1454].
4. Solo K, Mehra M, Dhawan R, et al. Prevalence of prostate cancer (PC) clinical states (CS) in the United States: estimates using a dynamic progression model. J Clin Oncol 2011;29(Suppl 15):4637.
5. Perlmutter MA, Lepor H. Androgen deprivation therapy in the treatment of advanced prostate cancer. Rev Urol 2007;9(Suppl 1):S3–8.
6. Cookson MS, Aus G, Burnett AL, et al. Variation in the definition of biochemical recurrence in patients treated for localized prostate cancer: the American Urological Association Prostate Guidelines for Localized Prostate Cancer Update Panel report and recommendations for a standard in the reporting of surgical outcomes. J Urol 2007;177:540–5.
7. Smith MR, Manola J, Kaufman DS, et al. Celecoxib versus placebo for men with prostate cancer and a rising serum prostate-specific antigen after radical prostatectomy and/or radiation therapy. J Clin Oncol 2006;24:2723–8.
8. Paller C, Ye X, Wozniak PJ, et al. A randomized phase II study of pomegranate extract for men with rising prostate-specific antigen following initial therapy for localized prostate cancer. Prostate Cancer Prostatic Dis 2013;16(1):50–5.
9. Kestin LL, Vicini FA, Martinez AA. Practical application of biochemical failure definitions: what to do and when to do it. Int J Radiat Oncol Biol Phys 2002; 53:304–15.
10. Kuban DA, Levy LB, Potters L, et al. Comparison of biochemical failure definitions for permanent prostate brachytherapy. Int J Radiat Oncol Biol Phys 2006;65:1487–93.
11. Horwitz EM, Thames HD, Kuban DA, et al. Definitions of biochemical failure that best predict clinical failure in patients with prostate cancer treated with external

beam radiation alone: a multi-institutional pooled analysis. J Urol 2005;173: 797–802.

12. Kupelian PA, Mahadevan A, Reddy CA, et al. Use of different definitions of biochemical failure after external beam radiotherapy changes conclusions about relative treatment efficacy for localized prostate cancer. Urology 2006; 68:593–8.

13. Pound CR, Partin AW, Eisenberger MA, et al. Natural history of progression after PSA elevation following radical prostatectomy. JAMA 1999;281:1591–7.

14. Freedland SJ, Humphreys EB, Mangold LA, et al. Risk of prostate cancer-specific mortality following biochemical recurrence after radical prostatectomy. JAMA 2005;294:433–9.

15. Antonarakis ES, Feng Z, Trock BJ, et al. The natural history of metastatic progression in men with prostate-specific antigen recurrence after radical prostatectomy: long-term follow-up. BJU Int 2012;109:32–9.

16. Zhou P, Chen MH, McLeod D, et al. Predictors of prostate cancer-specific mortality after radical prostatectomy or radiation therapy. J Clin Oncol 2005;23: 6992–8.

17. Bolla M, van Poppel H, Tombal B, et al. Postoperative radiotherapy after radical prostatectomy: a randomised controlled trial (EORTC trial 22911). Lancet 2005; 366:572–8.

18. Thompson IM, Tangen CM, Paradelo J, et al. Adjuvant radiotherapy for pathological T3N0M0 prostate cancer significantly reduces risk of metastases and improves survival: long-term followup of a randomized clinical trial. J Urol 2009; 181:956–62.

19. Wiegel T, Bottke D, Steiner U, et al. Phase III postoperative adjuvant radiotherapy after radical prostatectomy compared with radical prostatectomy alone in pT3 prostate cancer with postoperative undetectable prostate-specific antigen: ARO 96-02/AUO AP 09/95. J Clin Oncol 2009;27:2924–30.

20. Stephenson AJ, Scardino PT, Kattan MW, et al. Predicting the outcome of salvage radiation therapy for recurrent prostate cancer after radical prostatectomy. J Clin Oncol 2007;25:2035–41.

21. Trock BJ, Han M, Freedland SJ, et al. Prostate cancer-specific survival following salvage radiotherapy vs observation in men with biochemical recurrence after radical prostatectomy. JAMA 2008;299:2760–9.

22. Pearse M, Choo R, Danjoux C, et al. Prospective assessment of gastrointestinal and genitourinary toxicity of salvage radiotherapy for patients with prostate-specific antigen relapse or local recurrence after radical prostatectomy. Int J Radiat Oncol Biol Phys 2008;72:792–8.

23. Feng M, Hanlon AL, Pisansky TM, et al. Predictive factors for late genitourinary and gastrointestinal toxicity in patients with prostate cancer treated with adjuvant or salvage radiotherapy. Int J Radiat Oncol Biol Phys 2007;68: 1417–23.

24. Elliott SP, Meng MV, Elkin EP, et al. Incidence of urethral stricture after primary treatment for prostate cancer: data from CaPSURE. J Urol 2007;178:529–34. http://dx.doi.org/10.1016/j.juro.2007.03.126 [discussion: 534].

25. Loblaw DA, Virgo KS, Nam R, et al. Initial hormonal management of androgen-sensitive metastatic, recurrent, or progressive prostate cancer: 2006 update of an American Society of Clinical Oncology practice guideline. J Clin Oncol 2007;25:1596–605.

26. Brawer MK. Radiation therapy failure in prostate cancer patients: risk factors and methods of detection. Rev Urol 2002;4(Suppl 2):S2–11.

27. Zagars GK, Pollack A, von Eschenbach AC. Prostate cancer and radiation therapy: the message conveyed by serum prostate-specific antigen. Int J Radiat Oncol Biol Phys 1995;33:23–35. http://dx.doi.org/10.1016/0360-3016(95)00154-Q.
28. Zelefsky MJ, Leibel SA, Gaudin PB, et al. Dose escalation with three-dimensional conformal radiation therapy affects the outcome in prostate cancer. Int J Radiat Oncol Biol Phys 1998;41:491–500.
29. Stephenson AJ, Eastham JA. Role of salvage radical prostatectomy for recurrent prostate cancer after radiation therapy. J Clin Oncol 2005;23:8198–203. http://dx.doi.org/10.1200/JCO.2005.03.1468.
30. Kaplan ID, Prestidge BR, Bagshaw MA, et al. The importance of local control in the treatment of prostatic cancer. J Urol 1992;147:917–21.
31. Fuks Z, Leibel SA, Wallner KE, et al. The effect of local control on metastatic dissemination in carcinoma of the prostate: long-term results in patients treated with 125I implantation. Int J Radiat Oncol Biol Phys 1991;21:537–47.
32. Holzman M, Carlton CE Jr, Scardino PT. The frequency and morbidity of local tumor recurrence after definitive radiotherapy for stage C prostate cancer. J Urol 1991;146:1578–82.
33. Bianco FJ Jr, Scardino PT, Stephenson AJ, et al. Long-term oncologic results of salvage radical prostatectomy for locally recurrent prostate cancer after radiotherapy. Int J Radiat Oncol Biol Phys 2005;62:448–53. http://dx.doi.org/10.1016/j.ijrobp.2004.09.049.
34. Ward JF, Sebo TJ, Blute ML, et al. Salvage surgery for radiorecurrent prostate cancer: contemporary outcomes. J Urol 2005;173:1156–60. http://dx.doi.org/10.1097/01.ju.0000155534.54711.60.
35. Cooperberg MR, Grossfeld GD, Lubeck DP, et al. National practice patterns and time trends in androgen ablation for localized prostate cancer. J Natl Cancer Inst 2003;95:981–9.
36. Agarwal PK, Sadetsky N, Konety BR, et al. Treatment failure after primary and salvage therapy for prostate cancer: likelihood, patterns of care, and outcomes. Cancer 2008;112:307–14. http://dx.doi.org/10.1002/cncr.23161.
37. Kirk D. Immediate vs deferred hormone treatment for prostate cancer: How safe is androgen deprivation? Br J Urol 2000;86:S220.
38. Immediate versus deferred treatment for advanced prostate cancer: initial results of the Medical Rersearch Council Trial: the Medical Research Council Prostate Cancer Working Party Investigators. Br J Urol 1997;79:235.
39. Pinover WH, Horwitz EM, Hanlon AL, et al. Validation of a treatment policy for patients with prostate specific antigen failure after three-dimensional conformal prostate radiation therapy. Cancer 2003;97:1127–33. http://dx.doi.org/10.1002/cncr.11166.
40. Moul JW, Wu H, Sun L, et al. Early versus delayed hormonal therapy for prostate specific antigen only recurrence of prostate cancer after radical prostatectomy. J Urol 2008;179:S53–9. http://dx.doi.org/10.1016/j.juro.2008.03.138.
41. Siddiqui SA, Boorjian SA, Inman B, et al. Timing of androgen deprivation therapy and its impact on survival after radical prostatectomy: a matched cohort study. J Urol 2008;179:1830–7 [discussion: 1837].
42. Crook JM, O'Callaghan CJ, Duncan G, et al. Intermittent androgen suppression for rising PSA level after radiotherapy. N Engl J Med 2012;367:895–903.
43. Hussain MH, Tangen C, Higano C, et al. Intermittent (IAD) versus continuous androgen deprivation (CAD) in hormone sensitive metastatic prostate cancer (HSM1PC) patients (pts): results of S9346 (INT-0162), an international phase III trial. J Clin Oncol 2012;30(Suppl) [abstract 4].

44. Calais da Silva FE, Bono AV, Whelan P, et al. Intermittent androgen deprivation for locally advanced and metastatic prostate cancer: results from a randomised phase 3 study of the South European Uroncological Group. Eur Urol 2009;55: 1269–77.

45. Keizman D, Carducci MA. Intermittent androgen deprivation–questions remain. Nat Rev Urol 2009;6:412–4. http://dx.doi.org/10.1038/nrurol.2009.145.

46. Keizman D, Huang P, Antonarakis ES, et al. The change of PSA doubling time and its association with disease progression in patients with biochemically relapsed prostate cancer treated with intermittent androgen deprivation. Prostate 2011;71:1608–15.

47. Braga-Basaria M, Dobs AS, Muller DC, et al. Metabolic syndrome in men with prostate cancer undergoing long-term androgen-deprivation therapy. J Clin Oncol 2006;24:3979–83.

48. Smith MR, Lee H, McGovern F, et al. Metabolic changes during gonadotropin-releasing hormone agonist therapy for prostate cancer: differences from the classic metabolic syndrome. Cancer 2008;112:2188–94. http://dx.doi.org/10.1002/cncr.23440.

49. Sharifi N, Gulley JL, Dahut WL. Androgen deprivation therapy for prostate cancer. JAMA 2005;294:238–44.

50. Smith MR, Egerdie B, Hernández Toriz N, et al. Denosumab in men receiving androgen-deprivation therapy for prostate cancer. N Engl J Med 2009;361: 745–55.

51. Muller M, Grobbee DE, den Tonkelaar I, et al. Endogenous sex hormones and metabolic syndrome in aging men. J Clin Endocrinol Metab 2005;90:2618–23.

52. Keating NL, O'Malley AJ, Smith MR. Diabetes and cardiovascular disease during androgen deprivation therapy for prostate cancer. J Clin Oncol 2006;24: 4448–56. http://dx.doi.org/10.1200/JCO.2006.06.2497.

53. Schweizer MT, Yang T, Wang H, et al. Association of metastasis-free survival (MFS) with overall survival (OS) in men with PSA-recurrent prostate cancer treated with deferred androgen-deprivation therapy. Genitourinary Cancers Symposium. 2013; [abstract 109].

54. Paller C, Xie J, Olatoye D, et al. The effect of PSA frequency and duration on PSA doubling time (PSADT) calculations in men with biochemically recurrent prostate cancer (BRPC) after definitive local therapy. J Clin Oncol 2012; 30(Suppl 15):99246.

55. Antonarakis ES, Zahurak ML, Lin J, et al. Changes in PSA kinetics predict metastasis-free survival in men with PSA-recurrent prostate cancer treated with nonhormonal agents: combined analysis of 4 phase II trials. Cancer 2012;118:1533–42.

56. Smith MR, Manola J, Kaufman DS, et al. Rosiglitazone versus placebo for men with prostate carcinoma and a rising serum prostate-specific antigen level after radical prostatectomy and/or radiation therapy. Cancer 2004; 101:1569–74.

57. Zietman AL, Coen JJ, Dallow KC, et al. The treatment of prostate cancer by conventional radiation therapy: an analysis of long-term outcome. Int J Radiat Oncol Biol Phys 1995;32:287–92.

58. D'Amico AV, Chen MH, Catalona WJ, et al. Surrogate end point for prostate cancer-specific mortality after radical prostatectomy or radiation therapy. J Natl Cancer Inst 2003;95:1376–83.

59. Antonarakis ES, Chen Y, Elsamanoudi SI, et al. Long-term overall survival and metastasis-free survival for men with prostate-specific antigen-recurrent

prostate cancer after prostatectomy: analysis of the Center for Prostate Disease Research National Database. BJU Int 2011;108:378–85.

60. D'Amico AV, Cote K, Loffredo M, et al. Determinants of prostate cancer-specific survival after radiation therapy for patients with clinically localized prostate cancer. J Clin Oncol 2002;20:4567–73.
61. Buyyounouski MK, Hanlon AL, Horwitz EM, et al. Interval to biochemical failure highly prognostic for distant metastasis and prostate cancer-specific mortality after radiotherapy. Int J Radiat Oncol Biol Phys 2008;70:59–66.

Management of Hormone-Sensitive Metastatic Prostate Cancer

Neeraj Agarwal, MD[a], Maha Hussain, MD[b],*

KEYWORDS

- Hormone-sensitive metastatic prostate cancer • Androgen signaling inhibitor
- Treatment • Future directions

KEY POINTS

- Targeting gonadal androgen synthesis (often in conjunction with blockade of androgen receptor) is the cornerstone of treatment of hormone-sensitive metastatic prostate cancer.
- Responses are not durable and almost all patients progress, with a median duration of approximately 18 months.
- Over the last decade, it has been recognized that despite the failure of androgen deprivation therapy, most tumors maintain some dependence on androgen or androgen receptor signaling for proliferation.
- Novel agents targeting these pathways continue to be developed.
- An area of active investigation is the identification and validation of biomarkers predicting response to therapy.

INTRODUCTION

More than 238,590 men were diagnosed with prostate cancer in 2013, with 29,720 estimated to die of their disease, as a result of progression to metastatic disease.[1] Although most men with metastatic prostate cancer develop metastatic disease after failing definitive therapy for their localized disease, about 5% have metastatic disease at the time of initial diagnosis. In the 1940s, Huggins and Hodges were the first to show that castration induces significant palliation in metastatic prostate cancer. Since then, targeting gonadal androgen synthesis (often in conjunction with blockade of androgen

Disclosure: None of the authors has any conflict of interest to disclose.
[a] Division of Medical Oncology, Huntsman Cancer Institute, University of Utah, 2000 Circle of Hope, Suite 2123, Salt Lake City, UT 84112, USA; [b] Division of Hematology/Oncology, Department of Internal Medicine, University of Michigan Comprehensive Cancer Center, University of Michigan, 7303 Cancer Center, 1500 E Medical Center Drive, Ann Arbor, MI 48109, USA
* Corresponding author.
E-mail address: mahahuss@med.umich.edu

receptor [AR]) has become the cornerstone of treatment of hormone-sensitive metastatic prostate cancer (HSPC). However, responses are not durable, and almost all patients progress, with a median duration of approximately 18 months.[2] Over the last decade, it has been recognized that despite the failure of androgen deprivation therapy (ADT), most tumors maintain some dependence on androgen or AR signaling for proliferation.[3] Many patients with metastatic prostate cancer respond to secondary hormone manipulation, after disease progression on ADT.[4]

ANDROGEN SYNTHESIS AND AR

The regulation of androgen production by the testicles originates in the hypothalamus, where the pulsatile release of gonadotropin-releasing hormone (GnRH) leads to the release of leutinizing hormone (LH) and follicle-stimulating hormone (FSH) from pituitary into the blood stream (**Fig. 1**).[5] Under the effect of LH, androgens are produced in the Leydig cells of the testes (most serum testosterone) and testosterone is converted to dihydrotestosterone (DHT) by 5α–reductase within the prostate. Another source of circulating androgens are the adrenal glands, where androgens, mainly 5-dehydroepiandrosterone (DHEA), DHEA sulfate, and androstenedione are synthesized in the zona reticularis. The first step in steroid biosynthesis is the formation of cholesterol from acetyl coenzyme A and squalene (**Fig. 2**). Cholesterol is then converted to pregnenolone and then to progesterone. The pivotal enzymes in androgen synthesis are the CYP17 enzymes (CYP17 hydroxylase, CYP17,20 lyase) located in the Leydig cells of the testes and the zona fasciculata and reticularis of the adrenal glands. CYP17 catalyzes the conversion of pregnenolone and progesterone to the weak androgen steroids, DHEA, and androstenedione, respectively. Both DHEA and androstenedione are converted to testosterone and then to DHT, reactions that are catalyzed by other enzymes.

AR is a steroid hormone receptor located in the cytoplasm that remains bound to heat shock proteins. The functional domains of AR include the C-terminal ligand-binding domain (LBD), a DNA-binding domain, and the N-terminal domain (NTD). When activated, the LBD results in the nuclear translocation of AR. The NTD is essential for the transcriptional activity of the AR in response to a ligand, as well as in the absence of a ligand.[6] When testosterone and DHT bind with LBD, AR dissociates from heat shock protein and undergoes homodimerization and tyrosine kinase phosphorylation, followed by translocation to the nucleus. Within the nucleus, AR binds to androgen response elements in the promoter and enhancer regions of the target gene. This event is followed by the recruitment of several coactivator and corepressor proteins and the formation of an active transcription complex, which induces transcription of several genes involved in cell cycle regulation and proliferation.[7]

MOLECULAR MECHANISM UNDERLYING PROSTATE CANCER PROGRESSION DESPITE ONGOING ADT
AR-Dependent Mechanisms

Several mechanisms have been identified to explain the persistent growth and proliferation of prostate cancer despite ongoing ADT.[4,8] Although ADT reduces the level of serum androgens to very low levels, it does not eliminate them completely. In patients on ADT, the adrenal glands are the major source of androgens. In addition, there is evidence that prostate cancer cells can initiate aberrant androgen signaling, as well as synthesize sufficient amounts of intratumoral androgens to allow continued androgen signaling and tumor growth in a castrate patient.[9] The concentrations of intratumoral testosterone in metastatic prostate tumors in men with

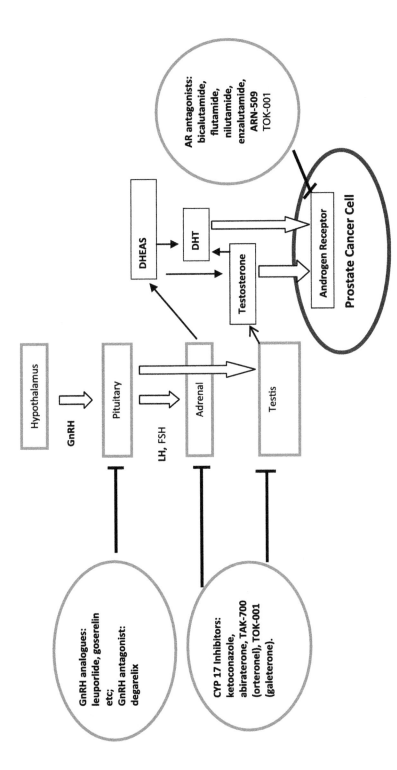

Fig. 1. Hypothalamic-pituitary-adrenal and hypothalamic-pituitary-testicular axis, along with drugs inhibiting these pathways. Thick arrows denote stimulation, flat lines denote inhibition, and thin arrows denote synthesis.

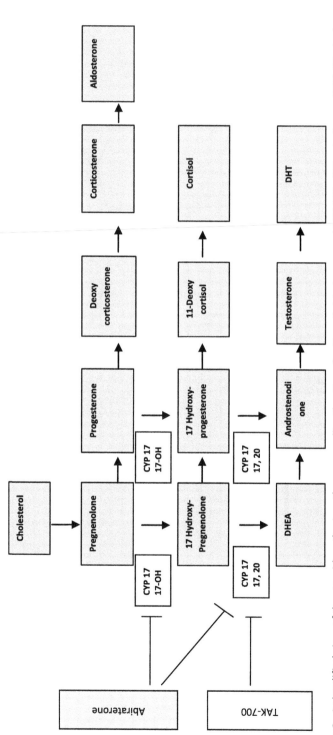

Fig. 2. A simplified view of the steroid synthesis pathway, as well as the sites of action of abiraterone and TAK-700. CYP, cytochrome P450 17 α-hydroxylase-C17, 20-lyase.

castration-resistant prostate cancer (CRPC) are 2 to 3 times higher than in men who have never received ADT, despite the fact that those not receiving ADT have higher serum testosterone levels.[4,10] After receiving 9 months of neoadjuvant deprivation therapy, men with localized prostate cancer did not have a reduction in the expression of many androgen-responsive genes, including the AR and prostate-specific antigen (PSA), although intratumoral testosterone and DHT levels were reduced by 75%.[11] Many enzymes involved in androgen synthesis are highly upregulated in CRPC compared with those with androgen-sensitive prostate cancer.[10] Castrate-resistant cell lines synthesized a 5-fold higher concentration of testosterone than androgen-dependent cell lines and were capable of directly converting radioactive cholesterol into testosterone in vitro.[12] These data indicate that castration, based on serum testosterone levels, is not synonymous with androgen ablation in the prostate tumor microenvironment. Prostate cancer cells can adapt to castration by intratumoral synthesis or conversion of adrenal androgens to testosterone and DHT and subsequently derive a growth advantage. One known (but rare) mechanism is the mutation of the AR gene, resulting in promiscuous ARs, which are activated by antiandrogens (such as bicalutamide) and other endogenous steroids (such as progesterone or deoxycorticosterone).[3,13]

Other mechanisms underlying prostate cancer progression, despite ongoing ADT, include increased AR gene expression, either because of AR gene amplification; an increased rate of transcription of AR gene, or from the increased stability of the AR transcript.[12,14] Somatic AR mutations, developing under the selection pressure of ADT, is another mechanism underlying continued progression of prostate cancer.[15] Antiandrogen therapy–associated AR mutants may provide the basis for the antiandrogen withdrawal syndrome, in which tumors regress and PSA declines on cessation of treatment.[16] This may be a reason why prostate cancer progressing on 1 AR antagonist may show favorable response to another.[17] Sequencing studies have shown prevalence of mutation in both LBD and NTD of the AR coding region.[13] One emerging and recently reported mechanism is AR gene rearrangement, resulting in constitutively active truncated AR splice variants that lack the AR LBD.[18]

These data establish enzymes of the androgen synthesis pathway and AR signaling as valid targets in addition to standard ADT to optimize outcomes in HSPC.

AR-Independent Mechanisms

Although androgen signaling plays an important role, all of the hallmarks of cancer may be invoked to drive the progression of prostate cancer in men being treated with ADT.[19] It is now recognized that stromal-epithelial cross talk in the prostate cancer microenvironment is critical for prostate cancer progression.[20,21] Hedgehog signaling, Src family kinases, fibroblast growth factors, transforming growth factor β, integrins, vascular endothelial growth factor, insulinlike growth factor, and interleukin 6 are important components and potential targets for drug development. Other important pathways include those that inhibit apoptosis and promote survival, including the mitogen-activated protein kinases and phosphoinositide 3-kinase-Akt pathways. Chromosomal rearrangements or deletions in prostate cancer may result in the overexpression of oncogenes by the androgen or other steroid receptors, providing an opportunity to target gene fusions, such as those involving the members of the ETS and RAF kinase families. Other pathways implicated in the progression of prostate cancer include a dysfunctional epigenetic environment, c-MET-hepatocyte growth factor receptor pathway, cytoprotective chaperone networks, and alternative mitogenic growth factor pathways, such as the epidermal growth factor pathway. These molecular pathways can be singularly differentially upregulated or in combination with other pathways and are responsible for the biological heterogeneity in prostate cancer, as well as the variable response to targeted therapies.[20,21]

These data establish AR-dependent, as well as AR-independent, molecular pathways as valid targets in prostate cancer in addition to standard ADT to optimize outcomes in HSPC. This review focuses on targeting androgen-dependent pathways in men with HSPC.

DRUGS TARGETING ANDROGEN SYNTHESIS AND AR SIGNALING IN METASTATIC PROSTATE CANCER

GnRH agonists and antagonists, which target the hypothalamic-pituitary-gonadal axis, and antiandrogens (AR receptor blockers) are routinely used for the treatment of hormone-sensitive prostate cancer. Several novel agents, which disrupt androgen synthesis, AR signaling, or both, are in development. Many of these agents have recently been shown to be efficacious in the castration refractory setting, and have the potential to improve outcomes in the hormone-sensitive setting when used in combination with standard ADT.

Targeting Hypothalamic-Pituitary-Testicular Axis

GnRH is a peptide hormone that is synthesized in hypothalamic neurons and then intermittently secreted into the hypophysioportal circulation in a pulsatile fashion. GnRH selectively stimulates gonadotroph cells within the anterior pituitary to release gonadotropins (ie, LH and FSH). Secretion of gonadotropins requires intermittent stimulation by GnRH, because continuous stimulation leads to desensitization of gonadotropic cells and inhibition of gonadotropin release.[22]

GnRH analogues or agonists
Unlike natural GnRH peptide, synthetic GnRH analogues or agonists have a higher affinity for gonatroph cells. In addition, they are less susceptible to enzymatic degradation. Binding of synthetic GnRH agonists with gonadotroph cells initially results in the release of LH and FSH. Receptor desensitization results in the inhibition of LH and FSH release. The initial stimulation of LH release results in a transient increase in testosterone from the testis, a phenomenon known as testosterone flare.[22,23] The GnRH agonists in current use include leuprolide, buserelin, goserelin, histrelin, and triptorelin and are generally used in long-lasting depot forms. GnRH agonists form the backbone of treatment of metastatic prostate cancer by inducing reversible medical castration, as shown in multiple clinical trials (described later).

GnRH antagonist
Degarelix (Firmagon, Ferring Pharmaceuticals, Parsippany, NJ, USA) has been developed as a pure GnRH antagonist, which does not cause an initial stimulation of gonadotroph cells and subsequently, a testosterone flare. In a phase 3 trial,[24] 610 men with prostate cancer were randomized to one of the 3 following regimens: a starting dose of 240 mg of degarelix, given subcutaneously for 1 month, followed by subcutaneous maintenance doses of 80 mg or 160 mg monthly, or intramuscular leuprolide at a dose of 7.5 mg monthly. Therapy was maintained for the 12-month study. Men with prostate cancer of all stages in whom ADT was indicated (except in the neoadjuvant setting) were eligible. Degarelix was not inferior to leuprolide at maintaining low testosterone levels over the treatment period. However, degarelix induced testosterone and PSA suppression significantly faster than leuprolide. The adverse effect profiles were similar for both agents, except for local injection site reactions, which were more frequent with degarelix than with leuprolide (40% vs <1%).

Targeting Androgen Synthesis

Ketoconazole has been historically used as a nonspecific inhibitor of enzymes of the androgen synthesis pathway. Abiraterone, a more specific inhibitor of CYP17 enzymes, has been recently approved for the treatment of CRPC. TAK-700 (orteronel, Millennium Pharmaceuticals, The Takeda Oncology Company, Cambridge, MA, USA), a selective 17,20 hydroxylase inhibitor, and TOK-001 (Galeterone, Tokai Pharmaceuticals, Cambridge, MA, USA), a dual inhibitor of CYP17 and AR are in development.

Ketoconazole

It has a weak and nonspecific inhibitory effect on several enzymes involved in androgen synthesis, including CYP17. However, it had no impact on survival.[25] The advent of effective novel CYP17 inhibitors has made ketoconazole a suboptimal treatment option.[26]

Abiraterone acetate

Abiraterone acetate (Zytiga, Johnson & Johnson, New Brunswick, NJ, USA), a pregnenolone analogue, is an orally administered small molecule that irreversibly inhibits CYP17. In a phase 3 trial, 1195 patients with metastatic CRPC who received previous docetaxel or 2 lines of chemotherapy were randomized in a 2:1 fashion to receive 5 mg of prednisone twice daily with either 1000 mg of abiraterone acetate (797 patients) or placebo (398 patients).[27] After a median follow-up of 12.8 months, median overall survival (OS), the primary end point, was longer in the abiraterone acetate-prednisone group than in the placebo-prednisone group (14.8 months vs 10.9 months, $P<.001$), leading to US Food and Drug Administration approval for this indication. Adverse effects were associated with secondary mineralocorticoid excess, including hypertension, hypokalemia, and edema, which were manageable by the addition of a mineralocorticoid antagonist or corticosteroid. Abiraterone acetate has also been evaluated in a separate phase 3 trial of 1088 chemotherapy-naive men with progressive CRPC.[28] In this trial, there was improved radiographic progression-free survival (PFS) with abiraterone over placebo (16.5 months vs 8.3 months, $P<.001$), leading to the regulatory approval of abiraterone in the prechemotherapy setting as well.

Resistance to abiraterone may be mediated by amplification of CYP17 (suggesting a potential role for dose escalation of abiraterone), as well as AR splice variants.[29]

TAK-700 (orteronel)

TAK-700, a CYP17 inhibitor with a potentially greater 17,20 lyase selectivity (ie, for androgen as opposed to corticosteroid synthesis), is under development.[30] Updated data from the phase 2 portion of a phase 1/2 study of TAK-700 in chemonaive patients with metastatic CRPC were reported.[31] Ninety-seven patients were treated with TAK-700 in 4 different dose cohorts: 300 mg twice daily (n = 23), 400 mg twice daily + prednisone 5 mg twice daily (n = 24), 600 mg twice daily + prednisone (n = 26), or 600 mg 4 times a day (n = 24). The most common adverse effects were fatigue (76%), nausea (47%), and constipation (38%), and the most common adverse effects of grade 3 or higher were fatigue (12%) and hypokalemia (8%). The PSA response rates ($\geq$50%) at 12 weeks were 63%, 50%, 41%, and 60% in the 300 mg twice daily, 400 and 600 mg twice daily + prednisone, and 600 mg 4 times a day groups, respectively. Of 51 RECIST (Response Evaluation Criteria In Solid Tumors)-evaluable patients, 10 had partial responses (of whom 5 were confirmed), 22 had stable disease, and 15 had progressive disease. At 12 weeks, the median serum testosterone levels were decreased from baseline in all groups: (ng/dL, 12 weeks/baseline) 0.98/8.50 (300 mg twice daily), 0.30/9.90 (400 mg twice daily + prednisone), 0.07/7.33 (600 mg twice daily + prednisone), 0.49/6.31 (600 mg 4 times a day). Similarly, at 12 weeks, the median dehydroepiandrosterone sulfate level decreased from baseline in all groups: (μg/dL, 12 weeks/baseline) 8.65/53.0 (300 mg twice daily), 0.10/36.3 (400 mg twice daily + prednisone), 0.10/51.7 (600 mg twice daily + prednisone), 5.30/31.5 (600 mg 4 times a day). Overall, the mean circulating tumor cell (CTC) numbers decreased from 16.6 (per 7.5 mL blood) at baseline to 3.9 at 12 weeks. TAK-700 300 mg or greater twice daily appeared active and well tolerated in patients with metastatic CRPC, with similar efficacy, with and without prednisone.

In a phase 2 study in nonmetastatic CRPC with biochemical recurrence alone, 38 patients were treated with TAK-700 300 mg twice daily without prednisone.[32] Treatment without prednisone was feasible and with manageable toxicities. After 3 months of treatment, 16% achieved a PSA level of 0.2 ng/mL of lower, 76% achieved a PSA decrease of 50% or greater and 32% achieved a PSA reduction of 90% or more. The median time to PSA progression was 14.8 months. TAK-700 without prednisone suppressed adrenal androgens by 85% to 90%. Only 1 patient had laboratory values consistent with a hypoadrenal state, for which he received corticosteroid replacement.

Recently, 2 phase 3 randomized, placebo-controlled trials with TAK-700 have completed accrual in patients with CRPC. Both trials are comparing the efficacy of prednisone 5 mg by mouth twice a day, with or without TAK-700 (400 mg orally twice daily) in predocetaxel and postdocetaxel settings, respectively.

Targeting AR

In addition to enzalutamide (Xtandi, Medivation Inc, San Francisco, CA, USA), a novel AR antagonist with downstream effects on androgen signaling, which was recently approved for CRPC, there are other novel drugs in this class that are in various phases of clinical development, including ARN-509 (Johnson & Johnson, New Brunswick, NJ, USA), TOK-001, and EPI-001.

Antiandrogens

Antiandrogens work by competitively inhibiting the binding of testosterone and DHT with the AR. Only nonsteroidal antiandrogens (eg, bicalutamide, flutamide, and nilutamide) are approved in the United States. In the setting of metastatic prostate cancer, antiandrogens are used as follows: in conjunction with a GnRH agonist initially to prevent testosterone flare, continuously as combined androgen blockade (CAB) therapy (as described later), or after the onset of castration refractory disease, as a part of secondary hormonal manipulation. Monotherapy with antiandrogens (without GnRH agonist) is not recommended because of concerns for inferior survival compared with GnRH agonist therapy alone.[33]

Enzalutamide (MDV3100)

Enzalutamide is a novel AR antagonist that binds to AR with a higher affinity than bicalutamide, blocks nuclear translocation of AR, binding to androgen response elements, recruitment of coactivators by the AR. In addition, enzalutamide does not generally confer agonist activity, or any effects on androgen synthesis.[4] In a phase 1/2 study of 140 patients with progressive, metastatic CRPC,[34] the maximum tolerated dose of enzalutamide for sustained treatment was 240 mg daily. Antitumor effects were seen at all doses, including decreases in serum PSA level of 50% or greater in 56% patients, soft tissue responses in 22% of patients, stabilization of bone disease in 56% of patients, and conversion from unfavorable to favorable CTC counts in 49% of patients. Enzalutamide was generally well tolerated, with fatigue as the most common dose-dependent grade 3 to 4 side effect. These data led to the initiation of placebo-controlled phase 3 trials (without prednisone) in chemonaive and postdocetaxel patients with metastatic CRPC. A 4.8-month advantage in median OS was reported in the postdocetaxel trial (18.4 vs 13.6 months, P<.001), translating into a 37% reduction in the risk of death (hazard ratio [HR] = 0.631). Enzalutamide crosses the blood-brain barrier and leads to sensitization to seizures a few patients. Seizures were reported in 5 of 800 patients (0.6%) receiving enzalutamide and have been hypothesized to be caused by inhibition of the γ-aminobutyric acid–gated chloride channel.[35]

ARN-509

ARN-509 has a mechanism of action similar to enzalutamide. In a phase 1/2 study of 24 men with metastatic CRPC, ARN-509 was well tolerated with promising PSA responses (55% patients had ≥50% PSA declines) and with pharmacodynamic evidence of AR antagonism. Of the 7 dose levels investigated, a dose of 240 mg daily was selected for the phase 2 portion, which planned to enroll patients with nonmetastatic and metastatic CRPC.[36]

TOK-001 (galeterone)

TOK-001 is an oral steroid analogue that inhibits CYP17, blocks AR, and reduces AR levels. In a phase 1 study of chemotherapy-naive men with CRPC, TOK-001 was well tolerated and showed clinical activity. Of 49 patients, 22% showed a decline in PSA level of more than 50%, and an additional 26% had PSA declines of 30% to 50%.[37] Based on these preliminary results, a phase 2 study is planned to begin accruing in 2013.

EPI-001

EPI-001 is a small molecule inhibitor of the NTD of the AR, which confers transcriptional activity. EPI-001 has shown substantial preclinical activity, warranting further clinical development of this class of agents.[38]

SYSTEMIC THERAPY FOR HSPC
Castration Versus CAB Therapy

Several meta-analyses have shown a modest 2% to 5% improvement in 5-year survival with CAB over castration, although with increased toxicity.[39–41] One of largest meta-analyses included the individual level data of 8275 patients from 27 trials.[39,42] Trials that used steroidal as well as nonsteroidal antiandrogens in their CAB regimens were included. Although there was an overall trend toward improved 5-year survival with CAB over castration, this did not reach statistical significance (P = .11). When trials using steroidal and nonsteroidal antiandrogens were analyzed separately, CAB with nonsteroidal antiandrogens (flutamide and nilutamide) were associated with a statistically significant 8% decrease in the risk of death compared with castration alone (95% confidence interval [CI] 3–13; P = .005, 2-sided), equating to a 2.9% increase in 5-year survival. On the other hand, CAB using steroidal antiandrogens, when compared with castration alone, was associated with a significant 13% increase in the risk of death (95% CI 0–27; P = .04, 2-sided), as well as a 2.8% reduction in 5-year survival rates.[42]

The American Society of Clinical Oncology guidelines state that CAB should be considered as an option and be discussed with patients, with the emphasis that improvement in OS may occur at the cost of higher toxicity.[23] These data provide a compelling rationale for developing more efficacious treatment regimens to improve survival outcome in these patients.

Intermittent ADT Versus Continuous ADT

Preclinical work conducted in the 1980s and early 1990s led to the hypothesis that intermittent ADT may delay the onset of castration resistance by reducing selection pressure on castrate resistance clones.[43] The probability of the onset of androgen-independent prostate cancer in androgen-dependent Shionogi carcinoma mice was greatly increased in an androgen-depleted atmosphere and was perceived to have occurred as a result of diminished androgen-induced differentiation of parent tumor stem cells.[44]

The clinical use of intermittent endocrine therapy in advanced prostate cancer was first reported in 1986,[45] when it was shown that patients with advanced prostate cancer could remain in symptomatic remission for considerable periods, despite interruptions in endocrine therapy with diethylstilbestrol. During the 1990s, intermittent androgen suppression was reported to significantly delay the onset of androgen independence in mouse models, when compared with continuous androgen suppression.[46]

These and other reports provided the rationale for designing an international phase 3 trial (S9346, INT-0162), comparing intermittent ADT with continuous ADT, in newly diagnosed HSPC.[47] Men with HSPC who had a PSA level of 5 ng/mL or greater were treated for 7 months with goserelin, plus bicalutamide. Men who achieved a PSA of 4 ng/mL or less on months 6 and 7 were stratified by previous neoadjuvant ADT/finasteride, performance status, and extent of disease (minimal vs extensive) and then randomized to continuous androgen deprivation (CAD) or intermittent androgen deprivation (IAD) with goserelin plus bicalutamide. The primary objective was to assess whether OS was noninferior with IAD, when compared with CAD. Over a period of 13 years (May, 1995 to September, 2008), 3040 men with HSPC were accrued. After 7 months of CAD, 1535 men achieved a PSA level of 4.0 ng/mL or less, after which they were randomized to CAD (n = 759) or IAD (n = 770). The grade 3 and 4 adverse effects were similar in both groups. After a median follow-up of 9.2 years, the median OS and 10-year OS from study entry were 3.6 years and 17%, respectively. From the time of randomization, the median and 10-year OS in the CAD arm were 5.8 years and 29%, respectively, compared with 5.1 years and 23%, respectively, in the IAD arm (HR [IAD/CAD] = 1.09 [95% CI 0.95, 1.24]). The preliminary report on quality-of-life outcomes showed significantly more impotence, less libido, and diminished emotional function with CAD over IAD.[48] The study conclusion was that survival with IAD was not comparable with CAD, and thus, CAD continues to be the standard of care for men with HSPC. However, patients with HSPC who are interested in IAD should be counseled regarding the outcomes from this trial.

Combining Chemotherapy with Castration in HSPC

In the 1980s, it was hypothesized that if cytotoxic chemotherapy was given early in the course of HSPC, and in combination with castration, androgen-resistant clones in heterogeneous prostate tumors would concomitantly be inhibited, with subsequent improvement in response rates, PFS, and OS.[49] In addition, in metastatic prostate cancer, many chemotherapeutic agents, used either as single agents or in combination with other agents, were reported to have response rates as high as 30% to 40%.[50] In a combined chemohormonal trial, 25 men with new HSPC were treated with bilateral orchiectomy, estrogen, and chemotherapy with 5-fluorouracil and cyclophosphamide.[51] The encouraging response rates provided the rationale for a larger, SWOG (Southwest Oncology Group) 8219 trial.[49] This randomized study of 143 men with new HSPC compared endocrine therapy (diethylstilbestrol or bilateral orchiectomy) alone, followed by cyclophosphamide and doxorubicin chemotherapy at progression, versus initial combined chemoendocrine therapy with all these agents. However, there was no difference in PFS or OS between the 2 groups. Later, in a phase 2 study (SWOG 0032), estramustine, etoposide, and paclitaxel were combined with ADT in 41 men with high-risk HSPC, which was defined as the presence of visceral disease or bone metastases to both the axial and the appendicular skeleton.[52] The median PFS and the OS for the evaluable population were 13 months and 38 months, respectively.

The interest in using combined chemohormonal therapy for the treatment of HSPC was renewed when docetaxel was reported to improve OS in the CRPC setting.[53–55] These data led to the initiation of an intergroup phase 3 study (ECOG [Eastern Cooperative Oncology Group] 3805/CHAARTED [Chemohormonal Therapy Versus Androgen Ablation Randomized Trial for Extensive Disease]) comparing androgen ablation therapy, with or without chemotherapy with docetaxel, with prednisone in men with HSPC.[56,57] This trial has recently completed accrual, and is expected to define the role of upfront chemotherapy, in combination with ADT in HSPC. The results of another phase 3 trial, evaluating the role of docetaxel, in addition to ADT in HSPC, were recently reported. In this study, 385 men were randomized (1:1) to ADT (surgical or medical castration with or without nonsteroidal antiandrogens) alone or to ADT with docetaxel. OS, the primary end point, was not improved with the addition of docetaxel.[58] STAMPEDE (Systemic Therapy in Advancing or Metastatic Prostate Cancer: Evaluation of Drug Efficacy)[59] is an ongoing multiarm, multistage, adaptively randomized, controlled trial of men with locally advanced or metastatic prostate cancer beginning long-term ADT. Originally, the trial was designed to randomize men to one of the following arms: ADT alone, or ADT plus one of the following: docetaxel, zoledronic acid, celecoxib, zoledronic acid plus docetaxel, or zoledronic acid plus celecoxib. Later, 2 additional treatment arms were added: ADT plus abiraterone, and ADT plus radiation therapy to the prostate. The primary end point is OS. Recently, accrual was discontinued on the 2 arms containing celecoxib, because of lack of benefit.

PREDICTING RESPONSE TO ADT IN HSPC

Prostate cancer is a heterogeneous disease, as indicated by variable responses and outcomes in men receiving identical treatments (eg, the duration of response to ADT in men with HSPC can vary from months to years). This characteristic suggests the need for an individualized treatment approach, which uses biomarkers to select patients predicted to have a poor response to therapy and who may be candidates for more aggressive initial treatment. In this context, biomarkers can be prognostic, correlating with the outcome independent of treatment effects, or predictive, predicting the degree of benefit or toxicity from a given treatment. Although ADT has been used to treat metastatic prostate cancer for many decades, there are no established predictive biomarkers for response to ADT. Various components of the AR signaling pathway, genetic polymorphisms in androgen regulatory and metabolic pathways, and other molecular markers, have emerged as potential biomarkers of response and survival (summarized in **Box 1**).[60] A transcription-based AR activity signature, developed from an androgen-sensitive prostate cancer cell (LNCaP), has been shown to accurately predict AR activity in multiple prostate cancer cell lines, as well as reflect hormone status and intraprostatic prostatic DHT levels.[61] AR gene amplification can directly contribute to the development of ADT failure, by allowing cells to resume hormone-dependent growth in the presence of low concentrations of androgen.[62] AR variants have been identified in metastases obtained by rapid autopsy from patients

Box 1
Potential biomarkers of response to ADT and survival[a]

Potential biomarkers of response to ADT

  Androgens and AR

  • Serum testosterone, dehydrotestosterone, androstenediol, dehydroepiandrosterone

  • AR messenger RNA expression

  • AR protein expression

  • AR protein localization

  • AR gene amplification

  • AR gene mutations

  • AR splice variants

  Genetic polymorphisms in androgen regulatory and metabolic pathway

  • Hormones (LHRH, LH)

  • Receptors (LHRHR, LHR)

  • Enzymes (androgen biosynthesis and metabolism, estrogen biosynthesis)

  • Transporter and binding proteins (testosterone transporter, SHBG)

  • Hormone response elements (androgen response elements, estrogen response elements)

  Other molecular biomarkers

  • Chromosomal alterations (TPMRSS2:ERG fusion gene)

Potential biomarkers of survival (biomarkers of outcome)

• Gleason grading score

• Serum PSA

• CRP

• BMI

• Markers of bone metabolism

• CTCs

[a] Only those biomarkers discussed in the text are mentioned in Box 1.

treated with antiandrogens and by the lymph node excision from hormone-naive patients.[13] In hormone-naive samples, few mutations occurred, suggesting these mutations to be random passenger mutations, and not rendering a significant growth advantage. NTD mutations were shared across treatment groups, and likely provide a general growth advantage, regardless of past treatment. In contrast, mutations in the LBD were case specific, and uniquely correlated with the type of antiandrogen used, thus indicating that these antagonists select for distinct variants of mutated AR.[13]

Genetic polymorphisms have been reported in androgen regulatory pathways (luteinizing hormone-releasing hormone [LHRH], luteinizing hormone receptor [LHR], AR, and steroid hormone binding globulin [SHBG]), as well as in androgen biosynthesis and metabolic pathways (CYP19A1, HSDCB1, HSD17B4, SLC01B3). These polymorphisms are known to influence disease-specific survival, and response to ADT.[60] The TMPRSS2-ERG fusion gene is the most frequent genomic rearrangement found in prostate cancer and is a fusion of the ETS transcription factor family gene (ERG), with the promoter of the highly expressed transmembrane protease serine 2

(TMPRSS2) gene. TMPRSS 2:ERG expression is restored in the castration refractory setting and may contribute to the progression of prostate cancer, despite low androgen levels.[63] However, TMPRSS2: ERG fusion did not consistently predict PSA response to ADT or abiraterone.[64–67] In recent years, CTCs have emerged as a prognostic marker and have been shown to predict response to therapy in the castration-resistant setting.[68] The recent approval of a prognostic test based on CTC enumeration in CRPC is encouraging.[69] However, CTCs as prognostic and predictive biomarkers in the setting of HSPC have not been widely tested, and more sensitive technologies may be needed in this setting.

Serum PSA level predicts survival in men with HSPC who are on treatment with ADT. Based on the data from a phase 3 international trial (S9346, INT-0162) of more than 1000 patients with new M1 prostate cancer undergoing ADT (with goserelin and bicalutamide), serum PSA level after 7 months of therapy predicted survival.[70] The median survival was 13 months for patients with a PSA level greater than 4 ng/mL, 44 months for a PSA level of 0.2 to 4 ng/mL, and 75 months for a PSA level of 0.2 ng/mL or less. In a landmark analysis[71] of a total of 1078 patients with HSPC receiving ADT (SWOG 9346 trial) and 597 patients with CRPC receiving chemotherapy (SWOG 9916 trial), PSA progression correlated with OS in both HSPC and CRPC, although the correlation was stronger in HSPC. Other studies[72,73] have also reported the extent of the PSA nadir and time to PSA nadir as predictors of survival in men with HSPC receiving ADT.

Other biomarkers shown to correlate with outcomes in HSPC being treated with ADT include C-reactive protein (CRP), body mass index (BMI), and markers of bone metabolism.[60] In men with HSPC receiving ADT, CRP predicted cancer-specific survival, independent of PSA.[74] In phase 3 randomized studies coordinated by SWOG,[75] a higher BMI (but not obesity) was associated with improved PFS and OS in HSPC, but not in CRPC. Markers of bone metabolism have been shown to correlate with the duration of response to ADT in HSPC and had prognostic value in the castration-resistant setting.[76,77]

ONGOING STUDIES OF ADT IN COMBINATION WITH NOVEL AGENTS IN HSPC AND FUTURE DIRECTIONS

Based on data from more than 1000 patients with new HSPC undergoing ADT (goserelin in combination with bicalutamide) on the SWOG-9346 study, a failure to achieve a PSA of 4 ng/mL or less (or to be experiencing an increase in PSA) after 7 months of combined ADT is a powerful negative predictor of survival.[71] The median OS for this group of patients was 20 months from the start of ADT. In contrast, the median OS for patients who achieved undetectable PSA levels of 0.2 ng/mL or less (45% of patients) at month 7 had a median OS of 82 months from the start of ADT. These data provide the rationale for testing strategies to optimize the androgen blockade in new HSPC. SWOG 1216 is an intergroup phase 3 randomized trial comparing ADT plus TAK-700 versus ADT plus bicalutamide in new HSPC, and is accruing men with HSPC. OS is the primary end point (**Table 1**).

Insulinlike growth factor 1 receptor (IGF-IR) and its ligands IGF-I and IGF-II have been implicated in the development, maintenance, and progression of prostate cancer. Increased IGF-I and IGF-IR activity are associated with an increased risk of developing prostate cancer, progression to metastatic disease, and development of castration resistance.[78,79] Anti-IGF-IR antibodies, IGF-IR kinase inhibitors, and antisense oligonucleotides to IGF-IR have been shown to inhibit prostate cancer growth in vitro and in animal models.[80–82] A fully human monoclonal antibody, IMC-A12 (ImClone Systems), specific to IGF-IR, significantly inhibited growth of

Table 1
Randomized, phase 3 clinical trials in HSPC

Year of Most Recent Update (Reference)	Intervention	Number of Patients	Primary Question	Outcome	Identifier
1989[2]	Leuprolide with and without flutamide	603	Does maximal androgen blockade improve the effectiveness of ADT?	Improved PFS and OS with CAB vs leuprolide alone	SWOG8494, INT-0036, NCT: not available
1998[94]	Bilateral orchiectomy with or without flutamide	1387	Does OS improve with CAB over castration alone?	No difference in PFS and OS	SWOG8894, INT-0105, NCT: not available
2012[47]	Intermittent ADT vs continuous ADT with goserelin and bicalutamide	3040	Is OS with IAD noninferior to that with CAD?[a]	OS with IAD was not comparable with that with CAD	SWOG9346, INT-0162, NCT: not available
2012[60]	Androgen ablation therapy with or without chemotherapy with docetaxel with prednisone	780	Does early chemotherapy improve OS of patients commencing ADT for HSPC?	Completed accrual (results awaited)	ECOG 3805/CHAARTED, NCT00309985
2013[94]	ADT plus TAK-700 vs ADT plus bicalutamide	1486	Does OS improve with concomitant inhibition of CYP 17,20 lyase along with ADT over CAB?	Accruing	SWOG1216, NCT01809691
2013[58]	ADT with or without docetaxel	385	Does addition of docetaxel to ADT improve OS?	No difference in OS	NCT00104715
2013[59]	ADT alone, or ADT plus one of the following: docetaxel, celecoxib, zoledronic acid, celecoxib, zoledronic acid plus docetaxel, zoledronic acid plus celecoxib, abiraterone, or XRT to the prostate[b]	5000	Does addition of following interventions to ADT improve OS? docetaxel, zolendronic acid, celecoxib, abiraterone, or XRT to the prostate?	Accruing	NCT00268476

Abbreviation: NCT, ClinicalTrials.gov identifier.
[a] Coprimary end point was quality-of-life differences between CAD and IAD.
[b] Arms containing celecoxib were discontinued early because of lack of benefit.
Data from Refs. [1,47,57–59,93]

androgen-dependent and androgen-independent prostate xenografts.[83] In a phase 2 trial of men with asymptomatic CRPC,[84] treatment with IMC-A12 was well tolerated, with ~30% men experiencing disease stabilization for 6 months or more. In addition, a study of IMC-A12 in 180 men with new HSPC has recently completed accrual (SWOG0925).[85] The primary study objective is to compare the undetectable PSA rate (PSA<0.2 ng/mL) after 28 weeks of treatment (IMC-A12 administered every 2 weeks) between those randomized to an LHRH agonist and bicalutamide and those randomized to an LHRH agonist, bicalutamide and IMC-A12.

The T-lymphocyte checkpoint, CTLA-4, has been validated as a therapeutic target in advanced melanoma. Based on the preliminary evidence, that radiotherapy enhances the impact of subsequent immunotherapy, 2 placebo-controlled phase 3 trials evaluating the anti-CTLA-4 antibody, ipilimumab, after radiation to a metastatic site, have completed accrual.[86,87] A phase 2 study of ipilimumab plus ADT, is accruing men with new HSPC. The primary end points are the proportion of men achieving a PSA level of 0.2 ng/mL or lower at month 7 of treatment, and overall PSA response.[88]

Overexpression of the oncogene Bcl-2 is a known mechanism by which prostate cancer adapts and progresses on ADT.[89] AT-101 (R-(-)-gossypol acetic acid), a small molecule Bcl-2 inhibitor, was shown to increase apoptosis in prostate cancer xenograft mouse models, when used concomitantly with androgen blockade, and has the potential to delay the onset of castration resistance when used in combination with ADT in new HSPC.[90] A phase 2 trial of AT-101 in combination with ADT has completed accrual of 55 men with HSPC.[91] The primary end point was the percentage of patients with undetectable PSA (<0.2 ng/mL) after 7 months of therapy with this combination regimen. Although the final results are pending, in a preliminary report, 26% of patients achieved an undetectable PSA at 7 months of treatment.[92]

Metastatic prostate cancer is a biologically heterogeneous and invariably fatal disease. Various molecular pathways have been identified, which underlie the progression of HSPC to castration refractoriness, and novel agents targeting these pathways continue to be developed. An area of active investigation is the identification and validation of biomarkers predicting response to therapy. The development of novel combination regimens with the concomitant development of biomarkers is imperative for improvising survival outcomes, and requires close collaboration between laboratory and clinical investigation, as well as a commitment to clinical trials.

REFERENCES

1. Siegel R, Naishadham D, Jemal A. Cancer Statistics 2013. CA Cancer J Clin 2013;63(1):11–30.
2. Crawford ED, Eisenberger MA, McLeod DG, et al. A controlled trial of leuprolide with and without flutamide in prostatic carcinoma. N Engl J Med 1989;321(7): 419–24.
3. Taplin ME, Rajeshkumar B, Halabi S, et al. Androgen receptor mutations in androgen-independent prostate cancer: Cancer and Leukemia Group B Study 9663. J Clin Oncol 2003;21(14):2673–8.
4. Chen Y, Clegg NJ, Scher HI. Anti-androgens and androgen-depleting therapies in prostate cancer: new agents for an established target. Lancet Oncol 2009; 10(10):981–91.
5. Sharifi N, Auchus RJ. Steroid biosynthesis and prostate cancer. Steroids 2012; 77(7):719–26.
6. Sadar MD. Small molecule inhibitors targeting the "Achilles' heel" of androgen receptor activity. Cancer Res 2011;71(4):1208–13.

7. Taplin ME. Drug insight: role of the androgen receptor in the development and progression of prostate cancer. Nat Clin Pract Oncol 2007;4:236–44.

8. Reid AH, Attard G, Barrie E, et al. CYP17 inhibition as a hormonal strategy for prostate cancer. Nat Clin Pract Urol 2008;5(11):610–20.

9. Titus MA, Schell MJ, Lih FB, et al. Testosterone and dihydrotestosterone tissue levels in recurrent prostate cancer. Clin Cancer Res 2005;11(13):4653–7.

10. Montgomery RB. Maintenance of intratumoral androgens in metastatic prostate cancer: a mechanism for castration-resistant tumor growth. Cancer Res 2008;68:4447–54.

11. Mostaghel EA. Intraprostatic androgens and androgen-regulated gene expression persist after testosterone suppression: therapeutic implications for castration-resistant prostate cancer. Cancer Res 2007;67:5033–41.

12. Dillard PR, Lin MF, Khan SA. Androgen-independent prostate cancer cells acquire the complete steroidogenic potential of synthesizing testosterone from cholesterol. Mol Cell Endocrinol 2008;295(1–2):115–20.

13. Steinkamp MP, O'Mahony OA, Brogley M, et al. Treatment-dependent androgen receptor mutations in prostate cancer exploit multiple mechanisms to evade therapy. Cancer Res 2009;69(10):4434–42.

14. Edwards J, Krishna NS, Grigor KM, et al. Androgen receptor gene amplification and protein expression in hormone refractory prostate cancer. Br J Cancer 2003;89(3):552–6.

15. Feldman BJ, Feldman D. The development of androgen-independent prostate cancer. Nat Rev Cancer 2001;1(1):34–45.

16. Hara T, Miyazaki J, Araki H, et al. Novel mutations of androgen receptor: a possible mechanism of bicalutamide withdrawal syndrome. Cancer Res 2003;63(1):149–53.

17. Suzuki H, Okihara K, Miyake H, et al. Alternative nonsteroidal antiandrogen therapy for advanced prostate cancer that relapsed after initial maximum androgen blockade. J Urol 2008;180(3):921–7.

18. Li Y, Chan SC, Brand LJ, et al. Androgen receptor splice variants mediate enzalutamide resistance in castration-resistant prostate cancer cell lines. Cancer Res 2013;73(2):483–9.

19. Hanahan D, Weinberg RA. Hallmarks of cancer: the next generation. Cell 2011;144(5):646–74.

20. Karlou M, Tzelepi V, Efstathiou E. Therapeutic targeting of the prostate cancer microenvironment. Nat Rev Urol 2010;7(9):494–509.

21. Agarwal N, Sonpavde G, Sternberg CN. Novel molecular targets for the therapy of castration-resistant prostate cancer. Eur Urol 2012;61(5):950–60.

22. Conn PM, Crowley WF Jr. Gonadotropin-releasing hormone and its analogues. N Engl J Med 1991;324(2):93–103.

23. Loblaw DA, Virgo KS, Nam R, et al. Initial hormonal management of androgen-sensitive metastatic, recurrent, or progressive prostate cancer: 2006 update of an American Society of Clinical Oncology practice guideline. J Clin Oncol 2007;25(12):1596–605.

24. Klotz L, Boccon-Gibod L, Shore ND, et al. The efficacy and safety of degarelix: a 12-month, comparative, randomized, open-label, parallel-group phase III study in patients with prostate cancer. BJU Int 2008;102(11):1531–8.

25. Small EJ, Halabi S, Dawson NA, et al. Antiandrogen withdrawal alone or in combination with ketoconazole in androgen-independent prostate cancer patients: a phase III trial (CALGB 9583). J Clin Oncol 2004;22(6):1025–33.

26. Small EJ, Vogelzang NJ. Second-line hormonal therapy for advanced prostate cancer: a shifting paradigm. J Clin Oncol 1997;15(1):382–8.

27. de Bono JS, Logothetis CJ, Molina A, et al. Abiraterone and increased survival in metastatic prostate cancer. N Engl J Med 2011;364(21):1995–2005.

28. Ryan CJ, Smith MR, de Bono JS, et al. Abiraterone in metastatic prostate cancer without previous chemotherapy. N Engl J Med 2013;368(2):138–48.

29. Mostaghel EA, Marck BT, Plymate SR, et al. Resistance to CYP17A1 inhibition with abiraterone in castration-resistant prostate cancer: induction of steroidogenesis and androgen receptor splice variants. Clin Cancer Res 2011;17(18):5913–25.

30. Kaku T, Hitaka T, Ojida A, et al. Discovery of orteronel (TAK-700), a naphthylmethylimidazole derivative, as a highly selective 17,20-lyase inhibitor with potential utility in the treatment of prostate cancer. Bioorg Med Chem 2011;19(21):6383–99.

31. Agus DA, Stadler WM, Shevrin DH, et al. Safety, efficacy, and pharmacodynamics of the investigational agent orteronel (TAK-700) in metastatic castration-resistant prostate cancer (mCRPC): updated data from a phase I/II study. J Clin Oncol 2012;30(Suppl 5) [abstract 98].

32. Hussain M, Corn P, Michaelson D, et al. Activity and safety of the investigational agent orteronel in men with nonmetastatic castration-resistant prostate cancer and rising prostate-specific antigen: results of a phase 2 study. 27th Annual European Association of Urology. Paris. February 24–28, 2012. Poster 124.

33. Seidenfeld J, Samson DJ, Hasselblad V, et al. Single-therapy androgen suppression in men with advanced prostate cancer: a systematic review and meta-analysis. Ann Intern Med 2000;132(7):566–77.

34. Scher HI, Beer TM, Higano CS, et al. Antitumour activity of MDV3100 in castration-resistant prostate cancer: a phase 1-2 study. Lancet 2010;375(9724):1437–46.

35. Scher HI, Fizazi K, Saad F, et al. Increased survival with enzalutamide in prostate cancer after chemotherapy. N Engl J Med 2012;367(13):1187–97.

36. Rathkopf DE, Danila DC, Morris MJ, et al. Phase I/II safety and pharmacokinetic (PK) study of ARN-509 in patients with metastatic castration-resistant prostate cancer (mCRPC): phase I results of a Prostate Cancer Clinical Trials Consortium study. J Clin Oncol 2012;30(Suppl 5) [abstract 43].

37. Montgomery RB, Eisenberger MA, Rettig M, et al. Phase I clinical trial of galeterone (TOK-001), a multifunctional antiandrogen and CYP17 inhibitor in castration resistant prostate cancer (CRPC). J Clin Oncol 2012;30(Suppl) [abstract 4665].

38. Andersen RJ, Mawji NR, Wang J, et al. Regression of castrate-recurrent prostate cancer by a small-molecule inhibitor of the amino-terminus domain of the androgen receptor. Cancer Cell 2010;17(6):535–46.

39. Maximum androgen blockade in advanced prostate cancer: an overview of the randomised trials. Prostate Cancer Trialists' Collaborative Group. Lancet 2000;355(9214):1491–8.

40. Schmitt B, Bennett C, Seidenfeld J, et al. Maximal androgen blockade for advanced prostate cancer. Cochrane Database Syst Rev 2000;(2):CD001526.

41. Samson DJ, Seidenfeld J, Schmitt B, et al. Systematic review and meta-analysis of monotherapy compared with combined androgen blockade for patients with advanced prostate carcinoma. Cancer 2002;95(2):361–76.

42. Klotz L, Schellhammer P, Carroll K. A re-assessment of the role of combined androgen blockade for advanced prostate cancer. BJU Int 2004;93(9):1177–82.

43. Isaacs JT, Coffey DS. Adaptation versus selection as the mechanism responsible for the relapse of prostatic cancer to androgen ablation therapy as studied in the Dunning R-3327-H adenocarcinoma. Cancer Res 1981;41(12 Pt 1):5070–5.

44. Bruchovsky N, Rennie PS, Coldman AJ, et al. Effects of androgen withdrawal on the stem cell composition of the Shionogi carcinoma. Cancer Res 1990;50(8): 2275–82.

45. Klotz LH, Herr HW, Morse MJ, et al. Intermittent endocrine therapy for advanced prostate cancer. Cancer 1986;58(11):2546–50.

46. Sato N, Gleave ME, Bruchovsky N, et al. Intermittent androgen suppression delays progression to androgen-independent regulation of prostate-specific antigen gene in the LNCaP prostate tumour model. J Steroid Biochem Mol Biol 1996;58(2):139–46.

47. Hussain M, Tangen CM, Berry DL, et al. Intermittent versus continuous androgen deprivation in prostate cancer. N Engl J Med 2013;368(14):1314–25.

48. Moinpour C, Berry DL, Ely B, et al. Preliminary quality-of-life outcomes for SWOG-9346: intermittent androgen deprivation in patients with hormone-sensitive metastatic prostate cancer (HSM1PC)–phase III. J Clin Oncol 2012; 30(Suppl) [abstract 4571].

49. Osborne CK, Blumenstein B, Crawford ED, et al. Combined versus sequential chemo-endocrine therapy in advanced prostate cancer: final results of a randomized Southwest Oncology Group study. J Clin Oncol 1990;8(10): 1675–82.

50. Tannock IF. Is there evidence that chemotherapy is of benefit to patients with carcinoma of the prostate? J Clin Oncol 1985;3(7):1013–21.

51. Mukamel E, Nissenkorn I, Servadio C. Early combined hormonal and chemotherapy for metastatic carcinoma of prostate. Urology 1980;16(3):257–60.

52. Smith DC, Tangen CM, Van Veldhuizen PJ Jr, et al. Phase II evaluation of early oral estramustine, oral etoposide, and intravenous paclitaxel combined with hormonal therapy in patients with high-risk metastatic prostate adenocarcinoma: Southwest Oncology Group S0032. Urology 2011;77(5):1172–6.

53. Petrylak DP, Tangen CM, Hussain MH, et al. Docetaxel and estramustine compared with mitoxantrone and prednisone for advanced refractory prostate cancer. N Engl J Med 2004;351(15):1513–20.

54. Tannock IF, de Wit R, Berry WR, et al. Docetaxel plus prednisone or mitoxantrone plus prednisone for advanced prostate cancer. N Engl J Med 2004; 351(15):1502–12.

55. Dorff TB, Tangen CM, Crawford ED, et al. Cooperative Group Trials–Southwest Oncology Group (SWOG) innovations in advanced prostate cancer. Ther Adv Med Oncol 2009;1(2):69–77.

56. Sweeney CJ. ECOG: CHAARTED–ChemoHormonal therapy versus androgen ablation randomized trial for extensive disease in prostate cancer. Clin Adv Hematol Oncol 2006;4(8):588–90.

57. NCT00309985: Androgen ablation therapy with or without chemotherapy in treating patients with metastatic prostate cancer (ClinicalTrials.gov).

58. Gravis G, Fizazi K, Joly F, et al. Androgen-deprivation therapy alone or with docetaxel in non-castrate metastatic prostate cancer (GETUG-AFU 15): a randomised, open-label, phase 3 trial. Lancet Oncol 2013;14(2):149–58.

59. Sydes MR, Parmar MK, Mason MD, et al. Flexible trial design in practice-stopping arms for lack-of-benefit and adding research arms mid-trial in STAMPEDE: a multi-arm multi-stage randomized controlled trial. Trials 2012;13:168.

60. Grivas PD, Robins DM, Hussain M. Predicting response to hormonal therapy and survival in men with hormone sensitive metastatic prostate cancer. Crit Rev Oncol Hematol 2013;85(1):82–93.

61. Mendiratta P, Mostaghel E, Guinney J, et al. Genomic strategy for targeting therapy in castration-resistant prostate cancer. J Clin Oncol 2009;27(12):2022–9.

62. Koivisto P, Kononen J, Palmberg C, et al. Androgen receptor gene amplification: a possible molecular mechanism for androgen deprivation therapy failure in prostate cancer. Cancer Res 1997;57(2):314–9.

63. Mehra R, Tomlins SA, Yu J, et al. Characterization of TMPRSS2-ETS gene aberrations in androgen-independent metastatic prostate cancer. Cancer Res 2008; 68(10):3584–90.

64. Danila DC, Anand A, Sung CC, et al. TMPRSS2-ERG status in circulating tumor cells as a predictive biomarker of sensitivity in castration-resistant prostate cancer patients treated with abiraterone acetate. Eur Urol 2011;60(5): 897–904.

65. Leinonen KA, Tolonen TT, Bracken H, et al. Association of SPINK1 expression and TMPRSS2:ERG fusion with prognosis in endocrine-treated prostate cancer. Clin Cancer Res 2010;16(10):2845–51.

66. Attard G, Swennenhuis JF, Olmos D, et al. Characterization of ERG, AR and PTEN gene status in circulating tumor cells from patients with castration-resistant prostate cancer. Cancer Res 2009;69(7):2912–8.

67. Karnes RJ, Cheville JC, Ida CM, et al. The ability of biomarkers to predict systemic progression in men with high-risk prostate cancer treated surgically is dependent on ERG status. Cancer Res 2010;70(22):8994–9002.

68. Balic M, Williams A, Lin H, et al. Circulating tumor cells: from bench to bedside. Annu Rev Med 2013;64:31–44.

69. Danila DC, Fleisher M, Scher HI. Circulating tumor cells as biomarkers in prostate cancer. Clin Cancer Res 2011;17(12):3903–12.

70. Hussain M, Tangen CM, Higano C, et al. Absolute prostate-specific antigen value after androgen deprivation is a strong independent predictor of survival in new metastatic prostate cancer: data from Southwest Oncology Group Trial 9346 (INT-0162). J Clin Oncol 2006;24(24):3984–90.

71. Hussain M, Goldman B, Tangen C, et al. Prostate-specific antigen progression predicts overall survival in patients with metastatic prostate cancer: data from Southwest Oncology Group Trials 9346 (Intergroup Study 0162) and 9916. J Clin Oncol 2009;27(15):2450–6.

72. Choueiri TK, Xie W, D'Amico AV, et al. Time to prostate-specific antigen nadir independently predicts overall survival in patients who have metastatic hormone-sensitive prostate cancer treated with androgen-deprivation therapy. Cancer 2009;115(5):981–7.

73. Huang SP, Bao BY, Wu MT, et al. Significant associations of prostate-specific antigen nadir and time to prostate-specific antigen nadir with survival in prostate cancer patients treated with androgen-deprivation therapy. Aging Male 2012; 15(1):34–41.

74. McArdle PA, Mir K, Almushatat AS, et al. Systemic inflammatory response, prostate-specific antigen and survival in patients with metastatic prostate cancer. Urol Int 2006;77(2):127–9.

75. Montgomery RB, Goldman B, Tangen CM, et al. Association of body mass index with response and survival in men with metastatic prostate cancer: Southwest Oncology Group trials 8894 and 9916. J Urol 2007;178(5):1946–51 [discussion: 1951].

76. Sharma J, Yiannoutsos CT, Hahn NM, et al. Prognostic value of suppressed markers of bone turnover (BTO) after 6 months of androgen deprivation therapy (ADT) in prostate cancer. J Clin Oncol 2011;29(Suppl) [abstract 4594].

77. Lara P, Ely B, Quinn DI, et al. SWOG 0421: prognostic and predictive value of bone metabolism biomarkers (BMB) in castration resistant prostate cancer (CRPC) patients (pts) with skeletal metastases treated with docetaxel (DOC) with or without atrasentan (ATR). J Clin Oncol 2012;30(Suppl) [abstract 4547].

78. Hellawell GO, Turner GD, Davies DR, et al. Expression of the type 1 insulin-like growth factor receptor is up-regulated in primary prostate cancer and commonly persists in metastatic disease. Cancer Res 2002;62(10):2942-50.

79. Krueckl SL, Sikes RA, Edlund NM, et al. Increased insulin-like growth factor I receptor expression and signaling are components of androgen-independent progression in a lineage-derived prostate cancer progression model. Cancer Res 2004;64(23):8620-9.

80. Blum G, Gazit A, Levitzki A. Development of new insulin-like growth factor-1 receptor kinase inhibitors using catechol mimics. J Biol Chem 2003;278(42):40442-54.

81. Burfeind P, Chernicky CL, Rininsland F, et al. Antisense RNA to the type I insulin-like growth factor receptor suppresses tumor growth and prevents invasion by rat prostate cancer cells in vivo. Proc Natl Acad Sci U S A 1996;93(14):7263-8.

82. Burtrum D, Zhu Z, Lu D, et al. A fully human monoclonal antibody to the insulin-like growth factor I receptor blocks ligand-dependent signaling and inhibits human tumor growth in vivo. Cancer Res 2003;63(24):8912-21.

83. Wu JD, Odman A, Higgins LM, et al. In vivo effects of the human type I insulin-like growth factor receptor antibody A12 on androgen-dependent and androgen-independent xenograft human prostate tumors. Clin Cancer Res 2005;11(8):3065-74.

84. Higano CS, Alumkal JJ, Ryan CJ, et al. A phase II study of cixutumumab (IMC-A12), a monoclonal antibody (MAb) against the insulin-like growth factor 1 receptor (IGF-IR), monotherapy in metastatic castration-resistant prostate cancer (mCRPC): feasibility of every 3-week dosing and updated results. Genitourinary Cancers Symposium San Francisco, California, March 5-7, 2010. Abstract no. 189.

85. NCT01120236: bicalutamide and goserelin or leuprolide acetate with or without cixutumumab in treating patients with newly diagnosed metastatic prostate cancer (ClinicalTrials.gov).

86. NCT00861614: a randomized, double-blind, phase 3 trial comparing ipilimumab vs. placebo following radiotherapy in subjects with castration resistant prostate cancer that have received prior treatment with docetaxel (ClinicalTrials.gov).

87. NCT01057810: randomized, double-blind, phase 3 trial to compare the efficacy of ipilimumab vs placebo in asymptomatic or minimally symptomatic patients with metastatic chemotherapy-naïve castration resistant prostate cancer (ClinicalTrials.gov).

88. NCT01377389: ipilimumab + androgen deprivation therapy in prostate cancer (ClinicalTrials.gov).

89. Shi Y, Chatterjee SJ, Brands FH, et al. Role of coordinated molecular alterations in the development of androgen-independent prostate cancer: an in vitro model that corroborates clinical observations. BJU Int 2006;97(1):170-8.

90. McGregor N, Patel L, Craig M, et al. AT-101 (R-(-)-gossypol acetic acid) enhances the effectiveness of androgen deprivation therapy in the VCaP prostate cancer model. J Cell Biochem 2010;110(5):1187-94.

91. NCT00666666:R-(-)-gossypol and androgen ablation therapy in treating patients with newly diagnosed metastatic prostate cancer (ClinicalTrials.gov).
92. Stein MN, Khan I, Hussain M, et al. Phase II study of AT-101 to abrogate Bcl-2-mediated resistance to androgen-deprivation therapy (ADT) in patients (pts) with newly diagnosed androgen-dependent metastatic prostate cancer (ADMPC). J Clin Oncol 2011;29(Suppl 7) [abstract 137].
93. Eisenberger MA, Blumenstein BA, Crawford ED, et al. Bilateral orchiectomy with or without flutamide for metastatic prostate cancer. N Engl J Med 1998;339(15): 1036–42.
94. 1809691: S1216, Phase III ADT+TAK-700 vs. ADT+Bicalutamide for Metastatic Prostate Cancer (ClinicalTrials.gov).

Management of Patients with Castration-Resistant Disease

Carmel Pezaro, MBChB, FRACP, DMedSc, Aurelius Omlin, MD,
David Lorente, MD, Johann de Bono, MBChB, FRCP, MSc, PhD, FMedSci*

KEYWORDS

- Castration-resistant prostate cancer • Novel therapies • Androgen receptor signaling

KEY POINTS

- Agents proven to improve survival for men with castration-resistant prostate cancer include docetaxel and cabazitaxel chemotherapies, androgen/androgen receptor targeting treatments with abiraterone and enzalutamide, sipuleucel-T immunotherapy, and the radionuclide ^{223}radium.
- Signaling through the androgen receptor continues to drive the progression of prostate cancer after development of castration resistance.
- Improvements in disease stratification and response assessment are needed to assist patient care and future drug development.
- Multiple promising treatments are in the later stages of clinical development.
- Participation in clinical trials should be encouraged as part of best standard of care for men with metastatic prostate cancer.

INTRODUCTION

The medical management of men with castration-resistant prostate cancer (CRPC) has changed dramatically in the last decade. Multiple successful phase III trials have been reported, and men can now access several agents developed to extend survival, delay morbidity caused by complications, and preserve quality of life. Strategies now proven to extend survival in CRPC include the taxane chemotherapies docetaxel and cabazitaxel, inhibition of androgen biosynthesis with the CYP-inhibitor abiraterone acetate (abiraterone), the second-generation androgen receptor (AR)

Disclosure: All authors are employees of the Institute for Cancer Research (ICR). The ICR has a commercial interest in abiraterone and PI3K and AKT inhibitors. J.S. de Bono has served as a paid consultant for Johnson & Johnson, Sanofi Aventis, Medivation, Astellas, AstraZeneca, Dendreon, Genentech, Pfizer, and GlaxoSmithKline.
Prostate Cancer Targeted Therapy Group and Drug Development Unit, The Royal Marsden NHS Foundation Trust, The Institute of Cancer Research, Downs Road, Sutton, Surrey SM2 5PT, UK
* Corresponding author. Prostate Cancer Targeted Therapies Group and Drug Development Unit, Royal Marsden NHS Foundation Trust and The Institute of Cancer Research, Downs Road, Sutton, Surrey SM2 5PT, UK.
E-mail address: johann.de-bono@icr.ac.uk

Hematol Oncol Clin N Am 27 (2013) 1243–1260
http://dx.doi.org/10.1016/j.hoc.2013.08.008
0889-8588/13/$ – see front matter Crown Copyright © 2013 Published by Elsevier Inc. All rights reserved.

antagonist enzalutamide, sipuleucel-T immunotherapy, and the α-emitting radionu-clide ^{223}radium. The introduction of these novel therapies has fostered interest in translational science and a deeper understanding of the underlying biology in CRPC. This article summarizes clinical data and unresolved issues in the use of current and emerging CRPC therapies.

OVERVIEW OF DRUG CLASSES

Drug-discovery programs do not always march alongside basic science. Sometimes clinical researchers declare that a compound works before the mechanism by which it is working has been fully elucidated. For this reason, assignment of agents into classes of activity for CRPC may change as our scientific understanding increases (**Fig. 1**).

Hormonal therapies remain a mainstay of treatment in advanced prostate cancer, even after development of castration resistance. Ongoing castration by means of bilateral orchiectomy or luteinizing hormone–releasing hormone (LHRH) analogue has

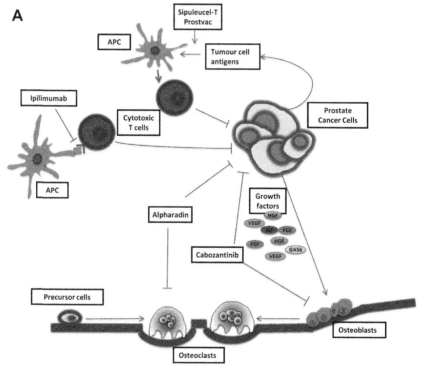

Fig. 1. Targets of current and emerging treatments for advanced prostate cancer. (*A*) Agents acting externally on the environment of prostate cancer. (*B*) Agents acting on internal targets of prostate cancer. Alpharadin (α-radiation emitting radioisotope); cabozantinib (cMET and VEGF receptor-2 inhibitor); sipuleucel-T and Prostvac (vaccine therapies); ipilimumab (anti–CTLA-4 antibody); abiraterone (CYP17 inhibitor); enzalutamide (antiandrogen, blocks AR shuttling into the nucleus, blocks interaction of activated AR with DNA); docetaxel and cabazitaxel (microtubule inhibitors, potentially also blocking AR shuttling into the nucleus); custirsen (clusterin inhibitor). APC, antigen-presenting cell; AR, androgen receptor; DHT, dihydrotestosterone; FGF, fibroblast growth factor; GAS6, Growth arrest–specific 6; HGF, hepatocyte growth factor; IGF-1, insulin like growth factor 1; T, testosterone; VEGF, vascular endothelial growth factor.

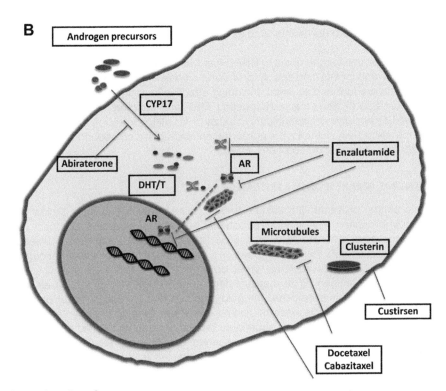

Fig. 1. (*continued*)

invariably been mandated in CRPC trials. In addition, there is compelling evidence to continue systemic castration for abiraterone, as the effect is overcome in the absence of LHRH analogue because of a compensatory LH surge.[1] Docetaxel clearance is reduced in the noncastrate setting, causing potentially greater toxicity than that demonstrated in CRPC trials.[2] Older second-line hormonal therapies such as estrogen preparations and first-generation AR antagonists continue to be used in select CRPC patients, but these strategies lack level III evidence and are not reviewed in this article.

Signaling through the AR remains a key driver of progression in CRPC. Adrenal androgen synthesis accounts for up to 20% of circulating androgens under normal circumstances and, along with intratumoral androgen production, contributes to progression of prostate cancer despite androgen-deprivation therapy. Abiraterone interferes with AR signaling by inhibiting the CYP17 enzyme, blocking androgen production from steroid precursors and thereby reducing androgen levels in the so-called super-castrate range. The second-generation AR antagonist enzalutamide binds to and inhibits AR function without demonstrable agonist activity in the setting of overexpressed or mutated AR.

The taxane chemotherapy agents docetaxel and cabazitaxel have proven utility in CRPC. However, it is no longer clear whether these drugs should be in a separate class as cytotoxics acting as microtubule stabilizers, or whether the activity of taxanes also occurs through inhibition of AR function.

Immune targeting is a current focus of treatment in CRPC, including the specific vaccine therapies sipuleucel-T and Prostvac-VF. There is also considerable interest in the use of agents that cause general modulation of the immune system through blockade of immune checkpoints such as CTLA4 and PD1 to decrease immune tolerance to cancer.

Identifying promising therapies in CRPC has been hampered by the lack of useful intermediate end points and falsely promising signals from phase II trials. Several novel agents are further discussed, including effective targeting of bone metastases with radium-223 (^{223}Ra), the multitargeting MET and vascular endothelial growth factor (VEGF) tyrosine kinase inhibitor cabozantinib, oligonucleotide therapy against the apoptosis protein clusterin, the purported antiangiogenic compound tasquinimod, and targeting of heat-shock proteins (HSPs).

SEQUENCING AND RESPONSE ASSESSMENT

Prostate cancer presents with unique disease characteristics that have clinical and research implications. The majority of patients with metastatic disease present with bone metastases, whereas less than 50% have measurable soft-tissue disease. Response assessments therefore depend on a combination of parameters that contain considerable uncertainty such as serial bone and computed tomography scans, prostate-specific antigen (PSA) measurements, and clinical variables such as pain. Overall survival (OS) is considered the gold-standard primary end point for phase III clinical trials, but in the presence of several survival-prolonging treatments it will be increasingly challenging to prove superiority of a novel treatment based on a survival advantage. Intermediate end points or markers of surrogacy for OS are urgently needed. Circulating tumor cells (CTCs) are a promising new technology in patients with advanced prostate cancer. Changes in CTC counts including conversion from unfavorable (CTC $\geq$5/7.5 mL plasma) to favorable (CTC <5) counts have been associated with longer OS.[3,4] In the COU-301 abiraterone trial CTC conversion was associated with improved OS as early as 4 weeks after initiation of treatment.[5] For CTCs to meet criteria for surrogacy, further confirmation from phase III clinical trials will be required. CTCs can also be molecularly characterized using AR amplification, phosphatase and tensin homologue (PTEN) and epidermal growth factor receptor (EGFR) assays, and for chromosomal rearrangements (eg, TMPRSS2-ERG rearrangements).[6,7]

The time between primary diagnosis of prostate cancer and the diagnosis of advanced metastatic disease is generally several years. Collection of fresh tumor tissue later in the disease is therefore important. However, the lack of easily accessible soft-tissue disease and the predominance of bone metastatic disease have made tumor biopsies difficult. Undirected bone marrow biopsies from the iliac crest may be technically feasible in men with prostate cancer, but the published positive yield of 25% was thought to be insufficient to recommend its routine use.[8] Serial bone marrow biopsies in a cohort of patients on abiraterone also proved feasible, but the rate of positive samples was 47% and only 44% of patients had tumor infiltration of 5% or greater.[9]

The availability of several novel treatment options that have different mechanisms of action raises the question of rational combination strategies and sequencing approaches. Combinations of novel agents in clinical trials in advanced prostate cancer are highlighted herein. At present there are no level I data available on sequencing of treatments in advanced prostate cancer, but several case series have been presented at recent oncology conferences. In a published cohort of 35 patients treated with docetaxel following treatment with abiraterone, PSA declines in PSA of at least 50% were reported in 9 patients (26%), with median OS of 12.5 months (95% confidence interval [CI] 10.6–19.4).[10] These data are retrospective and derived from a small set of patients, but seem to suggest a lower activity of docetaxel following abiraterone treatment, which may be explained by shared mechanisms of resistance when targeting the AR, or representing disease more resistant to treatment in general owing to the later stage in the cancer's evolution.

TARGETING OF ANDROGEN RECEPTOR
Abiraterone

Abiraterone (Zytiga; Janssen Pharmaceuticals) is a high-affinity, selective, irreversible inhibitor of cytochrome P450 CYP17, which mediates the conversion of cholesterol to androgen precursors. Abiraterone is structurally related to pregnenolone, a natural substrate of CYP17.

Abiraterone was developed as an acetate prodrug, which increases oral bioavailability. Early clinical trials determined that dosing with a high-fat diet increased drug absorption and exposure.[11]

Following promising early-phase data, abiraterone was compared with placebo in the phase III COU-AA-301 trial.[12] A cohort of 1195 men with progressive CRPC following docetaxel chemotherapy were randomized in a 2:1 ratio to receive abiraterone 1000 mg daily with prednisone 5 mg twice daily, or matched placebo and prednisone. The final analysis after a median follow-up of 20.2 months showed significantly longer survival with abiraterone in comparison with placebo (OS 15.8 vs 11.2 months; hazard ratio [HR] 0.74, 95% CI 0.64–0.86, $P<.001$).[13] All secondary end points, including time to PSA progression (8.5 vs 6.6 months, HR 0.63; $P<.001$), radiographic progression-free survival (PFS) (5.6 vs 3.6 months; HR 0.66, $P<.001$), and PSA response rate (29.5% vs 5.5%; $P<.001$) favored abiraterone treatment.

The randomized, double-blind, placebo-controlled phase III COU-AA-302 trial evaluated abiraterone in the chemotherapy-naïve setting. A total of 1088 prechemotherapy metastatic CRPC patients were randomized in a 1:1 ratio to receive abiraterone with prednisone or placebo with prednisone. Primary end points for this study were radiographic PFS and OS. The trial was halted following an interim analysis, performed after 43% of the expected OS events.[14] Radiographic PFS was significantly improved with abiraterone (16.5 vs 8.3 months; HR 0.53, 95% CI 0.45–0.62). There was a strong trend in OS (median not reached vs 27.2 months; HR 0.75, 95% CI 0.61–0.93); however, this did not meet the prespecified criteria for statistical significance at interim analysis. No new safety concerns were identified. Abiraterone is currently being tested in the treatment of men with hormone-sensitive prostate cancer as part of the STAMPEDE trial (NCT00268476), as well as in multiple combination studies (see www. clinicaltrials.gov for details).

CYP17 inhibition results in increased corticotropin levels via a negative feedback loop, causing raised levels of upstream adrenal steroids that prevent the development of adrenocortical insufficiency but can cause a syndrome of secondary mineralocorticoid excess.[11] On the COU-AA-301 trial mineralocorticoid-related adverse events were more frequently reported with abiraterone, including fluid retention (31% vs 22%), hypertension (10% vs 8%), and hypokalemia (17% vs 8%), although these were mostly graded as mild to moderate.[12] Mineralocorticoid antagonists (eplerenone) or low-dose glucocorticoids, which decrease corticotropin and steroids upstream of the CYP17 blockade, have been used for the treatment of hypertension or fluid retention secondary to abiraterone, although even these agents can bind and activate mutant AR.[15]

Enzalutamide

Enzalutamide (MDV3100; Xtandi; Astellas Pharma) is a small-molecule AR antagonist that also blocks the AR nuclear translocation and binding to DNA. Unlike bicalutamide, enzalutamide has no known agonist activity in models with AR overexpression.[16] Enzalutamide is administered orally without the need of concomitant steroids.

In a phase I/II study enzalutamide showed significant activity, with PSA declines of 50% or more in 62% of 65 chemotherapy-naïve patients and in 51% of 75 patients pretreated with docetaxel.[17] The main toxicities were fatigue, nausea, and loss of appetite. It was then evaluated in 2 large phase III trials, in the postchemotherapy (AFFIRM) and prechemotherapy (PREVAIL) settings.

The AFFIRM trial randomized 1199 men with CRPC previously treated with chemotherapy to receive enzalutamide 160 mg daily or placebo. The study was unblinded after an interim analysis showed a significant benefit for patients on enzalutamide, with a median OS improvement of 4.8 months (18.4 vs 13.6 months; HR 0.63, 95% CI 0.53–0.75, $P<.001$).[18] All secondary end points, including PSA response rate (54% vs 2%; $P<.001$), soft-tissue response (29% vs 4%; $P<.001$), time to PSA progression (8.3 vs 3 months; $P<.001$), radiographic PFS (8.3 vs 2.9 months; $P<.001$) and quality-of-life measures significantly favored the enzalutamide arm.

The main reported adverse events on the enzalutamide arm of AFFIRM were fatigue, diarrhea, and hot flashes. Seizures were reported in 5 patients (0.6%), most of whom had predisposing or concomitant risks. The AFFIRM investigators recommended enzalutamide avoidance in patients with a history of seizure and caution in patients with predisposing risk factors (stroke, alcoholism, brain metastases) or who used medication known to lower the seizure threshold.

The PREVAIL trial (NCT01212991) randomized 1680 asymptomatic or mildly symptomatic chemotherapy-naïve CRPC patients in a 1:1 ratio to enzalutamide or placebo, with primary end points of OS and PFS. Accrual was completed in June 2012, and results are awaited.

Novel Hormonal Therapies

TAK-700

TAK-700 (orteronel; Millennium Pharmaceuticals) is a selective inhibitor of the 17,20-lyase, with less affinity for the 17α-hydroxylase. Although it has a theoretical advantage that it may not require concomitant steroids, current phase III trials mandate the use of concomitant prednisolone. Orteronel showed activity in a phase I/II trial of men with CRPC.[19] PSA declines of at least 50% were achieved in 41% to 63% of the 97-patient expansion cohort, with higher PSA response rates seen with schedules that omitted prednisolone. The safety profile appeared acceptable, with main grade-3 adverse events of fatigue (12%) and hypokalemia (8%). Two large randomized phase III trials are currently evaluating orteronel in the prechemotherapy (NCT01193244) and postchemotherapy (NCT01193257) setting.

VT 464

VT 464 (Viamet) is another selective oral CYP17 inhibitor with selectivity for 17,20-lyase, which potentially avoids the need for concomitant steroids.[20] It is currently undergoing phase I development.

ARN-509

ARN-509 (Janssen Pharmaceuticals) is a small-molecule androgen-signaling inhibitor that, though it has a structure and mechanism of action similar to those of enzalutamide, has been purported to have reduced distribution to the brain in preclinical models.[21] This could be associated with a lower risk of seizures than enzalutamide, allowing higher clinical dose escalation. In preclinical models ARN-509 appeared to have greater efficacy than enzalutamide.[21] A phase I trial of 30 patients with metastatic CRPC showed PSA declines of 50% or more in 43% participants, with fatigue (38%), nausea (29%), and pain (24%) as the most common adverse events of grades 1 to 2.[22] ARN-509 continues to undergo phase I/II testing.

ODM-201
Additional second-generation antiandrogens are in clinical development, including ODM-201 (Orion Pharma), which showed high rates of PSA decline in phase I testing, including in docetaxel-pretreated patients.[23]

TOK-700
TOK-700 (galeterone; Tokai Pharmaceuticals) is a novel, orally available agent that combines CYP17-lyase inhibition with binding and inhibition of the AR and AR degradation. TOK-700 was evaluated in a phase I dose-escalation trial ARMOR1, presented at the 2012 American Association for Cancer Research annual meeting.[24] Treatment was well tolerated, with fatigue, transaminase elevations, and gastrointestinal symptoms as main adverse events. Almost 50% of patients showed a decline in PSA levels of at least 30%, and 22% showed a decline of 50% or greater.

IMMUNOTHERAPY
Sipuleucel-T

Sipuleucel-T (Provenge; Dendreon Corp) was the first immunotherapy to be approved by the US Food and Drug Administration (FDA) in 2010 for the treatment of prostate cancer. Sipuleucel-T consists of activated antigen-presenting cells (APCs) derived from autologous peripheral blood mononuclear cells. Each APC collection is by a leukapheresis procedure, which usually requires insertion of a "long-line" central venous catheter. Sipuleucel-T is administered as 3 infusions over a 1-month period, and leukapheresis is performed before each of these infusions. The APCs are stimulated ex vivo using a recombinant protein PA2024, which consists of prostatic acid phosphatase fused to granulocyte-macrophage colony-stimulating factor (GM-CSF). Within approximately 3 days of the leukapheresis, the stimulated APCs are reinfused.

In the phase III IMPACT trial, 512 patients with CRPC, bone or lymph node metastases, and a chemotherapy-free interval of at least 3 months were randomized in a 2:1 ratio to sipuleucel-T or placebo treatment. The trial reported an OS benefit of 4.1 months for sipuleucel-T (25.8 vs 21.7 months; HR 0.78, 95% CI 0.61–0.98, $P = .03$).[25] Other efficacy measures, such as PFS and PSA decline of at least 50%, were equal in both treatment arms. Although prior chemotherapy treatment was not excluded, it is noteworthy that more than 80% of patients were chemotherapy-naïve. In addition, the patients' characteristics indicate a highly selected population, with Gleason score of 7 or less in 75% patients, while 43% of patients had low-volume bone-only metastases and 52% were free of pain at study entry. The most common sipuleucel-T related adverse events were influenza-like symptoms, including chills (51%), fever (23%), fatigue (16%), nausea (14%) and headaches (11%), mostly of mild to moderate grade, which occurred within 24 hours of infusion and generally resolved within 48 hours.

A smaller randomized trial of 127 patients failed to meet the primary end point of time to tumor progression but reported a survival benefit similar to that of the IMPACT trial (25.9 vs 21.4 months; HR 1.70 for placebo, 95% CI 1.13–2.56),[26] as did the integrated analysis of the D9901 and D9902A randomized phase II clinical trials.[27] A randomized phase II clinical trial, in which patients with detectable serum PSA 3 to 4 months following radical prostatectomy were randomized in a 2:1 ratio between sipuleucel-T or placebo, showed no difference in the primary end point of time to biochemical progression (18.0 vs 15.4 months; HR = 0.936, $P = .737$).[28] The lack of predictive biomarkers, the high cost of treatment, and the complexity of treatment preparation and administration may limit the use of this treatment. Ongoing phase II clinical trials of sipuleucel-T will investigate the coadministration of immunomodulatory agents such as cyclophosphamide (NCT01420965) or the immune response regulator indoximod (NCT01560923), and also investigate concurrent versus sequential administration of abiraterone (NCT01487863).

Prostvac

Prostvac (Bavarian Nordic) is a recombinant vaccinia-viral expression cassette expressing PSA and costimulatory molecules (B7.1, ICAM-1, and Lfa-3), which is administered subcutaneously. A phase II clinical trial included 125 chemotherapy-naïve patients without visceral metastases and a Gleason score of 7 or less, who were randomized 2:1 to Prostvac plus GM-CSF or placebo. Although PFS was similar in both arms, the median OS was significantly longer with Prostvac than with placebo (25.1 vs 16.6 months; HR 0.56, 95% CI 0.37–0.85).[29] A large 3-arm phase III clinical trial will randomize chemotherapy-naïve men with asymptomatic or minimally symptomatic CRPC between Prostvac ± GM-CSF or placebo (NCT01322490).

Ipilimumab

Ipilimumab (Yervoy; Bristol-Myers Squibb) is a monoclonal antibody against the cytotoxic T-lymphocyte antigen CTLA-4. Activation of T cells by APC requires interaction between the major histocompatibility complex and the T-cell receptor plus simultaneous interaction with a costimulatory molecule (CD28) on T cells. CTLA-4 (CD152) is a T-cell membranous protein and CD28 homologue, which acts as an inhibitor of T-cell activation. Phase I clinical trial data confirmed the safety and tolerability of ipilimumab 3 mg/kg in patients with advanced prostate cancer, and showed 50% or greater declines in PSA in 2 of 14 patients.[30] A phase I clinical trial combining ipilimumab 10 mg/kg with a poxviral-based vaccine targeting PSA and T-cell costimulatory molecule expression proved the feasibility of the combination approach, and reported PSA declines of at least 50% in 6 of 30 patients.[31] Phase III trials of ipilimumab 10 mg/kg versus placebo have been conducted in asymptomatic or minimally symptomatic CRPC patients (NCT01057810) and in symptomatic patients following palliative radiotherapy (NCT00861614), and several phase II clinical trials of ipilimumab in combination with androgen deprivation (NCT01498978; NCT01377389) or abiraterone (NCT01688492) are ongoing.

Targeting the interaction between the programmed death 1 (PD-1) receptor on cytotoxic T cells and its ligand PD-L1 has recently been shown to induce prolonged stabilization of disease and some durable tumor regressions in advanced solid tumors.[32] A 3-arm randomized phase II clinical trial of sipuleucel-T, CT-011 (a PD-1 inhibitor), and cyclophosphamide in advanced prostate cancer is ongoing (NCT01420965).

CHEMOTHERAPY
Docetaxel

The TAX-327 study was published in 2004 and proved that survival could be improved for men with CRPC. TAX-327 enrolled 1006 men and randomized participants equally between open-label mitoxantrone, weekly docetaxel, or 3-weekly docetaxel.[33] All participants received continuous low-dose prednisone 10 mg/d. Compared with mitoxantrone, 3-weekly docetaxel was superior in the primary end point of OS, producing a median improvement of 2.4 months (HR 0.76, 95% CI 0.62–0.94, $P = .009$). Docetaxel treatment was associated with higher rates of PSA declines of at least 50% (45% vs

32%; P<.001), and was also superior in the secondary end points of pain reduction (35% vs 22%; P = .01) and improvement in quality of life (22% vs 13%; P = .009). The combination of a modest survival gain with palliation of symptoms resulted in docetaxel becoming a standard of care for men with CRPC, and subsequent treatments have been defined in the prechemotherapy or postchemotherapy space.

The toxicity profile of docetaxel is well understood and managed after a decade of research and widespread clinical use. Although grade-3 to -4 neutropenia was reported in 32% of patients in TAX-327, only 1 patient suffered a treatment-related death during the study and the rate of serious adverse events was similar across all treatment arms.[33] The most common nonhematologic adverse events of alopecia, diarrhea, nail changes, and sensory neuropathies were generally mild and manageable.

Since TAX-327 was published, many attempts have been made to improve docetaxel further using combination treatment. Thus far no combination has improved survival over single-agent docetaxel and, indeed, some combinations have been inferior. Optimal schedule and duration of docetaxel continue to be debated, but no formal randomized studies have been undertaken. The timing of docetaxel also continues to be investigated. A small phase III trial reported in 2012 found a PFS advantage without impacting OS, by delivering docetaxel concurrently with initiation of androgen-deprivation therapy rather than traditional sequencing after failure of androgen-deprivation therapy,[34] and this will be further examined in the STAMPEDE trial (NCT00268476) and the ECOG-E3805 CHAARTED trial (NCT00309985).

Docetaxel was initially believed to cause cytotoxicity in CRPC through the standard taxane chemotherapy mechanism of inhibition of microtubule function. More recent preclinical evidence has suggested that the mechanism of action may be more complex and may include inhibition of AR function.[35]

Cabazitaxel

Cabazitaxel (Jevtana; Sanofi Aventis) is another member of the taxane chemotherapy family. Structurally, cabazitaxel differs from docetaxel by way of substitution of 2 methoxy side chains in place of hydroxyl groups.[36] Cabazitaxel was selected for clinical development after demonstrating comparable antitumor activity in docetaxel-sensitive cell lines, with greater cytotoxicity in models rendered docetaxel-resistant because of P-glycoprotein overexpression[37] or multidrug resistance.[38,39] Early clinical testing suggested activity in CRPC, and led to the phase III TROPIC study in 755 men with progressive CRPC after treatment with docetaxel.[40] Participants were randomized between open-label 3-weekly mitoxantrone or cabazitaxel 25 mg/m^2 in combination with low-dose prednisone. Cabazitaxel treatment resulted in a median 2.4-month improvement in OS (HR 0.74, 95% CI 0.64–0.86, P<.0001). Cabazitaxel was also superior for secondary activity end points of PSA and soft-tissue responses (PSA responses: 39.2% vs 17.8%, P = .0002; soft tissue: 14.4% vs 4.4%, P = .0005) but, unlike docetaxel, was not superior to mitoxantrone for pain palliation. Preplanned analysis suggested maintenance of cabazitaxel benefit across examined subgroups.

Although a member of the same family, the toxicity profile of cabazitaxel is different from that of docetaxel. Bone marrow suppression was significant, and febrile neutropenia occurred in 28 (8%) of patients in the cabazitaxel arm in TROPIC. Neutropenia and a 6% rate of grade-3 to -4 diarrhea contributed to on-trial mortality of 5%. Concern about the high treatment-associated toxicity prompted the phase III PRO-SELICA study, which is an open-label noninferiority study comparing cabazitaxel 25 mg/m^2 with 20 mg/m^2 (NCT01308580).

Cabazitaxel combination studies are now in progress, including a phase III combination study adding the clusterin inhibitor custirsen (NCT01083615), and several earlier-phase combination studies. A phase III head-to-head first-line comparison with docetaxel is also under way (FIRSTANA, NCT01308567).

Other Chemotherapies

Mitoxantrone

Mitoxantrone was used as a comparator in both seminal chemotherapy studies. The evidence for mitoxantrone efficacy in CRPC came from a phase III trial that demonstrated superior pain palliation when compared with single-agent prednisone.[41] The trial failed to show any improvement in survival, but was not powered to do so.

Satraplatin

Oral satraplatin chemotherapy was tested against placebo in a second-line chemotherapy phase III study.[42] Satraplatin treatment was associated with significantly decreased risk of clinical and/or radiologic disease progression (HR 0.67, $P<.001$), but did not alter the coprimary end point of OS. Selecting the subgroup of patients with DNA-repair defects could improve the clinical benefit observed with platinum therapies and might culminate in improvement of OS.

NOVEL THERAPIES

^{223}Radium

^{223}Ra chloride (Alpharadin, Bayer) is a novel α-emitting radionuclide that is preferentially integrated into areas of new bone formation such as bone metastases, and causes DNA double-strand breaks, resulting in irreparable cellular damage.[43,44] A randomized phase II trial showed that ^{223}Ra led to reduction in levels of bone-derived alkaline phosphatase and a suggested delay in time to skeletal-related events (SRE).[45] The definitive phase III ALSYMPCA trial randomized 921 patients in a 2:1 ratio to ^{223}Ra (50 kBq/kg intravenously delivered 4-weekly, maximum 6 treatments) or matching placebo.[46] Eligible patients had progressive CRPC with symptomatic bone metastases and had either previously received docetaxel or, in 40% participants, refused or were judged unsuitable for docetaxel. ^{223}Ra was superior for the primary end point of OS, with a median improvement of 3.6 months in comparison with placebo (HR = 0.695, $P = .00007$). Secondary efficacy end points of time to first SRE and quality-of-life measures also favored ^{223}Ra treatment.[47] ^{223}Ra appeared to be well tolerated, with low frequencies of myelosuppression, including grade-3 to -4 neutropenia and thrombocytopenia in 2.2% and 6.3% of participants, respectively.

Cabozantinib

Cabozantinib (XL-184; Cometriq, Exelixis) is an oral tyrosine kinase inhibitor targeting MET and VEGF receptor 2 as well as RET, KIT, AXL, and FLT3. Preclinical studies in several cancer models demonstrated inhibition of tumor growth.[48] Prostate cancer cells, osteoblasts, and osteoclasts have all been shown to express MET.[49] MET expression has also been associated with migration of cancer cells into bone marrow.[50]

Cabozantinib was recently shown to delay time to progression in medullary thyroid cancer in the phase III EXAM trial.[51] In CRPC, a large multicohort phase II trial demonstrated high rates of clinical activity.[52] An expansion cohort of 93 patients with progressive CRPC on or shortly after discontinuing docetaxel were treated with cabozantinib 100 mg daily, and 49% of patients achieved durable pain palliation while 60% met predefined criteria for bone-scan response.[53] Of the 59 patients in this cohort with unfavorable baseline CTC counts, 39% converted to favorable counts and 92% had CTC declines of 30% or greater. The common side effects were comparable with those shown by other tyrosine kinase inhibitors, with grade-3 to -4 events including fatigue (28%), anorexia (6%), diarrhea (11%), hand-foot syndrome (5%), hypertension (9%), and venous thrombosis (6%). A further 51 patients were treated at a lower starting dose of 40 mg/d, and comparable clinical efficacy was reported in this cohort.[54]

Two phase III trials will examine the use of cabozantinib in minimum third-line CRPC patients: COMET-1 is a placebo-controlled trial with an OS end point (NCT01605227), whereas COMET-2 is a smaller trial with blinded randomization between cabozantinib and mitoxantrone chemotherapy using a pain-response end point (NCT01522443). In addition, several combination trials, such as with abiraterone plus cabozantinib (NCT01574937), are ongoing or planned in less heavily treated patients.

Custirsen

Clusterin is an antiapoptotic protein that is induced by stress and appears to confer treatment resistance. Custirsen (OGX-011; OncoGenex Technologies) is a second-generation antisense oligonucleotide that inhibits clusterin expression. In preclinical studies custirsen treatment improved tumor-cell death and enhanced chemosensitivity.[55–57] A phase I trial used an innovative neoadjuvant design, and showed 90% inhibition of clusterin levels in prostate and lymph node tissues and a dose-dependent increase in apoptosis.[58]

Two randomized phase II trials in CRPC have been reported. The first enrolled 82 men to treatment with docetaxel with or without custirsen.[59] Although the PSA and soft-tissue responses appeared similar, survival data were encouraging, with median OS of 23.9 months for the combination treatment compared with 16.9 months with docetaxel alone. In the second-line phase II trial 42 patients with progressive CRPC on or within 6 months of docetaxel treatment were randomized between docetaxel retreatment or mitoxantrone, combined with custirsen and prednisone.[60] Docetaxel retreatment with custirsen resulted in PSA declines of at least 50% in 40% of the cohort. In both arms, low serum clusterin levels during treatment appeared to be associated with improved survival, although this finding requires validation in larger trial populations. Phase III trials are being conducted, testing the addition of custirsen to first-line docetaxel (NCT01188187) and to second-line cabazitaxel (NCT01578655).

Tasquinimod

Tasquinimod (ABR-215050; Active Biotech) is an oral analogue of quinoline-3-carboxamide. The mechanisms for the purported antiangiogenic and tumor-inhibitory effects of tasquinimod are not fully elucidated, but one proposed target is the immunomodulatory protein S100A9.[61] A randomized phase II trial was conducted using a primary end point of PFS at 6 months. Although the trial was reported as positive, with 69% of the enrolled 134 tasquinimod patients progression-free at 6 months compared with 37% of the 67 placebo patients ($P<.001$), it is notable that 86 patients in the tasquinimod arm withdrew from treatment but were still considered in the primary end-point assessment. The benefit from tasquinimod will be further examined in a 1200-patient phase III trial in men with minimally symptomatic metastatic CRPC (NCT01234311). The study has been designed with a PFS end point, which may be difficult to interpret in an era of multiple survival-prolonging therapies.

OGX-427

OGX-427 (OncoGenex Technologies) is a second-generation antisense oligonucleotide against HSP-27. HSP-27 regulates cell signaling and survival pathways. In prostate cancer models, androgen-bound AR induced HSP-27 phosphorylation, which then complexed with AR, and enhanced AR stability, shuttling, and transcriptional activity.[62] A phase I trial suggested OGX-427 activity in CRPC patients, including PSA declines of at least 30% in 3 of 16 and 5 of 9 eligible patients in single-agent and docetaxel-combination cohorts, respectively, as well as radiographic responses and CTC conversions.[63] Preliminary data from a randomized phase II study of prednisone with or without OGX-427 in men with chemotherapy-naïve CRPC were reported at American Society of Clinical Oncology 2012 meeting.[64] Of the 32 evaluable men, PSA declines of 50% or more were observed in 41% of men who received OGX-427, compared with 20% with prednisone alone, with CTC conversion in 50% and 30%, respectively, and radiographic partial responses in 3 of 8 evaluable men who received OGX-427. A randomized phase II study in men with disease progression on abiraterone is planned (NCT01681433).

Other Promising Novel Therapies

AR is a client of multiple HSPs. HSPs are chaperones that regulate binding of ligands to the AR and several other proteins involved in mitogenic signaling, and may be therapeutic targets.[65] Phase II clinical trials with HSP90 inhibitors alone (NCT01270880) or in combination with abiraterone (NCT01685268) are currently recruiting patients.

Recent evidence has uncovered a reciprocal feedback mechanism between AR and the critical PTEN-PI3K-AKT-mTOR signaling pathway.[66] These findings provide the rationale for clinical trials using combinations of AR-targeting drugs with inhibitors of the PI3K-AKT-mTOR pathway.

The pathogenesis of prostate cancer appears to involve key molecular events, including PTEN loss and *ERG* gene rearrangements, which may stratify patients clinically.[67] *ERG* interacts with DNA-repair enzymes including poly(ADP-ribose) polymerase (PARP).[68] The PARP inhibitor olaparib (AZD-2281; Astra Zeneca) showed evidence of activity in men with familial prostate cancer and DNA-repair defects,[69] and is currently being tested in a phase II trial in men with sporadic prostate cancer (NCT01682772).

RESISTANCE MECHANISMS

Unlike breast cancer, in which several distinct molecularly defined subgroups have been identified, prostate cancer is commonly treated as a homogeneous disease apart from the small subset of patients who have neuroendocrine differentiation. Better disease characterization and the development of predictive biomarkers is of vital importance to enable patient selection for treatments and new drug development.

Several mechanisms of treatment resistance have been described, and mainly relate to AR-targeting agents such as the CYP17 inhibitors, AR antagonists, and, possibly, taxanes. Key mechanisms of resistance, which also highlight the continued importance of AR signaling, are:

- AR mutations
- AR amplification
- AR splice variants
- Tissue steroidogenesis
- Activation of alternative signaling pathways
- Ligand-independent AR activation

The observation of antiandrogen withdrawal responses, whereby stopping first-generation antiandrogens resulted in PSA declines, was explained on a molecular level by the discovery of mutations in the AR that turn these antiandrogens into AR agonists.[70–72] Preclinical data also confirmed that the commonly used steroidal agents prednisolone, eplerenone, and spironolactone could activate mutated AR.[15] These data may explain the post hoc analysis of the enzalutamide phase III clinical trial that showed shorter median OS for patients on corticosteroids (12.3 months on enzalutamide vs 9.3 months on placebo; $P = .0116$, HR 0.70) compared with patients not on corticosteroids (not reached on enzalutamide vs 15.8 months on placebo; $P<.0001$, HR 0.59), even after controlling for other disease variables.[73]

The impact and clinical relevance of other proposed mechanisms of resistance are less well established. AR amplifications may result in increased sensitivity to low levels of androgens.[74] AR splice variants (AR-V) are AR proteins that generally lack the ligand-binding domain but may be involved in the progression of prostate cancer through ligand-independent activation of AR signaling.[75,76] Continued AR signaling may also be the result of intratumoral conversion of cholesterol and weak adrenal androgens such as dehydroepiandrosterone and androstenedione to dihydrotestosterone.[77]

SUMMARY

Six systemic therapies have now been proved to improve survival in men with CRPC, including docetaxel and cabazitaxel chemotherapies, AR targeting with the CYP17 inhibitor abiraterone and AR antagonist enzalutamide, sipuleucel-T immunotherapy, and the radionuclide ^{223}Ra. The ongoing challenge facing the oncology community is the rational selection and best sequencing of these and other novel agents to provide the best outcome for individual patients. Innovations in molecular stratification and biomarkers for treatment response will greatly enhance our ability to minimize ineffective therapies and more efficiently develop new therapies against this common and burdensome disease.

REFERENCES

1. O'Donnell A, Judson I, Dowsett M, et al. Hormonal impact of the 17alpha-hydroxylase/C(17,20)-lyase inhibitor abiraterone acetate (CB7630) in patients with prostate cancer. Br J Cancer 2004;90(12):2317–25.
2. Franke RM, Carducci MA, Rudek MA, et al. Castration-dependent pharmacokinetics of docetaxel in patients with prostate cancer. J Clin Oncol 2010;28(30): 4562–7.
3. de Bono JS, Scher HI, Montgomery RB, et al. Circulating tumor cells predict survival benefit from treatment in metastatic castration-resistant prostate cancer. Clin Cancer Res 2008;14(19):6302–9.
4. Scher HI, Jia X, de Bono JS, et al. Circulating tumour cells as prognostic markers in progressive, castration-resistant prostate cancer: a reanalysis of IMMC38 trial data. Lancet Oncol 2009;10(3):233–9.
5. Scher HI, Heller G, Molina A, et al. Evaluation of circulating tumor cell (CTC) enumeration as an efficacy response biomarker of overall survival (OS) in metastatic castration-resistant prostate cancer (mCRPC): planned final analysis (FA) of COU-AA-301, a randomized double-blind, placebo-controlled phase III study of abiraterone acetate (AA) plus prednisone (P) post docetaxel. J Clin Oncol 2011;29(Suppl) [abstract LBA4517].
6. Shaffer DR, Leversha MA, Danila DC, et al. Circulating tumor cell analysis in patients with progressive castration-resistant prostate cancer. Clin Cancer Res 2007;13(7):2023–9.
7. Attard G, Swennenhuis JF, Olmos D, et al. Characterization of ERG, AR and PTEN gene status in circulating tumor cells from patients with castration-resistant prostate cancer. Cancer Res 2009;69(7):2912–8.

8. Ross RW, Halabi S, Ou SS, et al. Predictors of prostate cancer tissue acquisition by an undirected core bone marrow biopsy in metastatic castration-resistant prostate cancer—a Cancer and Leukemia Group B study. Clin Cancer Res 2005;11(22):8109–13.

9. Efstathiou E, Titus M, Tsavachidou D, et al. Effects of abiraterone acetate on androgen signaling in castrate-resistant prostate cancer in bone. J Clin Oncol 2012;30(6):637–43.

10. Mezynski J, Pezaro C, Bianchini D, et al. Antitumour activity of docetaxel following treatment with the CYP17A1 inhibitor abiraterone: clinical evidence for cross-resistance? Ann Oncol 2012;23(11):2943–7.

11. Attard G, Reid AH, Yap TA, et al. Phase I clinical trial of a selective inhibitor of CYP17, abiraterone acetate, confirms that castration-resistant prostate cancer commonly remains hormone driven. J Clin Oncol 2008;26(28):4563–71.

12. de Bono JS, Logothetis CJ, Molina A, et al. Abiraterone and increased survival in metastatic prostate cancer. N Engl J Med 2011;364(21):1995–2005.

13. Fizazi K, Scher HI, Molina A, et al. Abiraterone acetate for treatment of metastatic castration-resistant prostate cancer: final overall survival analysis of the COU-AA-301 randomised, double-blind, placebo-controlled phase 3 study. Lancet Oncol 2012;13(10):983–92.

14. Ryan CJ, Smith MR, De Bono JS, et al. Abiraterone in metastatic prostate cancer without previous chemotherapy. N Engl J Med 2013;368(2):138–48.

15. Richards J, Lim AC, Hay CW, et al. Interactions of abiraterone, eplerenone, and prednisolone with wild-type and mutant androgen receptor: a rationale for increasing abiraterone exposure or combining with MDV3100. Cancer Res 2012;72(9):2176–82.

16. Tran C, Ouk S, Clegg NJ, et al. Development of a second-generation antiandrogen for treatment of advanced prostate cancer. Science 2009;324(5928):787–90.

17. Scher HI, Beer TM, Higano CS, et al. Antitumour activity of MDV3100 in castration-resistant prostate cancer: a phase 1-2 study. Lancet 2010;375(9724):1437–46.

18. Scher HI, Fizazi K, Saad F, et al. Increased survival with enzalutamide in prostate cancer after chemotherapy. N Engl J Med 2012;367(13):1187–97.

19. Agus DB, Stadler WM, Shevrin DH, et al. Safety, efficacy, and pharmacodynamics of the investigational agent orteronel (TAK-700) in metastatic castration-resistant prostate cancer (mCRPC): updated data from a phase I/II study. J Clin Oncol 2012;30(Suppl 5) [abstract 98].

20. Eisner JR, Abbott DH, Bird IM, et al. VT-464: a novel, selective inhibitor of P450c17(CYP17)-17,20 lyase for castration-refractory prostate cancer (CRPC). J Clin Oncol 2012;30(Suppl 5) [abstract 198].

21. Clegg NJ, Wongvipat J, Joseph JD, et al. ARN-509: a novel antiandrogen for prostate cancer treatment. Cancer Res 2012;72(6):1494–503.

22. Rathkopf DE, Morris MJ, Danila DC, et al. A phase I study of the androgen signaling inhibitor ARN-509 in patients with metastatic castration-resistant prostate cancer (mCRPC). J Clin Oncol 2012;30(Suppl) [abstract 4548].

23. Massard C, James N, Culine S, et al. ARADES trial: a first-in-man, open-label, phase I/II safety, pharmacokinetic, and proof-of-concept study of ODM-201 in patients (pts) with progressive metastatic castration-resistant prostate cancer (mCRPC). ESMO Congress. 2012. [abstract LBA25_PR].

24. Taplin ME, Chu F, Morrison JP, et al. ARMOR1: safety of galeterone (TOK-001) in a Phase 1 clinical trial in chemotherapy naïve patients with castration resistant

prostate cancer (CRPC). AACR Annual Meeting. Chicago; 31 March–4 April. 2012. [abstract CT07].

25. Kantoff PW, Higano CS, Shore ND, et al. Sipuleucel-T immunotherapy for castration-resistant prostate cancer. N Engl J Med 2010;363(5):411–22.

26. Small EJ, Schellhammer PF, Higano CS, et al. Placebo-controlled phase III trial of immunologic therapy with sipuleucel-T (APC8015) in patients with metastatic, asymptomatic hormone refractory prostate cancer. J Clin Oncol 2006;24(19): 3089–94.

27. Higano CS, Schellhammer PF, Small EJ, et al. Integrated data from 2 randomized, double-blind, placebo-controlled, phase 3 trials of active cellular immunotherapy with sipuleucel-T in advanced prostate cancer. Cancer 2009;115(16):3670–9.

28. Beer TM, Bernstein GT, Corman JM, et al. Randomized trial of autologous cellular immunotherapy with sipuleucel-T in androgen-dependent prostate cancer. Clin Cancer Res 2011;17(13):4558–67.

29. Kantoff PW, Schuetz TJ, Blumenstein BA, et al. Overall survival analysis of a phase II randomized controlled trial of a Poxviral-based PSA-targeted immunotherapy in metastatic castration-resistant prostate cancer. J Clin Oncol 2010; 28(7):1099–105.

30. Small EJ, Tchekmedyian NS, Rini BI, et al. A pilot trial of CTLA-4 blockade with human anti-CTLA-4 in patients with hormone-refractory prostate cancer. Clin Cancer Res 2007;13(6):1810–5.

31. Madan RA, Mohebtash M, Arlen PM, et al. Ipilimumab and a poxviral vaccine targeting prostate-specific antigen in metastatic castration-resistant prostate cancer: a phase 1 dose-escalation trial. Lancet Oncol 2012;13(5):501–8.

32. Brahmer JR, Tykodi SS, Chow LQ, et al. Safety and activity of anti-PD-L1 antibody in patients with advanced cancer. N Engl J Med 2012;366(26):2455–65.

33. Tannock IF, de Wit R, Berry WR, et al. Docetaxel plus prednisone or mitoxantrone plus prednisone for advanced prostate cancer. N Engl J Med 2004; 351(15):1502–12.

34. Gravis G, Fizazi K, Joly Lobbedez FJ, et al. Survival analysis of a randomised Phase III trial comparing androgen deprivation therapy (ADT) plus docetaxel versus ADT alone in hormone-sensitive metastatic prostate cancer (GETUG-AFU 15/0403). ESMO Congress. 2012. [abstract 8930].

35. Darshan MS, Loftus MS, Thadani-Mulero M, et al. Taxane-induced blockade to nuclear accumulation of the androgen receptor predicts clinical responses in metastatic prostate cancer. Cancer Res 2011;71(18):6019–29.

36. Galsky MD, Dritselis A, Kirkpatrick P, et al. Cabazitaxel. Nat Rev Drug Discov 2010;9(9):677–8.

37. Mita AC, Denis LJ, Rowinsky EK, et al. Phase I and pharmacokinetic study of XRP6258 (RPR 116258A), a novel taxane, administered as a 1-hour infusion every 3 weeks in patients with advanced solid tumors. Clin Cancer Res 2009; 15(2):723–30.

38. Bissery MC. Preclinical evaluation of new taxoids. Curr Pharm Des 2001;7(13): 1251–7.

39. Yap TA, Pezaro CJ, de Bono JS. Cabazitaxel in metastatic castration-resistant prostate cancer. Expert Rev Anticancer Ther 2012;12(9):1129–36.

40. de Bono JS, Oudard S, Ozguroglu M, et al. Prednisone plus cabazitaxel or mitoxantrone for metastatic castration-resistant prostate cancer progressing after docetaxel treatment: a randomised open-label trial. Lancet 2010;376(9747):1147–54.

41. Tannock IF, Osoba D, Stockler MR, et al. Chemotherapy with mitoxantrone plus prednisone or prednisone alone for symptomatic hormone-resistant prostate

cancer: a Canadian randomized trial with palliative end points. J Clin Oncol 1996;14(6):1756–64.

42. Sternberg CN, Whelan P, Hetherington J, et al. Phase III trial of satraplatin, an oral platinum plus prednisone vs. prednisone alone in patients with hormone-refractory prostate cancer. Oncology 2005;68(1):2–9.

43. Henriksen G, Breistol K, Bruland OS, et al. Significant antitumor effect from bone-seeking, alpha-particle-emitting (223)Ra demonstrated in an experimental skeletal metastases model. Cancer Res 2002;62(11):3120–5.

44. Ritter MA, Cleaver JE, Tobias CA. High-LET radiations induce a large proportion of non-rejoining DNA breaks. Nature 1977;266(5603):653–5.

45. Nilsson S, Franzen L, Parker C, et al. Bone-targeted radium-223 in symptomatic, hormone-refractory prostate cancer: a randomised, multicentre, placebo-controlled phase II study. Lancet Oncol 2007;8(7):587–94.

46. Parker C, Nilsson S, Heinrich D, et al. Updated analysis of the phase III, double-blind, randomized, multinational study of radium-223 chloride in castration-resistant prostate cancer (CRPC) patients with bone metastases (ALSYMPCA). J Clin Oncol 2012;30(Suppl) [abstract LBA4512].

47. Parker C, Nilsson S, Heinrich D, et al. Alpha emitter radium-223 and survival in metastatic prostate cancer. N Engl J Med 2013;369(3):213–23.

48. Yakes FM, Chen J, Tan J, et al. Cabozantinib (XL184), a novel MET and VEGFR2 inhibitor, simultaneously suppresses metastasis, angiogenesis, and tumor growth. Mol Cancer Ther 2011;10(12):2298–308.

49. Inaba M, Koyama H, Hino M, et al. Regulation of release of hepatocyte growth factor from human promyelocytic leukemia cells, HL-60, by 1,25-dihydroxyvita-min D3, 12-O-tetradecanoylphorbol 13-acetate, and dibutyryl cyclic adenosine monophosphate. Blood 1993;82(1):53–9.

50. Ono K, Kamiya S, Akatsu T, et al. Involvement of hepatocyte growth factor in the development of bone metastasis of a mouse mammary cancer cell line, BALB/c-MC. Bone 2006;39(1):27–34.

51. Schoffski P, Elisei R, Müller S, et al. An international, double-blind, randomized, placebo-controlled phase III trial (EXAM) of cabozantinib (XL184) in medullary thyroid carcinoma (MTC) patients (pts) with documented RECIST progression at baseline. J Clin Oncol 2012;30(Suppl) [abstract 5508].

52. Hussain M, Smith MR, Sweeney C, et al. Cabozantinib (XL184) in meta-static castration-resistant prostate cancer (mCRPC): results from a phase II randomized discontinuation trial. J Clin Oncol 2011;29(Suppl) [abstract 4516].

53. Smith MR, Sweeney C, Rathkopf DE, et al. Cabozantinib (XL184) in chemotherapy-pretreated metastatic castration resistant prostate cancer (mCRPC): results from a phase II nonrandomized expansion cohort (NRE). J Clin Oncol 2012;30(Suppl) [abstract 4513].

54. De Bono JS, Smith MR, Rathkopf DE, et al. Cabozantinib (XL184) at 40mg in pa-tients with metastatic castration resistant prostate cancer (mCRPC): results of a Phase 2 non-randomised expansion cohort (NRE). ESMO Congress. 2012. [abstract 8970].

55. Miyake H, Chi KN, Gleave ME. Antisense TRPM-2 oligodeoxynucleotides che-mosensitize human androgen-independent PC-3 prostate cancer cells both in vitro and in vivo. Clin Cancer Res 2000;6(5):1655–63.

56. Zellweger T, Miyake H, Cooper S, et al. Antitumor activity of antisense clusterin oligonucleotides is improved in vitro and in vivo by incorporation of 2′-O-(2-me-thoxy)ethyl chemistry. J Pharmacol Exp Ther 2001;298(3):934–40.

57. Sowery RD, Hadaschik BA, So AI, et al. Clusterin knockdown using the antisense oligonucleotide OGX-011 re-sensitizes docetaxel-refractory prostate cancer PC-3 cells to chemotherapy. BJU Int 2008;102(3):389–97.
58. Chi KN, Eisenhauer E, Fazli L, et al. A phase I pharmacokinetic and pharmacodynamic study of OGX-011, a 2′-methoxyethyl antisense oligonucleotide to clusterin, in patients with localized prostate cancer. J Natl Cancer Inst 2005;97(17):1287–96.
59. Chi KN, Hotte SJ, Yu EY, et al. Randomized phase II study of docetaxel and prednisone with or without OGX-011 in patients with metastatic castration-resistant prostate cancer. J Clin Oncol 2010;28(27):4247–54.
60. Saad F, Hotte S, North S, et al. Randomized phase II trial of Custirsen (OGX-011) in combination with docetaxel or mitoxantrone as second-line therapy in patients with metastatic castrate-resistant prostate cancer progressing after first-line docetaxel: CUOG trial P-06c. Clin Cancer Res 2011;17(17):5765–73.
61. Bjork P, Bjork A, Vogl T, et al. Identification of human S100A9 as a novel target for treatment of autoimmune disease via binding to quinoline-3-carboxamides. PLoS Biol 2009;7(4):e97.
62. Zoubeidi A, Zardan A, Beraldi E, et al. Cooperative interactions between androgen receptor (AR) and heat-shock protein 27 facilitate AR transcriptional activity. Cancer Res 2007;67(21):10455–65.
63. Hotte SJ, Yu EY, Hirte HW, et al. Phase I trial of OGX-427, a 2′methoxyethyl antisense oligonucleotide (ASO), against heat shock protein 27 (Hsp27): final results. J Clin Oncol 2010;28(15S) [abstract 3077].
64. Chi KN, Hotte SJ, Ellard S, et al. A randomized phase II study of OGX-427 plus prednisone (P) versus P alone in patients (pts) with metastatic castration resistant prostate cancer (CRPC). J Clin Oncol 2012;30(Suppl 5) [abstract 121].
65. Ni L, Yang CS, Gioeli D, et al. FKBP51 promotes assembly of the Hsp90 chaperone complex and regulates androgen receptor signaling in prostate cancer cells. Mol Cell Biol 2010;30(5):1243–53.
66. Carver BS, Chapinski C, Wongvipat J, et al. Reciprocal feedback regulation of PI3K and androgen receptor signaling in PTEN-deficient prostate cancer. Cancer Cell 2011;19(5):575–86.
67. Reid AH, Attard G, Ambroisine L, et al. Molecular characterisation of ERG, ETV1 and PTEN gene loci identifies patients at low and high risk of death from prostate cancer. Br J Cancer 2010;102(4):678–84.
68. Brenner JC, Ateeq B, Li Y, et al. Mechanistic rationale for inhibition of poly(ADP-ribose) polymerase in ETS gene fusion-positive prostate cancer. Cancer Cell 2011;19(5):664–78.
69. Fong PC, Boss DS, Yap TA, et al. Inhibition of poly(ADP-ribose) polymerase in tumors from BRCA mutation carriers. N Engl J Med 2009;361(2):123–34.
70. Taplin ME, Bubley GJ, Shuster TD, et al. Mutation of the androgen-receptor gene in metastatic androgen-independent prostate cancer. N Engl J Med 1995;332(21):1393–8.
71. Taplin ME, Bubley GJ, Ko YJ, et al. Selection for androgen receptor mutations in prostate cancers treated with androgen antagonist. Cancer Res 1999;59(11):2511–5.
72. Steinkamp MP, O'Mahony OA, Brogley M, et al. Treatment-dependent androgen receptor mutations in prostate cancer exploit multiple mechanisms to evade therapy. Cancer Res 2009;69(10):4434–42.
73. Scher HI, Fizazi K, Saad F, et al. Association of baseline corticosteroid with outcomes in a multivariate analysis of the Phase 3 AFFIRM study of enzalutamide

(ENZA), an androgen receptor signaling inhibitor (ARSI). ESMO Congress. 2012. [abstract 899PD].

74. Kawata H, Ishikura N, Watanabe M, et al. Prolonged treatment with bicalutamide induces androgen receptor overexpression and androgen hypersensitivity. Prostate 2010;70(7):745–54.

75. Hornberg E, Ylitalo EB, Crnalic S, et al. Expression of androgen receptor splice variants in prostate cancer bone metastases is associated with castration-resistance and short survival. PLoS One 2011;6(4):e19059.

76. Guo Z, Yang X, Sun F, et al. A novel androgen receptor splice variant is up-regulated during prostate cancer progression and promotes androgen depletion-resistant growth. Cancer Res 2009;69(6):2305–13.

77. Locke JA, Guns ES, Lubik AA, et al. Androgen levels increase by intratumoral de novo steroidogenesis during progression of castration-resistant prostate cancer. Cancer Res 2008;68(15):6407–15.

Optimizing Bone Health and Minimizing Skeletal Morbidity in Men with Prostate Cancer

Rana R. McKay, MD, Mary-Ellen Taplin, MD, Toni K. Choueiri, MD*

KEYWORDS

- Prostate cancer • Androgen deprivation therapy • Osteoporosis • Bone metastases
- Skeletal-related events • Bisphosphonate • Zoledronic acid • Denosumab

KEY POINTS

- Patients with prostate cancer are at increased risk of skeletal complications.
- Treatment-related osteoporosis is an established risk for patients receiving androgen deprivation therapy.
- Several agents, including bisphosphonates, receptor activator of nuclear factor-κβ ligand inhibitors, and selective estrogen receptor modulators, have shown benefit in the management of treatment-related osteoporosis.
- Patients with bone metastases from prostate cancer are at increased risk of skeletal-related events (SREs).
- Zoledronic acid and denosumab are effective in preventing SREs in patients with castration-resistant prostate cancer with bone metastases.
- Radium-223, a radiopharmaceutical that targets bone, is effective at preventing SREs and improving survival in patients with metastatic castration-resistant prostate cancer.
- Systemic agents, including abiraterone and enzalutamide, are active in preventing SREs, given efficacy in disease control.

INTRODUCTION

Prostate cancer is the most common cancer in men in the United States, with a lifetime risk of 16%, and is the second leading cause of death in this population.[1] Patients on androgen deprivation therapy (ADT) or those with bone metastases are susceptible to skeletal complications. Therefore, optimizing bone health is critical in the management of patients with prostate cancer.

Disclosures: There are no funding or other individual acknowledgments or disclosures.
Lank Center for Genitourinary Oncology, Department of Medical Oncology, Dana-Farber Cancer Institute, Brigham and Women's Hospital, Harvard Medical School, 450 Brookline Avenue, Boston, MA 02215, USA
* Corresponding author.
E-mail address: toni_choueiri@DFCI.harvard.edu

Hematol Oncol Clin N Am 27 (2013) 1261–1283
http://dx.doi.org/10.1016/j.hoc.2013.08.009
0889-8588/13/$ – see front matter © 2013 Elsevier Inc. All rights reserved.

hemonc.theclinics.com

NORMAL BONE PHYSIOLOGY

Normal bone remodeling is the process by which bone is renewed to maintain strength and mineral homeostasis.[2] It involves the coordinated actions of osteoclasts, responsible for bone resorption, and osteoblasts, which mediate bone formation (**Fig. 1**).[2]

The receptor activator of nuclear factor-κβ ligand (RANKL) is a critical cytokine in the remodeling process. RANKL, which is released from osteoblasts and bone marrow stromal cells, binds to RANK receptors on monocyte/macrophage precursor cells, thus promoting osteoclast differentiation, activation, and survival.[2] Subsequently, mature, multinucleated osteoclasts adhere to the bone matrix.[2] They undergo structural changes to form resorption lacunae and export acid and lytic enzymes into the lacunae, which leads to hydroxyapatite decalcification and bone degradation.[2] Osteoprotegerin (OPG), which is secreted from osteoblasts and stromal cells, competitively blocks RANKL binding to its cellular receptor RANK.[3] The RANKL/RANK/OPG regulatory axis results in tight coupling of the process of bone remodeling. Certain hormones, cytokines, and humoral factors influence bone homeostasis. Proresorptive factors include parathyroid hormone (PTH), PTH-related protein (PTHrP), interleukin 1 (IL-1), IL-6, tumor necrosis factor (TNF), prostaglandin E_2, and vitamin D.[4]

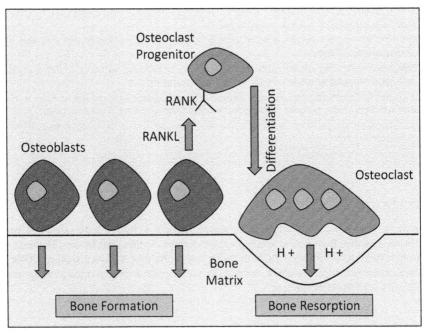

Fig. 1. Normal bone physiology. The skeleton is a metabolically active organ that undergoes continuous remodeling, a dynamic process of bone resorption by osteoclasts and bone formation by osteoblasts. Osteoblasts and bone marrow stromal cells release RANKL, which binds to RANK on mononuclear osteoclast precursor cells. This process promotes osteoclast differentiation and activation. Mature, multinucleated osteoclasts bind to the bone matrix, forming resorption lacunae, into which they secrete acid and lytic enzymes, leading to bone resorption. Osteoblasts, which arise from osteoprogenitor cells, form a cell layer over the bone surface, on which the matrix is formed and subsequently mineralized to become bone.[2]

Osteoblasts arise from osteoprogenitor cells, which are induced to differentiate under the influence of bone morphogenetic proteins (BMPs), estrogens, calcitonin, transforming growth factor β (TGF-β) and platelet-derived growth factor (PDGF).[4] The Wnt signaling pathway and runt-related transcription factor 2 are critical for the initiation of osteoblast differentiation.[5] Mature osteoblasts form the connective tissue matrix, which mineralizes to become bone.[4] Thus, the coupling of osteoclast and osteoblast function maintains bone homeostasis.

TREATMENT-RELATED OSTEOPOROSIS

ADT is the mainstay of systemic treatment of prostate cancer. The intended therapeutic effect of ADT is severe hypogonadism, a common cause of osteoporosis in men.[6] Based on retrospective SEER (Surveillance Epidemiology and End Results)/Medicare claims data, in men diagnosed with prostate cancer between 2000 and 2002, approximately 45% were exposed to ADT at some point after their diagnosis.[7] In addition, the prevalence of ADT is increasing in the United States.[8]

Bone mineral density (BMD), a surrogate for fracture risk, decreases in men receiving ADT. A rapid loss of BMD occurs within the first 12 months of therapy.[9–11] Based on a review of data from clinical trials and retrospective studies, rates of bone loss in the lumbar spine ranged from 2% to 8% and from 1.8% to 6.5% in the femoral neck during the initial 12 months of ADT.[12] Typically, men 50 years and older not receiving ADT lose BMD at a rate of 0.5% per year.[13] BMD continues to decline with ADT treatment beyond 12 months.[9,10,14]

In addition to decreased BMD, ADT use in men is associated with an increased risk of clinical osteoporosis-related bone fractures. In a SEER/Medicare claims study of more than 50,000 men diagnosed with prostate cancer,[15] of men surviving at least 5 years after diagnosis, men who received ADT had a significantly higher fracture rate compared with men not receiving ADT (19.4% vs 12.6%; $P<.001$). The risk of fracture increased with longer duration of therapy. This study included patients with both metastatic and nonmetastatic disease. In another Medicare claims study of more than 11,000 patients,[16] men with nonmetastatic prostate cancer receiving gonadotropin-releasing hormone (GnRH) agonist therapy were more likely to develop fractures than a control group of men with nonmetastatic prostate cancer not receiving GnRH-agonist treatment (relative risk [RR] 1.21; 95% confidence internal [CI] 1.14–1.29; $P<.001$). Patients receiving less than 1 year of therapy were not at increased fracture risk. Based on retrospective data, there is evidence to suggest that skeletal fracture is an independent negative predictor of survival in patients with prostate cancer (both nonmetastatic and metastatic).[17]

Testosterone and estrogen are essential in regulating bone integrity in men. The direct effect of estrogen on osteocytes, osteoclasts, and osteoblasts leads to inhibition of bone remodeling, decreased bone resorption, and maintenance of bone formation, respectively.[18] In a study examining the relative contributions of testosterone versus estrogen toward regulating bone metabolism in men, estrogen accounted for 70% of the total effect of sex steroids on bone resorption in older men.[19] Based on results from a prospective study, older men with low estradiol were at greater risk for low BMD and increased fracture.[20]

Given that testosterone undergoes peripheral aromatization to form estradiol, men treated with ADT also have low estrogen states. In a prospective study of men initiating ADT for nonmetastatic prostate cancer, there was a 73% decrease in serum estradiol from baseline pretreatment levels to after 48 weeks of treatment.[21] Low estrogen states are associated with an imbalance between bone resorption and formation, resulting in decreased BMD and increased risk of fracture.[22–24]

BONE METASTASES IN PROSTATE CANCER

The skeleton is the most frequent site of metastases in advanced prostate cancer, with estimates of involvement between 80% and 90% in castration-resistant prostate cancer (CRPC).[25] The most common sites of involvement include the vertebral column, pelvis, ribs, long bones, and skull. Although prostate cancer causes radiographically dense osteoblastic lesions, the woven bone produced by osteoblasts is structurally weak.[26] Pain is a common symptom associated with the presence of bone metastases. In addition, patients are at risk of skeletal-related events (SREs), including pathologic fractures, spinal cord compression, need for skeletal radiation, need for surgery to the bone, and, in some cases, hypercalcemia. The rate of SREs in patients with bone metastases and CRPC ranges from 40% to 50%.[27,28]

Bone metastases in prostate cancer promote increased osteoblast and osteoclast activity, as made evident by increased biochemical markers of bone turnover.[29] It is postulated that interactions between tumor cells and the bone microenvironment result in a vicious cycle of bone destruction and aggressive tumor growth (**Fig. 2**).[30] Production of interleukins, prostaglandins, and parathyroid hormone-related protein (PTH-rP) by tumor cells stimulates osteolysis, leading to the release of factors and

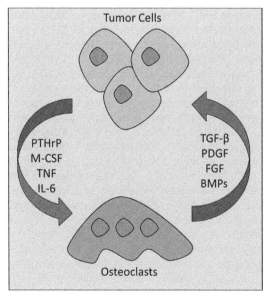

Fig. 2. The vicious cycle of bone metastases. Interactions between tumor cells and the bone microenvironment cause bone destruction via osteoclast activation and tumor growth. Tumor cells secrete cytokines and factors that activate osteoblasts to produce RANKL and downregulate OPG. This situation leads to activation of osteoclast precursors and subsequent osteolysis. The process of bone resorption releases TGF-β, PDGF, fibroblast growth factor (FGF), and BMPs, which promote tumor cell proliferation and further production of proresorptive factors, including PTH-rP, macrophage colony-stimulating factor (M-CSF), TNF, IL-6. This process leads to a vicious cycle of osteolysis and tumor growth.

cytokines derived from the bone matrix. These factors, including TGF-β and PDGF, induce tumor cell proliferation, leading to propagation of the vicious cycle of tumor growth and bone destruction.[30]

OSTEOCLAST-TARGETED THERAPIES
Bisphosphonates

Bisphosphonates are stable analogues of a naturally occurring inorganic pyrophosphate (**Fig. 3**). Bisphosphonates have 2 additional side-chains (R_1 and R_2), which are not present on pyrophosphate. In general, a hydroxyl substitution at R_1 enhances the affinity of bisphosphonates for calcium, whereas the presence of a nitrogen atom in R_2 enhances the potency of the compound and determines the mechanism of action.[31] **Table 1** highlights the potency of available bisphosphonates based on in vitro assays.[32]

Bisphosphonates bind to hydroxyapatite crystals on exposed bone. They are released in the acidic environment of the resorption lacunae and are taken up by osteoclasts via endocytosis.[33] Non-nitrogen–containing bisphosphonates incorporate into adenosine triphosphate and induce osteoclast apoptosis.[33] Nitrogen-containing bisphosphonates induce changes in the cytoskeleton of osteoclasts, including loss of the ruffled border, leading to osteoclast inactivation and apoptosis.[34] This action is mainly the result of inhibition of farnesyl pyrophosphate synthase, an enzyme in the mevalonate pathway, which plays a key role in cholesterol biosynthesis.[34] In addition to their inhibitory effect on osteoclasts, bisphosphonates seem to have a beneficial effect on osteoblasts.[35]

Bisphosphonates have poor oral bioavailability, with absorption of only about 1% of an oral dose (**Table 2**).[32] Approximately 50% of the absorbed bisphosphonate is rapidly cleared by the kidney, with a half-life of approximately 1 hour, and the remaining 50% is taken up by bone, and may persist there for years.[32]

Therapy with bisphosphonates is associated with adverse side effects, including hypocalcemia, renal impairment, osteonecrosis of the jaw (ONJ), and acute phase reactions.[36] Bisphosphonates with greater potency and those administered intravenously (IV) have a greater potential for adverse events.[36] Bisphosphonates require dose modification for renal impairment and are not recommended for patients with a

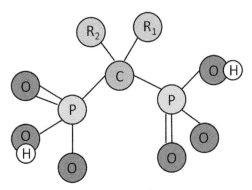

Fig. 3. Basic structure of a bisphosphonate. Bisphosphonates are synthetic analogues to naturally occurring inorganic pyrophosphate. The 2 phosphate groups (PO_3) bound to a carbon determine the name bisphosphonate. The R_1 side chain mainly influences pharmacokinetics of the drug, whereas the R_2 side chain determines mechanism of action and potency.[31]

Table 1
Potency of bisphosphonates[32]

Agent	Relative Potency
Non–Nitrogen-Containing Bisphosphonates	
First generation	
Etidronate	1
Clodronate	10
Nitrogen-Containing Bisphosphonates	
Second generation	
Alendronate	100
Pamidronate	100–1000
Third generation	
Neridronate	100
Risedronate	1000–10,000
Ibandronate	1000–10,000
Zoledronate	>10,000

creatinine clearance rate less than 30 mL/min, given risk of hypocalcemia and worsening renal failure. ONJ is a well-recognized complication of bisphosphonate treatment. In patients with bone metastases receiving higher doses of IV therapy, the incidence is approximately 1% to 12%.[37] The Southwest Oncology Group is investigating the incidence, risk factors, and outcomes associated with ONJ in a prospective trial seeking to enroll a total of 7200 patients.[38] Risk factors for the development of ONJ include head and neck radiotherapy, periodontal disease, and dental extractions.[37] About 30% of patients treated with IV zoledronic acid are at risk of an acute phase reaction, associated with fevers, myalgias, and nausea, which can occur within the first several days following administration, but diminishes in duration and intensity.[39]

Table 2
Pharmacokinetics of zoledronic acid and denosumab[32,41]

Drug	Mechanism of Action	Bioavailability	Half-Life (d)	Clearance	Dose Modification
Zoledronic acid	Binds to hydroxyapatite crystals on exposed bone	1% (oral), 100% (IV)	Triphasic	Renal	Yes[a]
Denosumab	Monoclonal antibody to RANKL	62% (subcutaneous)	25	Reticuloendothelial system	No[b]

[a] Dose modification is based on renal function. Trials of zoledronic acid in men with prostate cancer excluded patients with creatinine clearance rate <30 mL/min. Use is not recommended in patients with creatinine clearance rate <30 mL/min or on dialysis given risk of hypocalcemia and worsening renal function.
[b] No adjustment is necessary when administered every 6 months. Once-monthly dosing has not been evaluated in patients with renal impairment. Patients with creatinine clearance rate <30 mL/min or on dialysis require close monitoring because of increased risk of hypocalcemia.

Receptor Activator of Nuclear Factor-κβ Ligand Inhibitors

Denosumab is a fully human monoclonal antibody administered subcutaneously that has high affinity and specificity for RANKL. It mimics the action of OPG by binding RANKL and reducing the activity of osteoclasts. Unlike bisphosphonates, denosumab does not accumulate in bone and has a longer circulatory half-life (>25 days) (see **Table 2**).[40] Although there are no recommendations for dose adjustment for renal insufficiency, patients with severe renal insufficiency are more prone to hypocalcemia.[41] In addition, use of monthly denosumab is not advised when creatinine clearance rate is less than 30 mL/min, given limited studies in this patient population.

MANAGEMENT OF TREATMENT-RELATED OSTEOPOROSIS
Defining Osteoporosis

The definition and diagnosis of osteoporosis in men relies, at least in part, on female standards.[42] The World Health Organization (WHO) recommends using the same classification of BMD to define osteoporosis in men, aged 50 years and older, as in women[43]:

- Normal is defined as a T-score greater than −1.0.
- Osteopenia is defined as a T-score between −1.0 and −2.5.
- Osteoporosis is defined as a T-score of less than or equal to −2.5.

The T-score is reported as the number of standard deviations (SDs) that a patient's BMD value is higher or lower than the reference value for a healthy 30-year-old adult. Fracture risk increases approximately 2-fold for every SD decrease in BMD.[44]

Who to Consider for Screening and Treatment?

The National Comprehensive Cancer Network guidelines recommend screening and treatment of osteoporosis in men with prostate cancer according to the National Osteoporosis Foundation (NOF) guidelines for the general population (**Table 3**). In the past, BMD was the primary factor used to assess fracture risk, although most fractures occurred in men with BMD measurements not in the osteoporotic range.[45] Given that there was a need for more sensitive risk determination, in 2008 the WHO introduced the Fracture Risk Assessment Tool (FRAX), which estimates the 10-year

Table 3 NOF screening and treatment recommendations[87]	
Screening recommendations	All men age 70 y or older
	Adults who have a fracture after age 50 y
	Adults with a condition or taking a medicine associated with low bone mass or bone loss
	Anyone being considered for pharmacologic therapy for osteoporosis
	Anyone being treated for osteoporosis, to monitor treatment effect
Men ≥50 y of age presenting with the following should be considered for treatment	Hip or vertebral fracture (both clinical or radiological)
	T-score ≤−2.5 at the femoral neck or spine after evaluation to exclude secondary causes
	Low bone mass as defined by T-score between −1.0 and −2.5 at the femoral neck or spine and 10-y probability of a hip fracture ≥3% or a 10-y probability of a major osteoporosis-related fracture ≥20% based on the US-adapted WHO/FRAX algorithm (http://www.shef.ac.uk/FRAX/)

probability of hip fracture and major osteoporotic fracture for untreated patients between ages 40 and 90 years using clinical risk factors for fracture and femoral neck BMD if available (http://www.shef.ac.uk/FRAX/). The FRAX algorithm is integrated into the NOF recommendations for treatment. Application of the NOF treatment guidelines to men in MrOS (Osteoporotic Fractures in Men Study)[46] estimated that 34% of US white men aged 65 years and older and 49% of men aged 75 years and older would be recommended for treatment. In a study of 363 men receiving ADT for prostate cancer,[47] the FRAX algorithm without BMD assessment estimated that 51.2% of men met criteria for pharmacologic intervention. The FRAX algorithm with BMD assessment estimated that 15% of men met criteria for pharmacologic intervention. Although the FRAX algorithm uses epidemiologic data from the general population, it is still a reasonable strategy to determine fracture risk in men receiving ADT for prostate cancer. To monitor effectiveness of treatment, the NOF recommends baseline BMD assessment with repeat testing every 2 years, recognizing that more frequent testing may be warranted in certain clinical situations.

Pharmacologic Interventions for Treatment-Related Osteoporosis

Several agents including bisphosphonates, RANKL inhibitors, and selective estrogen receptor modulators (SERMs) have shown benefit in the management of treatment-related osteoporosis (**Table 4**). The efficacy of bisphosphonates has been shown in small studies that reported improvement in BMD; however, these studies were not powered to assess fracture risk. Denosumab and toremifene have both been evaluated in phase 3 trials and showed improved BMD and decreased fracture risk. Despite efficacy of these treatments, the optimal agent, schedule, and duration of therapy remain in question.

Bisphosphonates

Although multiple bisphosphonates including neridronate (Nerixia), alendronate (Fosamax), pamidronate (Aredia), and zoledronic acid have been shown to decrease bone turnover and improve BMD in men receiving ADT, none has reported statistically significant improvement in the rates of fragility fractures.[10,21,48–52] These were smaller studies designed to primarily evaluate BMD as a surrogate end point. In a meta-analysis of 2634 men with prostate cancer (including both nonmetastatic and metastatic disease), treatment with bisphosphonate therapy had a substantial effect in preventing fractures (RR 0.80; P = .005) and osteoporosis (RR 0.39; $P<.00001$).[53] Given limited clinical data in men with ADT-associated bone loss, there still exists significant controversy regarding choice of agent, dose, and schedule. Compared with what is typically used for the prevention of SREs in patients with metastatic disease, dosing is appreciably less for the management of treatment-related osteoporosis.[54]

Receptor activator of nuclear factor-κβ ligand inhibitors

The Denosumab HALT (Hormone Ablation Bone Loss Trial) 138 study, a multicenter, double-blind, randomized, placebo-controlled trial, enrolled 1468 men receiving ADT at increased risk of fracture given age 70 years or older, low BMD defined as a T-score less than –1, or a history of an osteoporotic fracture.[55] Patients were randomly assigned to treatment with denosumab 60 mg subcutaneously every 6 months for 24 months or placebo. The primary end point was percent change in BMD at the lumbar spine at 24 months. A secondary end point included incidence of new vertebral fractures. The study reported statistically significant increased BMD at the lumbar spine (6.7% difference between groups), total hip (4.8% difference between groups), femoral neck (3.9% difference between groups), and distal third of the radius (5.5%

Table 4
Trials of osteoclast-targeted therapies for prevention of treatment-related fragility fractures

Trial	Number of Patients	Population	Treatment	Primary End Point	Outcome
Denosumab HALT 138[55]	1468	Men with nonmetastatic prostate cancer treated with ADT at high risk of fracture (age ≥70 y, low BMD, or history of osteoporotic fracture)	Denosumab 60 mg subcutaneous every 6 mo vs placebo × 2 y	Percent change in BMD at lumbar spine at 24 mo	Improvement in BMD at all sites and decreased incidence of new vertebral fractures (1.5% vs 3.9%; $P = .006$)
Toremifene[57]	1284	Men with nonmetastatic prostate cancer treated with ADT at high risk of fracture (age ≥70 y or low BMD)	Toremifene 80 mg orally daily vs placebo × 2 y	Incidence of new vertebral fractures	Improvement in BMD at all sites and decreased incidence of new vertebral fractures (2.5% vs 4.9%; $P = .05$)

difference between groups) at 24 months. In addition, patients who received denosumab had a decreased incidence of new vertebral fractures at 36 months (1.5% vs 3.9%; P = .006). The rates of adverse events were similar between the 2 groups. There was 1 person with hypocalcemia in the treatment arm and zero in the placebo arm. There were no documented cases of ONJ in either group.

SERMs

SERMs have shown benefit in men treated with ADT for prostate cancer secondary to their agonist activity at the estrogen receptor in bone.[56,57] In a phase 3, international, double-blind, randomized, placebo-controlled trial, 1284 men with nonmetastatic prostate cancer treated with ADT were randomized to toremifene (Fareston) or placebo for 2 years.[57] Patients were at high risk for fracture given age 70 years or older or osteopenia. The primary end point was incidence of new vertebral fractures. Men treated with toremifene had significantly fewer new vertebral fractures compared with placebo (2.5% vs 4.9%; RR 0.50; P = .05). In addition, toremifene significantly increased BMD at the lumbar spine, hip, and femoral neck compared with placebo ($P<.0001$). Treatment with toremifene was associated with an increased rate of venous thromboembolic events compared with placebo (2.6% vs 1.1%, respectively).

Calcium and Vitamin D Supplementation

Providing adequate calcium and vitamin D is recommended by the NOF. A meta-analysis of 11 trials, mostly in postmenopausal women, comparing calcium (500–1200 mg daily) plus vitamin D (300–1100 units daily) with placebo[58] showed that combined supplementation reduced the risk of total fractures (RR 0.88; 95% CI 0.78–0.99).

The NOF recommends at least 1200 mg daily of calcium for those older than 50 years. Calcium supplements are available in 2 formulations, including calcium carbonate, which requires gastric acid for optimal absorption, and calcium citrate, which does not require gastric acid for absorption and is recommended for patients receiving proton pump inhibitors.[59]

The NOF recommends at least 1000 IU units daily of vitamin D. All patients to be initiated on ADT should also be tested for vitamin D deficiency via measurement of serum 25-hydroxy vitamin D (25-OH-D).[60] Vitamin D supplements are available as ergocalciferol (D_2) or cholechalciferol (D_3). There is controversy regarding the choice of agent for supplementation. In a meta-analysis of 7 randomized trials evaluating serum 25-OH-D concentrations after supplementation with D_2 versus D_3,[61] D_3 was more efficacious at increasing serum 25-OH-D than D_2, with the greatest difference seen for weekly or monthly rather than daily dosing. Those with significant vitamin D deficiency (defined as 25-OH-D <20 ng/mL) should be aggressively repleted with vitamin D, typically 50,000 IU weekly for 8 weeks.[60]

Lifestyle Modifications

Lifestyle modifications are important in men receiving ADT for prostate cancer. These modifications include smoking cessation, moderating alcohol and caffeine consumption, and regular weight-bearing exercises and resistance training.[59] Fall prevention is also critical in reducing fracture risk.[59] Counseling patients on these modifications is essential in the care of men with prostate cancer treated with ADT and recommended interventions should be individualized.

Summary

Treatment-related osteoporosis can lead to increased morbidity in men treated with ADT for prostate cancer. Initial approaches for men receiving treatment with ADT include education regarding lifestyle modifications to decrease fracture risk and supplementation with calcium and vitamin D. The NOF screening and treatment guidelines (see **Table 3**), which use the FRAX algorithm and BMD assessments, can be used to inform screening and use of pharmacologic agents in patients with high fracture risk. For men who warrant treatment, consensus is lacking regarding the appropriate treatment agent, dose, schedule, and duration of therapy. Denosumab is the only commercially available agent shown to increase bone mass and prevent fracture in high-risk men receiving ADT for prostate cancer. Other pharmacologic agents to consider include bisphosphonates, such as zoledronic acid and alendronate. Repeat BMD assessment is recommended every 2 years, although more frequent testing may be warranted in selected individuals.

USE OF OSTEOCLAST-TARGETED THERAPIES IN METASTATIC CASTRATION-SENSITIVE PROSTATE CANCER

Although osteoclast-targeted therapies are beneficial in patients with CRPC metastatic to bone, their usefulness has not been clearly defined in patients with metastatic prostate cancer receiving first-line hormone therapy. Zoledronic acid is being evaluated in this setting in an ongoing clinical trial.[62] Use of denosumab in men with bone metastases from prostate cancer responding to hormone therapy has not been explored. Given high response rate and hence control of cancer, ADT alone may be effective at SRE prevention.

The Medical Research Council PR.05 study[63] is the only completed, randomized, placebo-controlled trial to evaluate the efficacy of a bisphosphonate in metastatic castration-sensitive prostate cancer. In this study, 311 men who were initiating or responding to first-line ADT were randomized to clodronate (Clasteon) (2080 mg orally daily) or placebo. The primary end point was symptomatic bone progression-free survival (PFS) or prostate cancer death. After a median follow-up of 59 months, the clodronate group showed improvements in symptomatic bone PFS (hazard ratio [HR] 0.79; 95% CI 0.61–1.02; $P = .066$) and overall survival (OS) (HR 0.80; 95% CI 0.62–1.03; $P = .082$); however, the results were not statistically significant. At long-term follow-up, treatment with clodronate was associated with statistically significant improved OS (8-year OS 22% vs 14%; HR 0.77; 95% CI 0.60–0.98; $P = .032$).[64] Treatment was not associated with improvement in pain or quality of life.

The CALGB/CTSU (Cancer and Leukemia Group B/Cancer Trials Support Unit) conducted a clinical trial investigating the use of zoledronic acid in men with metastatic castration-sensitive prostate cancer.[62] The CALBG/STSU 90202 trial was designed to randomize 680 men with metastatic prostate cancer recently initiated on ADT to receive zoledronic acid (4 mg IV every 4 weeks) or placebo. The primary end point was time to first SRE or prostate cancer death. Crossover to the treatment arm was required for men who developed CRPC or an SRE. As of 2012, the trial had stopped enrollment and follow-up was ongoing.

USE OF OSTEOCLAST-TARGETED THERAPIES IN METASTATIC CRPC

Patients with CRPC with bone metastases are at risk for significant skeletal morbidity. Although both clodronate and pamidronate have been evaluated in this setting, zoledronic acid is the only bisphosphonate that has shown benefit in preventing SREs in this high-risk population of men (**Table 5**).[65,66] In addition, denosumab has shown benefit in preventing SREs in men with CRPC with bone metastases.

Table 5
Trials of osteoclast-targeted therapies in CRPC

Trial	Number of Patients	Population	Treatment	Primary End Point	Outcome
Prevention of Bone Metastases in Patients with CRPC					
Denosumab 147[70]	1432	CRPC at high risk of developing metastases (PSA level ≥8 μg/L or PSA doubling time of ≤10 mo, or both)	Denosumab 120 mg subcutaneously vs placebo every 4 wk	BMFS	Increased BMFS (29.5 vs 25.2; P = .028) and delayed time to first bone metastases (32.2 vs 29.2 mo; P = .032)
Prevention of SREs in Patients with CRPC					
Zometa 039[28]	643	Men with CRPC and asymptomatic or minimally symptomatic bone metastases	Zoledronic acid IV (4 mg or 8 mg) vs placebo every 3 wk × 15 mo	Portion of men who experienced 1 SRE during the first 15 mo of therapy	Decreased frequency of SREs (33% vs 44%; P = .021) and increased time to develop SRE (363 vs 321 d; P = .002)
Denosumab 103[67]	1904	Men with CRPC with bone metastases	Denosumab 120 mg subcutaneously vs zoledronic acid 4 mg IV every 4 wk	Time to first on-study SRE	Increased time to first on-study SRE (20.7 vs 17.1 mo; P = .0008 for superiority)

Zoledronic Acid

The Zometa 039 trial[28] evaluated the efficacy of zoledronic acid in preventing SREs in patients with CRPC with bone metastases. The study randomized 643 men with CRPC and asymptomatic or minimally symptomatic bone metastases to zoledronic acid 4 mg IV, zoledronic acid 8 mg IV, or placebo every 3 weeks for 15 months. All men continued ADT and received any other therapy at the discretion of the treating physicians. The portion of men who experienced at least 1 SRE during the first 15 months of therapy was the primary end point of the trial. SREs were defined as pathologic bone fracture, spinal cord compression, surgery to bone, radiation to bone, or change in antineoplastic therapy to treat bone pain. The trial excluded patients with a serum creatinine rate greater than 3 mg/dL or significant hypocalcemia or hypercalcemia. All patients received calcium and vitamin D supplementation.

Given the observation of multiple cases of nephrotoxicity early in the trial, the infusion period was increased from 5 minutes to 15 minutes and the zoledronic acid dose in the 8 mg treatment group was reduced to 4 mg. After these modifications, the rate of renal toxicity between the zoledronic acid 4 mg group and placebo were similar. The statistical plan was amended to compare only the zoledronic acid 4 mg arm with placebo at the primary study analysis. In addition, a total of 8 patients in the zoledronic acid arms (4 in each) experienced grade 3 to 4 hypocalcemia.

At 15-month follow-up, the frequency of SREs was significantly reduced (33% vs 44%; $P = .021$) and the median time to develop an SRE was significantly longer (363 vs 321 days; $P = .002$) for those treated with zoledronic acid compared with placebo. Pain and analgesic scores were significantly higher in men who received placebo compared with zoledronic acid. The median OS was numerically longer in the zoledronic acid 4-mg group compared with the placebo group, although this was not statistically significant (546 vs 464 days; $P = .091$). The benefit in the incidence of SREs, time to SRE development, and pain was also observed at 24-month follow-up. Based on the results of this trial, zoledronic acid became the first osteoclast-targeted agent to be approved for men with bony metastatic CRPC.

Denosumab

The Denosumab 103 trial[67] was a multicenter, double-blind, randomized, study of men with CRPC and bone metastases. The study randomized 1904 men to either treatment with denosumab (120 mg subcutaneously every 4 weeks) or zoledronic acid (4 mg IV every 4 weeks). The primary end point was time to first on-study SRE, which was assessed for noninferiority. The same outcome was further assessed for superiority as a secondary end point. The trial excluded patients with a serum creatinine clearance rate less than 30 mL/min or significant hypocalcemia or hypercalcemia. It was strongly recommended that all patients take calcium and vitamin D supplementation.

At median on-study duration of 12.2 months for the denosumab arm and 11.2 months for the zoledronic acid arm, denosumab significantly prolonged the median time to first on-study SRE compared with zoledronic acid (20.7 vs 17.1 months; $P = .0002$ for noninferiority; $P = .008$ for superiority). OS and time to disease progression were similar between the treatment arms. In regards to adverse events, hypocalcemia occurred more frequently in the denosumab arm compared with the zoledronic acid arm (13% vs 5%; $P < .0001$). Although not statistically significant, there was a trend toward a higher rate of ONJ in the denosumab arm (2% vs 1%; $P = .09$).

Summary

Zoledronic acid and denosumab are beneficial in preventing SREs in men with CRPC with bone metastases. Denosumab showed a slightly greater benefit in prevention of SREs compared with zoledronic acid. In addition, the trials of zoledronic acid and denosumab for the prevention of SREs in men with metastatic CRPC were conducted in an era when patients with advanced prostate cancer had fewer treatment options for disease control. Because many new therapies for advanced prostate cancer have a beneficial impact on the rate of SREs, the choice of osteoclast-targeted agent, dose, schedule, duration of therapy, and role when used concurrently with anticancer agents in the modern treatment era remains an open question.

PREVENTION OF BONE METASTASES

Development of bone metastases is a clinical dilemma in patients with prostate cancer. Thus, investigation of strategies to prevent progression is logical. The efficacy of clodronate was evaluated in a phase 3 trial that failed to show improvement of bone-metastasis-free survival (BMFS) in patients with prostate cancer receiving ADT.[64,68] Although the Zometa 704 trial closed early because the event rate was lower than projected, based on the results of the European ZEUS (Zometa European Study) trial recently presented at the European Association of Urology Annual Congress, zoledronic acid had no impact in preventing bone metastases in high-risk patients receiving ADT.[69] Although no bisphosphonate has shown benefit in prevention of bone metastases, denosumab is the only drug shown to delay the onset of bone metastases in patients with CRPC.[70]

Zoledronic Acid

The potential for zoledronic acid prevention of bone metastases in nonmetastatic high-risk prostate cancer was investigated in the European ZEUS trial.[69] All patients in the trial had had previous local therapy and at least 1 high-risk feature, including PSA level of 20 ng/mL or greater at diagnosis, lymph node–positive disease, or Gleason score 8 to 10. Patients could have been on ADT or no hormonal therapy. In this study, 1433 men were randomized to standard treatment with or without zoledronic acid 4 mg IV every 3 months for 48 months. All patients received calcium and vitamin D supplementation. The primary end point was the proportion of patients who develop on-study bone metastases. At a median follow-up of 4.9 years in the zoledronic acid group and 4.8 years in the control group, the rates of development of bone metastases were 13.7% and 13.0%, respectively (P = .721). In addition, there was no difference in OS between the groups (P = .717). ONJ occurred in 9 patients in the zoledronic acid group and 1 patient in the control group.

Denosumab

Experimental and clinical evidence provides a strong rationale for denosumab inhibition of RANKL as a promising therapeutic agent for prevention of progression of prostate cancer in bone.[71] The Denosumab 147 trial is a phase 3, double-blind, randomized, placebo-controlled study of men with nonmetastatic CRPC at high-risk of bone metastases, defined as PSA level 8 µg/L or greater or PSA doubling time of 10 months or less, or both.[70] The study randomized 1432 patients to treatment with denosumab 120 mg subcutaneously or placebo every 4 weeks. The primary end point was BMFS. Patients were discontinued from treatment when bone metastasis occurred and received standard treatment at the discretion of the treating investigator.

Denosumab significantly increased BMFS by a median of 4.2 months compared with placebo (29.5 vs 25.2 months; $P = .028$). In addition, denosumab significantly delayed the time to first bone metastases (32.2 vs 29.2 months; $P = .032$). OS did not differ between groups (43.9 vs 44.8 months; $P = .91$). In a subgroup analysis of men with a PSA doubling time of less than 6 months,[72] denosumab prolonged BMFS by a median of 7.2 months with a 23% reduction in risk compared with placebo (25.9 vs 18.7 months; HR 0.77; 95% CI 0.64–0.93; $P = .0064$). Treatment with deno-sumab was associated with increased ONJ (5% vs 0%) and hypocalcemia (2% vs <1%) compared with placebo. This study failed to show an effect on quality of life, pain, and OS.

Given that the degree of benefit was similar between the premetastatic and meta-static setting, there is concern that the study included patients with established me-tastases that were undetectable by existing imaging studies. The appropriate sequence of denosumab in the treatment landscape for prostate cancer requires further investigation.

Summary

Prevention of bone metastases in patients with nonmetastatic CRPC remains an area for further investigation. Recently, zoledronic acid was shown to have no impact on preventing bone metastases in patients with high-risk prostate cancer. Denosumab is the only agent shown to delay the time to bone metastases; however, the magnitude of clinical benefit is less certain.

RADIOPHARMACEUTICALS

Radiopharmaceuticals have emerged as a treatment strategy for patients with CRPC and symptomatic bone metastases. These compounds are systemically administered agents that localize to sites of bone metastases and deliver focal radiation through β-emission (strontium-89 [Metastron], samarium-153 [Quadramet]) or α-emission (radium-223 [Xofigo]) (**Table 6**). Under ideal circumstances, the physical half-life of the isotopes should be long enough to enable sufficient therapeutic effect, but short enough to limit myelotoxicity.[73] In addition, the range of emission should be narrow to limit marrow toxicity. Strontium-89 and samarium-153 are used for the palliation of pain in patients with CRPC with symptomatic bone metastases. Radium-223 is the first radiopharmaceutical agent to show improved survival in patients with CRPC with symptomatic bone metastases.

Strontium-89 and samarium-153 are useful for the palliation of pain caused by bone metastases. They are contraindicated in patients with pathologic fractures, spinal cord compression, significant myelosuppression, or renal dysfunction.[73] Despite the bene-ficial palliative effect observed with strontium-89 and samarium-153, these agents have had limited clinical use, likely related to logistics of administration, myelotoxicity, availability of alternative treatment strategies, and other factors. Recently, the positive

Table 6
Physical characteristics of radiopharmaceuticals for prostate cancer[73]

Radiopharmaceutical	Half-Life (d)	Mean β Energy (MeV)	Mean α Energy (MeV)	Mean Tissue Penetration (mm)
Strontium-89	50.5	0.58	—	2.4
Samarium-153	1.9	0.22	—	0.6
Radium-223	11.4	—	5.64	<0.1

impact of radium-223 on OS is a landmark development, which may expand the usefulness of radiopharmaceuticals in the treatment of patients with symptomatic bone metastatic CRPC.

Strontium-89

The first use of a radiopharmaceutical was with strontium-89 in 1942. Strontium-89 is a calcium analogue with a long half-life (50.5 days) and relatively high-energy average β-emission (0.58 MeV).[73] The average soft tissue range of this agent is 2.4 mm.[73] It has been in use since 1993 for the palliation of pain associated with symptomatic bone metastases in patients with CRPC based on the results of several randomized clinical trials.[74,75]

A British trial of 284 men randomly assigned to treatment with strontium-89 or external beam radiation (focal or hemibody)[75] showed similar rates of pain control between the treatment arms; however, fewer patients reported new pain sites after strontium-89 treatment. A phase 3, placebo-controlled trial randomized 126 men treated with focal external beam radiation to treatment with strontium-89 or placebo.[74] Although there was no difference in OS between the 2 groups, patients given strontium-89 had decreased analgesic use, increased time to further radiation therapy, and decreased number of new painful sites.

Samarium-153

Samarium-153 binds to hydroxyapatite crystals in areas of high bone turnover and has low-energy average β-emission (0.22 MeV), with a short half-life (1.9 days).[73] The average soft tissue range of this agent is 0.6 mm.[73] The kidneys are the main route of elimination of unbound samarium-153, with complete excretion in 6 hours.[73]

Clinical benefit as shown by pain control was reported in clinical trials.[76,77] In a phase 3, double-blind, randomized, placebo-controlled trial,[77] 118 patients with symptomatic bone metastases, of whom 68% had prostate cancer, were randomized to 1 of 2 doses of samarium-153 (0.5 mCi/kg or 1.0 mCi/kg) or placebo. Compared with placebo, the higher dose of samarium-153 was associated with significantly less pain and decreased analgesic use. There was no difference in OS between the groups. Toxicity profiles were comparable with transient thrombocytopenia and leukopenia with samarium-153 treatment. Another phase 3, double-blind, placebo-controlled trial[76] randomized 152 men with bone metastatic CRPC to samarium-153 or a nonradioactive samarium placebo. Patients receiving samarium-153 had significant improvement of pain and decreased analgesic use, although there was no difference in OS between the treatment arms. Transient myelosuppression was the only significant adverse side effect.

Radium-223

Radium-223 is an α-emitting radioisotope that acts as a calcium mimic with natural bone-seeking proclivity.[73] In contrast to β-particles, α-particles provide more dense ionizing radiation in a narrow range of less than 0.1 mm, corresponding to 2 to 10 cell diameters, thus minimizing myelotoxicity.[78] The particles induce DNA double-strand breaks, leading to cell death at all stages of the cell cycle.[78] Radium-223 has a suitable half-life (11.4 days), and particles not taken up by bone are rapidly cleared to the gut and excreted.[73]

The efficacy of radium-223 was shown in the ALSYMPCA (Alpharadin in Symptomatic Prostate Cancer) trial.[79,80] This phase 3, international, double-blind, trial randomized 922 men with CRPC with bone metastases to radium-223 plus best supportive care or placebo plus best supportive care. Eligible patients had 2 or more symptomatic bone metastases, no known visceral metastases, and had either received previous docetaxel (Taxotere) or were unfit for docetaxel chemotherapy. Patients were randomized 2:1 to receive 6 injections of radium-223 (50 kBq/kg) at 4-week intervals. The primary end point was OS. Patients were stratified by previous docetaxel use, baseline alkaline phosphatase level, and current bisphosphonate use. Updated results were presented at the 2012 American Society of Clinical Oncology meeting. Based on data from a planned interim analysis of 809 patients, radium-223 significantly improved median OS (14 vs 11.2 months; P = .00185). In addition, SREs were lower and time to first SRE was significantly delayed in the treatment arm compared with placebo (13.6 vs 8.4 months; P = .00046). There was a low incidence of grade 3 to 4 myelosuppression (1.8% neutropenia and 0.8% thrombocytopenia).

NON-BONE–TARGETED THERAPIES DOCUMENTED TO DECREASE SRES

The development of novel therapeutics is transforming the treatment paradigm of advanced prostate cancer. Agents that are active in controlling the burden of disease and improving survival likely diminish the negative effects of bone metastases. SREs, which have classically been an end point of trials assessing efficacy of osteoclast-targeted agents, are being evaluated in trials of novel systemic agents. Abiraterone and enzalutamide have recently been shown to improve OS and have a beneficial impact on decreasing the rate of SREs in patients with metastatic CRPC. In addition to novel hormone therapies, other potential targets important in the development of bone metastases include MET, a receptor tyrosine kinase, and Src, a nonreceptor tyrosine kinase.[81,82]

Abiraterone

Abiraterone irreversibly inhibits the CYP17 enzyme, thus blocking androgen synthesis in the testis, adrenal glands, and prostatic tumor cells.[83] The activity of abiraterone was shown in a phase 3 trial in which 1195 men previously treated with docetaxel were randomly assigned to abiraterone plus prednisone or placebo plus prednisone.[83] After a median follow-up of 13 months, abiraterone significantly increased OS compared with placebo (median 14.8 vs 10.9 months; $P<.0001$). Abiraterone delayed the median time to SRE (25 vs 20.3 months; P = .0001) and significantly decreased pain compared with placebo.[84]

Enzalutamide

Enzalutamide is a novel androgen receptor (AR) signaling inhibitor that competitively inhibits binding of androgens to the AR, inhibits AR nuclear translocation, and inhibits association of the AR with DNA.[85] In a global, phase 3, double-blind, placebo-controlled trial, 1199 men with advanced prostate cancer previously treated with docetaxel were randomized to enzalutamide versus placebo in a 2:1 ratio.[86] The primary end point was OS. The study was stopped after a planned interim analysis at the time of 520 deaths. Treatment with enzalutamide was associated with improved OS (18.4 vs 13.6 months; $P<.0001$). In addition, time to first SRE was significantly longer in the treatment arm compared with placebo (8.3 vs 2.9 months; P = .001).

SUMMARY

Bone health is a critical issue in patients with prostate cancer. Strategies to reduce morbidity associated with treatment-related osteoporosis include lifestyle modifications, calcium and vitamin D supplementation, and pharmacologic intervention with osteoclast-targeted agents in patients with or at high risk for osteoporotic fractures. The mainstay of care for the management of bone metastases includes effective therapies to control the burden of disease, and in patients with CRPC, osteoclast-targeted agents. As improved therapeutics populate the treatment landscape, additional studies need to investigate the optimal dosing, schedule, duration, and role of osteoclast-targeted agents with concurrent administration of anticancer agents in the treatment of patients with metastatic disease.

REFERENCES

1. Siegel R, Naishadham D, Jemal A. Cancer statistics, 2012. CA Cancer J Clin 2012;62(1):10–29.
2. Boyle WJ, Simonet WS, Lacey DL. Osteoclast differentiation and activation. Nature 2003;423(6937):337–42.
3. Lacey DL, Boyle WJ, Simonet WS, et al. Bench to bedside: elucidation of the OPG-RANK-RANKL pathway and the development of denosumab. Nat Rev Drug Discov 2012;11(5):401–19.
4. Schoppet M, Preissner KT, Hofbauer LC. RANK ligand and osteoprotegerin: paracrine regulators of bone metabolism and vascular function. Arterioscler Thromb Vasc Biol 2002;22(4):549–53.
5. Gaur T, Lengner CJ, Hovhannisyan H, et al. Canonical WNT signaling promotes osteogenesis by directly stimulating Runx2 gene expression. J Biol Chem 2005; 280(39):33132–40.
6. Bilezikian JP. Osteoporosis in men. J Clin Endocrinol Metab 1999;84(10): 3431–4.
7. Gilbert SM, Kuo YF, Shahinian VB. Prevalent and incident use of androgen deprivation therapy among men with prostate cancer in the United States. Urol Oncol 2011;29(6):647–53.
8. Barry MJ, Delorenzo MA, Walker-Corkery ES, et al. The rising prevalence of androgen deprivation among older American men since the advent of prostate-specific antigen testing: a population-based cohort study. BJU Int 2006;98(5):973–8.
9. Daniell HW, Dunn SR, Ferguson DW, et al. Progressive osteoporosis during androgen deprivation therapy for prostate cancer. J Urol 2000;163(1):181–6.
10. Greenspan SL, Coates P, Sereika SM, et al. Bone loss after initiation of androgen deprivation therapy in patients with prostate cancer. J Clin Endocrinol Metab 2005;90(12):6410–7.
11. Mittan D, Lee S, Miller E, et al. Bone loss following hypogonadism in men with prostate cancer treated with GnRH analogs. J Clin Endocrinol Metab 2002; 87(8):3656–61.
12. Diamond TH, Higano CS, Smith MR, et al. Osteoporosis in men with prostate carcinoma receiving androgen-deprivation therapy: recommendations for diagnosis and therapies. Cancer 2004;100(5):892–9.
13. Guise TA, Oefelein MG, Eastham JA, et al. Estrogenic side effects of androgen deprivation therapy. Rev Urol 2007;9(4):163–80.
14. Lee H, McGovern K, Finkelstein JS, et al. Changes in bone mineral density and body composition during initial and long-term gonadotropin-releasing hormone agonist treatment for prostate carcinoma. Cancer 2005;104(8):1633–7.
15. Shahinian VB, Kuo YF, Freeman JL, et al. Risk of fracture after androgen deprivation for prostate cancer. N Engl J Med 2005;352(2):154–64.
16. Smith MR, Lee WC, Brandman J, et al. Gonadotropin-releasing hormone agonists and fracture risk: a claims-based cohort study of men with nonmetastatic prostate cancer. J Clin Oncol 2005;23(31):7897–903.

17. Oefelein MG, Ricchiuti V, Conrad W, et al. Skeletal fractures negatively correlate with overall survival in men with prostate cancer. J Urol 2002;168(3):1005–7.
18. Khosla S, Oursler MJ, Monroe DG. Estrogen and the skeleton. Trends Endocrinol Metab 2012;23(11):576–81.
19. Falahati-Nini A, Riggs BL, Atkinson EJ, et al. Relative contributions of testosterone and estrogen in regulating bone resorption and formation in normal elderly men. J Clin Invest 2000;106(12):1553–60.
20. Mellstrom D, Vandenput L, Mallmin H, et al. Older men with low serum estradiol and high serum SHBG have an increased risk of fractures. J Bone Miner Res 2008;23(10):1552–60.
21. Smith MR, McGovern FJ, Zietman AL, et al. Pamidronate to prevent bone loss during androgen-deprivation therapy for prostate cancer. N Engl J Med 2001; 345(13):948–55.
22. Amin S, Zhang Y, Felson DT, et al. Estradiol, testosterone, and the risk for hip fractures in elderly men from the Framingham Study. Am J Med 2006;119(5): 426–33.
23. Khosla S, Melton LJ 3rd, Atkinson EJ, et al. Relationship of serum sex steroid levels and bone turnover markers with bone mineral density in men and women: a key role for bioavailable estrogen. J Clin Endocrinol Metab 1998;83(7): 2266–74.
24. Rochira V, Balestrieri A, Madeo B, et al. Osteoporosis and male age-related hypogonadism: role of sex steroids on bone (patho)physiology. Eur J Endocrinol 2006;154(2):175–85.
25. Tannock IF, de Wit R, Berry WR, et al. Docetaxel plus prednisone or mitoxantrone plus prednisone for advanced prostate cancer. N Engl J Med 2004; 351(15):1502–12.
26. Keller ET, Brown J. Prostate cancer bone metastases promote both osteolytic and osteoblastic activity. J Cell Biochem 2004;91(4):718–29.
27. Norgaard M, Jensen AO, Jacobsen JB, et al. Skeletal related events, bone metastasis and survival of prostate cancer: a population based cohort study in Denmark (1999 to 2007). J Urol 2010;184(1):162–7.
28. Saad F, Gleason DM, Murray R, et al. A randomized, placebo-controlled trial of zoledronic acid in patients with hormone-refractory metastatic prostate carcinoma. J Natl Cancer Inst 2002;94(19):1458–68.
29. Cook RJ, Coleman R, Brown J, et al. Markers of bone metabolism and survival in men with hormone-refractory metastatic prostate cancer. Clin Cancer Res 2006; 12(11 Pt 1):3361–7.
30. Roodman GD. Mechanisms of bone metastasis. N Engl J Med 2004;350(16): 1655–64.
31. Rogers MJ, Watts DJ, Russell RG. Overview of bisphosphonates. Cancer 1997; 80(Suppl 8):1652–60.
32. Fleisch H. Bisphosphonates: mechanisms of action. Endocr Rev 1998;19(1): 80–100.
33. Papapoulos SE. Bisphosphonates: how do they work? Best Pract Res Clin Endocrinol Metab 2008;22(5):831–47.
34. van Beek ER, Cohen LH, Leroy IM, et al. Differentiating the mechanisms of antiresorptive action of nitrogen containing bisphosphonates. Bone 2003;33(5): 805–11.
35. Plotkin LI, Lezcano V, Thostenson J, et al. Connexin 43 is required for the anti-apoptotic effect of bisphosphonates on osteocytes and osteoblasts in vivo. J Bone Miner Res 2008;23(11):1712–21.

36. Perazella MA, Markowitz GS. Bisphosphonate nephrotoxicity. Kidney Int 2008; 74(11):1385–93.

37. Khan AA, Sandor GK, Dore E, et al. Bisphosphonate associated osteonecrosis of the jaw. J Rheumatol 2009;36(3):478–90.

38. Southwest Oncology Group. Osteonecrosis of the jaw in patients with cancer receiving zoledronic acid for bone metastases [ClinicalTrials.gov identifier NCT00874211]. US National Institutes of Health, ClinicalTrials.gov [online]. Available at: http://www.clinicaltrials.gov. Accessed December 5, 2012.

39. Dalle Carbonare L, Zanatta M, Gasparetto A, et al. Safety and tolerability of zo-ledronic acid and other bisphosphonates in osteoporosis management. Drug Healthc Patient Saf 2010;2:121–37.

40. Lee RJ, Saylor PJ, Smith MR. Contemporary therapeutic approaches target-ing bone complications in prostate cancer. Clin Genitourin Cancer 2010; 8(1):29–36.

41. Block GA, Bone HG, Fang L, et al. A single-dose study of denosumab in pa-tients with various degrees of renal impairment. J Bone Miner Res 2012;27(7): 1471–9.

42. Cummings SR, Cawthon PM, Ensrud KE, et al. BMD and risk of hip and nonver-tebral fractures in older men: a prospective study and comparison with older women. J Bone Miner Res 2006;21(10):1550–6.

43. Kanis JA, Melton LJ 3rd, Christiansen C, et al. The diagnosis of osteoporosis. J Bone Miner Res 1994;9(8):1137–41.

44. Marshall D, Johnell O, Wedel H. Meta-analysis of how well measures of bone mineral density predict occurrence of osteoporotic fractures. BMJ 1996; 312(7041):1254–9.

45. Schuit SC, van der Klift M, Weel AE, et al. Fracture incidence and association with bone mineral density in elderly men and women: the Rotterdam Study. Bone 2004;34(1):195–202.

46. Donaldson MG, Cawthon PM, Lui LY, et al. Estimates of the proportion of older white men who would be recommended for pharmacologic treatment by the new US National Osteoporosis Foundation guidelines. J Bone Miner Res 2010;25(7):1506–11.

47. Saylor PJ, Kaufman DS, Michaelson MD, et al. Application of a fracture risk algorithm to men treated with androgen deprivation therapy for prostate cancer. J Urol 2010;183(6):2200–5.

48. Diamond TH, Winters J, Smith A, et al. The antiosteoporotic efficacy of intrave-nous pamidronate in men with prostate carcinoma receiving combined androgen blockade: a double blind, randomized, placebo-controlled crossover study. Cancer 2001;92(6):1444–50.

49. Klotz LH, McNeill IY, Kebabdjian M, et al. A phase 3, double-blind, randomised, parallel-group, placebo-controlled study of oral weekly alendronate for the pre-vention of androgen deprivation bone loss in nonmetastatic prostate cancer: the Cancer and Osteoporosis Research with Alendronate and Leuprolide (CORAL) Study. Eur Urol 2013;63(5):927–35.

50. Michaelson MD, Kaufman DS, Lee H, et al. Randomized controlled trial of annual zoledronic acid to prevent gonadotropin-releasing hormone agonist-induced bone loss in men with prostate cancer. J Clin Oncol 2007;25(9): 1038–42.

51. Morabito N, Gaudio A, Lasco A, et al. Neridronate prevents bone loss in patients receiving androgen deprivation therapy for prostate cancer. J Bone Miner Res 2004;19(11):1766–70.

52. Smith MR, Eastham J, Gleason DM, et al. Randomized controlled trial of zole-dronic acid to prevent bone loss in men receiving androgen deprivation therapy for nonmetastatic prostate cancer. J Urol 2003;169(6):2008–12.
53. Serpa Neto A, Tobias-Machado M, Esteves MA, et al. Bisphosphonate ther-apy in patients under androgen deprivation therapy for prostate cancer: a systematic review and meta-analysis. Prostate Cancer Prostatic Dis 2012; 15(1):36–44.
54. Saylor PJ, Lee RJ, Smith MR. Emerging therapies to prevent skeletal morbidity in men with prostate cancer. J Clin Oncol 2011;29(27):3705–14.
55. Smith MR, Egerdie B, Hernandez Toriz N, et al. Denosumab in men receiving androgen-deprivation therapy for prostate cancer. N Engl J Med 2009;361(8): 745–55.
56. Smith MR, Fallon MA, Lee H, et al. Raloxifene to prevent gonadotropin-releasing hormone agonist-induced bone loss in men with prostate cancer: a randomized controlled trial. J Clin Endocrinol Metab 2004;89(8):3841–6.
57. Smith MR, Morton RA, Barnette KG, et al. Toremifene to reduce fracture risk in men receiving androgen deprivation therapy for prostate cancer. J Urol 2010; 184(4):1316–21.
58. Chung M, Lee J, Terasawa T, et al. Vitamin D with or without calcium supple-mentation for prevention of cancer and fractures: an updated meta-analysis for the U.S. Preventive Services Task Force. Ann Intern Med 2011;155(12): 827–38.
59. Gralow JR, Biermann JS, Farooki A, et al. NCCN Task Force Report: bone health in cancer care. J Natl Compr Canc Netw 2009;7(Suppl 3):S1–32 [quiz: S3–5].
60. Holick MF. Vitamin D deficiency. N Engl J Med 2007;357(3):266–81.
61. Tripkovic L, Lambert H, Hart K, et al. Comparison of vitamin D_2 and vitamin D_3 supplementation in raising serum 25-hydroxyvitamin D status: a systematic re-view and meta-analysis. Am J Clin Nutr 2012;95(6):1357–64.
62. Cancer and Leukemia Group B. Zoledronate in preventing skeletal (bone)-related events in patients who are receiving androgen deprivation therapy for prostate cancer and bone metastases [ClinicalTrials.gov identifier NCT00079001]. US National Institutes of Health, ClinicalTrials.gov [online]. Available at: http://www.clinicaltrials.gov. Accessed November 21, 2012.
63. Dearnaley DP, Sydes MR, Mason MD, et al. A double-blind, placebo-controlled, randomized trial of oral sodium clodronate for metastatic prostate cancer (MRC PR05 Trial). J Natl Cancer Inst 2003;95(17):1300–11.
64. Dearnaley DP, Mason MD, Parmar MK, et al. Adjuvant therapy with oral sodium clodronate in locally advanced and metastatic prostate cancer: long-term over-all survival results from the MRC PR04 and PR05 randomised controlled trials. Lancet Oncol 2009;10(9):872–6.
65. Ernst DS, Tannock IF, Winquist EW, et al. Randomized, double-blind, controlled trial of mitoxantrone/prednisone and clodronate versus mitoxantrone/predni-sone and placebo in patients with hormone-refractory prostate cancer and pain. J Clin Oncol 2003;21(17):3335–42.
66. Small EJ, Smith MR, Seaman JJ, et al. Combined analysis of two multicenter, randomized, placebo-controlled studies of pamidronate disodium for the pallia-tion of bone pain in men with metastatic prostate cancer. J Clin Oncol 2003; 21(23):4277–84.
67. Fizazi K, Carducci M, Smith M, et al. Denosumab versus zoledronic acid for treatment of bone metastases in men with castration-resistant prostate cancer: a randomised, double-blind study. Lancet 2011;377(9768):813–22.

68. Mason MD, Sydes MR, Glaholm J, et al. Oral sodium clodronate for nonmetastatic prostate cancer–results of a randomized double-blind placebo-controlled trial: Medical Research Council PR04 (ISRCTN61384873). J Natl Cancer Inst 2007;99(10):765–76.

69. Witjes W, Tammela T, Wirth M. Effectiveness of zoledronic acid for the prevention of bone metastases in high risk prostate cancer patients: a randomised, open label, multicenter study of the European Association of Urology (EAU) in cooperation with the Scandinavian Prostate Cancer Group (SPCG) and the Arbeitsgemeinschaft Urologische Onkologie (AUO). An initial report of the "ZEUS" study. ASCO Meeting Abstracts 2006;24(Suppl 18):14644.

70. Smith MR, Saad F, Coleman R, et al. Denosumab and bone-metastasis-free survival in men with castration-resistant prostate cancer: results of a phase 3, randomised, placebo-controlled trial. Lancet 2012;379(9810):39–46.

71. Guise TA, Mohammad KS, Clines G, et al. Basic mechanisms responsible for osteolytic and osteoblastic bone metastases. Clin Cancer Res 2006;12(20 Pt 2): 6213s–6s.

72. Saad F, Smith MR, Shore ND, et al. Effect of denosumab on prolonging bone-metastasis free survival (BMFS) in men with nonmetastatic castrate-resistant prostate cancer (CRPC) presenting with aggressive PSA kinetics. ASCO Meeting Abstracts 2012;30(Suppl 15):4510.

73. Goyal J, Antonarakis ES. Bone-targeting radiopharmaceuticals for the treatment of prostate cancer with bone metastases. Cancer Lett 2012;323(2):135–46.

74. Porter AT, McEwan AJ, Powe JE, et al. Results of a randomized phase-III trial to evaluate the efficacy of strontium-89 adjuvant to local field external beam irradiation in the management of endocrine resistant metastatic prostate cancer. Int J Radiat Oncol Biol Phys 1993;25(5):805–13.

75. Quilty PM, Kirk D, Bolger JJ, et al. A comparison of the palliative effects of strontium-89 and external beam radiotherapy in metastatic prostate cancer. Radiother Oncol 1994;31(1):33–40.

76. Sartor O, Reid RH, Hoskin PJ, et al. Samarium-153-Lexidronam complex for treatment of painful bone metastases in hormone-refractory prostate cancer. Urology 2004;63(5):940–5.

77. Serafini AN, Houston SJ, Resche I, et al. Palliation of pain associated with metastatic bone cancer using samarium-153 lexidronam: a double-blind placebo-controlled clinical trial. J Clin Oncol 1998;16(4):1574–81.

78. Nilsson S, Larsen RH, Fossa SD, et al. First clinical experience with alpha-emitting radium-223 in the treatment of skeletal metastases. Clin Cancer Res 2005;11(12):4451–9.

79. Parker C, Nilsson S, Heinrich D, et al. Updated analysis of the phase III, double-blind, randomized, multinational study of radium-223 chloride in castration-resistant prostate cancer (CRPC) patients with bone metastases (ALSYMPCA). J Clin Oncol 2012;30(Suppl) [abstract: LBA4512].

80. Sartor AO, Heinrich D, O'Sullivan JM, et al. Radium-223 chloride (Ra-223) impact on skeletal-related events (SREs) and ECOG performance status (PS) in patients with castration-resistant prostate cancer (CRPC) with bone metastases: interim results of a phase III trial (ALSYMPCA). J Clin Oncol 2012;30(Suppl) [abstract: 4551].

81. Peters S, Adjei AA. MET: a promising anticancer therapeutic target. Nat Rev Clin Oncol 2012;9(6):314–26.

82. Saad F, Lipton A. SRC kinase inhibition: targeting bone metastases and tumor growth in prostate and breast cancer. Cancer Treat Rev 2010;36(2):177–84.

83. de Bono JS, Logothetis CJ, Molina A, et al. Abiraterone and increased survival in metastatic prostate cancer. N Engl J Med 2011;364(21):1995–2005.
84. Logothetis CJ, Basch E, Molina A, et al. Effect of abiraterone acetate and prednisone compared with placebo and prednisone on pain control and skeletal-related events in patients with metastatic castration-resistant prostate cancer: exploratory analysis of data from the COU-AA-301 randomised trial. Lancet Oncol 2012;13(12):1210–7.
85. Arakawa H, Nakanishi T, Yanagihara C, et al. Enhanced expression of organic anion transporting polypeptides (OATPs) in androgen receptor-positive prostate cancer cells: possible role of OATP1A2 in adaptive cell growth under androgen-depleted conditions. Biochem Pharmacol 2012;84(8):1070–7.
86. Lester JE, Dodwell D, Horsman JM, et al. Current management of treatment-induced bone loss in women with breast cancer treated in the United Kingdom. Br J Cancer 2006;94(1):30–5.
87. National Osteoporosis Foundation. Clinicians' guide to prevention and treatment of osteoporosis. Washington, DC: National Osteoporosis Foundation; 2010.

Index

Note: Page numbers of article titles are in **boldface** type.

Hematol Oncol Clin N Am 27 (2013) 1285–1295
http://dx.doi.org/10.1016/S0889-8588(13)00160-3
0889-8588/13/$ – see front matter © 2013 Elsevier Inc. All rights reserved.

hemonc.theclinics.com

Moving?

Make sure your subscription moves with you!

To notify us of your new address, find your **Clinics Account Number** (located on your mailing label above your name), and contact customer service at:

Email: journalscustomerservice-usa@elsevier.com

800-654-2452 (subscribers in the U.S. & Canada)
314-447-8871 (subscribers outside of the U.S. & Canada)

Fax number: 314-447-8029

Elsevier Health Sciences Division
Subscription Customer Service
3251 Riverport Lane
Maryland Heights, MO 63043

*To ensure uninterrupted delivery of your subscription, please notify us at least 4 weeks in advance of move.

Printed and bound by CPI Group (UK) Ltd, Croydon, CR0 4YY

03/10/2024

01040493-0003